MW00995949

After the Baby's Birth...
A Woman's Way to Wellness

A Complete Guide for Postpartum Women

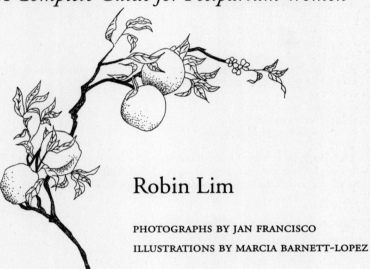

Robin Lim

PHOTOGRAPHS BY JAN FRANCISCO
ILLUSTRATIONS BY MARCIA BARNETT-LOPEZ

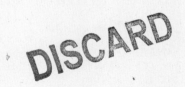
DISCARD

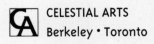

CELESTIAL ARTS
Berkeley • Toronto

Copyright © 1991, 2001 Robin Lim

All rights reserved. No part of this book may be reproduced in any form, except brief excerpts for the purpose of review, without written permission of the publisher.

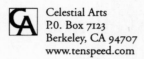 Celestial Arts
P.O. Box 7123
Berkeley, CA 94707
www.tenspeed.com

Photograph on page 238 © by Peggy O'Neil
Photographs on pages 5, 192, 278 (upper), and 322 © by Margo Berdeshevsky
Photographs on pages 27 and 318 by Joseph Yacoe
All other photographs © by Jan Francisco
Illustration on page iii by Lance Sims
Illustrations © by Marcia Barnett-Lopez. *Treasury of Chinese Design Motifs* and *Treasury of Japanese Design Motifs* by Dover Publications were used as reference materials.

Interior design by Courtnay Perry
Cover design by Nancy Austin
Cover photograph by George MacDonald

Distributed in Australia by Simon and Schuster Australia, in Canada by Ten Speed Press Canada, in New Zealand by Southern Publishers Group, in South Africa by Real Books, in Southeast Asia by Berkeley Books, and in the United Kingdom and Europe by Airlift Books.

Library of Congress Cataloging-in-Publication Data

Lim, Robin, 1956-
    After the baby's birth : a woman's way to wellness : a complete
guide for postpartum women / Robin Lim ; photographs by Jan Francisco ;
illustrations by Marcia Barnett-Lopez.— Rev. and updated ed.
       p. ; cm.
    Includes bibliographical references and index.
    ISBN 1-58761-110-4
    1. Postnatal care—Popular works. 2. Medicine, Ayurvedic.
    [DNLM: 1. Postnatal Care—Popular Works. 2. Infant Care—Popular
Works. WQ 150 L732a 2001]   1. Title.
    RG801 .L56 2001
    618.6—dc21

                              2001002970

This edition ISBN: 1-58761-110-4
First Celestial Arts ISBN: 0-89087-590-1

1 2 3 4 5—05 04 03 02 01

Printed in the United States

DEDICATED TO:

Our Lady, the Divine Mother of God,
who guides, protects, and lives
in the hearts of all mothers.

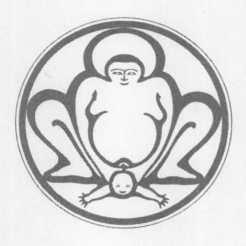

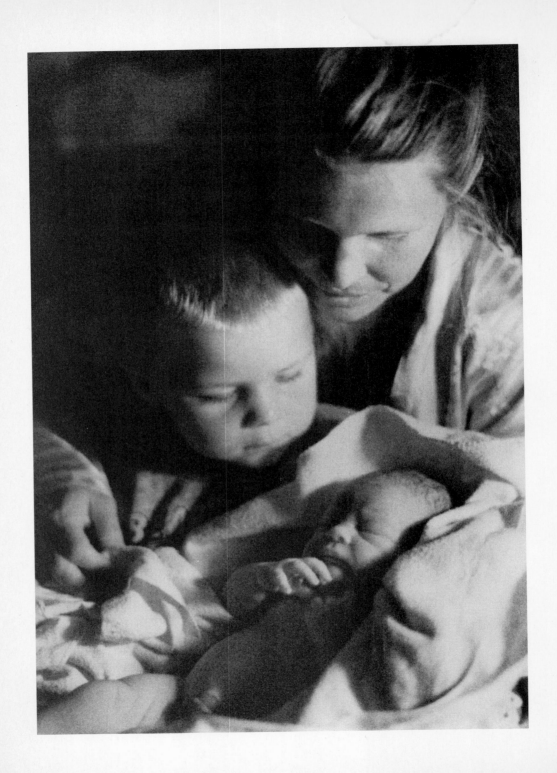

Contents

Acknowledgments for the Revised Edition

Worldwide, nearly 600,000 women between the ages of fifteen and forty-nine die every year as a result of complications arising from pregnancy and childbirth.[1] That is more than one mother lost per minute. These beautiful women will never experience the joys and challenges of postpartum. They will not hold their babies in their loving arms. I tell you about them here so that all of you mothers will acknowledge your own courage in embarking on this road. To endeavor to bring new human life onto this earth is a huge commitment. We do it in partnership with the very source of love, that beautiful creative force that made the universe. If we are blessed, we do it in partnership with the baby's father. Some of us have the help of community, the village, the extended family. Other new mothers are very alone. First and most profoundly, I wish to thank all mothers for their courage.

In the years since the original publication of *After the Baby's Birth…A Woman's Way to Wellness,* I moved to Asia and became a midwife there. It was the hundreds of women in Bali, Indonesia, and Baguio, Philippines, who asked me to receive their babies that taught me how precious each woman and each baby and each family is. I am full of gratitude for these teachers. I also wish to thank the women in Fairfield, Iowa, who called me to their homes, to their births.

For nurturing, I humbly thank my mother, Cresencia Munar Lim Jehle, my father, Robert A. Jehle, and my grandmother, Vicenta Munar Lim, who was herself a *hilot,* a midwife in the Philippines. Appreciation and hugs to the Hemmerle clan, for their supportive love. The Lim family of Baguio, Philippines, *maraming salamat.* I am forever grateful for my little sister/angel, the late Christine Jehle Kim.

June Whitson came to teach me the very "heart" of midwifery. Before her death from breast cancer, she made many trips to Indonesia to give her heart and hands in service to the women there. *Terima Kasih* Ibu June.

The breastfeeding chapter rocks because of Mary Kroeger, CNM, MPH; Judy Torgas; Gina Maria Catena, CNM; Ivana Kurtz, Toni Sugg, Déjà Bernhardt, and La Leche League International.

To Marie Zenack, who came to Indonesia to work, who called me to midwife her own daughter: As one of my most significant teachers in this life, you must be thanked for coauthoring chapter 18 with me.

To Jane Honikman of Postpartum Support International, my deepest gratitude for the years you yourself have given postpartum women.

viii

I wish to thank Gael Thompson and Joan Kelly for demonstrating that dance heals. Their influence and hearts are apparent in the movement and toning chapters.

To Jeannine Parvati Baker, always willing to hear me on the phone, providing me with inspiration and support. Thanks for blazing the trail with knowledge and love.

Eden Gabrielle Fromberg, doctor/healer/dear friend, who came to Bali and taught me how to patch up wounds. Her good heart is folded into these pages.

Grateful hugs go out to the doulas of the world, especially Debra Pascali-Bonaro (and everyone at MotherLove, Inc.), Marcie Freeman, Joanne Poole, and Kathy Deol.

Midwives, the guardians of birth, my profound gratitude pours out to each of you. I would especially like to thank Debby Lowry, Mary Jackson, Tina Garzero, Joanne Dugas, Anne Frye, Nancy Wainer, Nan Koehler, Pearl Breitbach, Dodie Neale, Faith Gibson, Elaine Mellon, Kate Bowland, Roxanne Potter, Mary Offerman, Melody Weig, Beverly Francis, Rahima Baldwin, Valerie El Halta, Raven Lang, Stephanie Struthmann, the late Sunny Supplee, Kadi Morningstar, Lori Arak, Elizabeth Davis, Kalanete, Ina May Gaskin, and Pamela Hunt. Each of you has helped me tremendously.

I pay special tribute to these wise women who have shared freely from their hearts: Hannelore Josam, Sophia Anastasia, Carolyn Sims, Sivan Wind, Karolynn Lucas, Ibu Rndi, Ni Ketut Rusni, Ni Wayan Li Wati, Made Wartini, Made Suastini, Wayan Rani, Nita Noor, Marietta Paragas and Shontoug Foundation, Debby Nofthaft, Marjan de Jong, Alesia Lloyd, Elizabeth Kelly, Nyoman Masni, Joy Alcos, Lonica Halley, Cindy Miller, Rebecca Buckley, Liz Asmus, Priya Chhalliyil, Remy Lim, Joyanna Cotter, Alice Walker, Mary Peterson, Jayne Sturgeon, Rebecca Bashara, Dr. Injil Abu Bakar, Gina Sitz, Anjalie Trice, Barbara Holden, Catherine Burtlow, Barbara Katz Rothman Ph.D., Michelle T. Verduzco, Rebecca S. Reeves, Kathleen Rutten, Lise Knouse, Aleshanee Akin, Colleen Inouye M.D., Andy Carmone, Shantel Aschenbrenner at Frontline Graphics, and Christina Wadsworth. I could not have done it without each of you.

Linda and Babu Walling, you taught me to believe in and build the "possible family" where extraordinary humans can grow up.

To Marina, Joseph, and Aluna Yacoe, thank you for being living proof that prayer heals.

Margo Berdeshevsky, you contributed images and imagination, it is no wonder we call you "Bird." Suzanne Arms, you have been a constant source of courage. Diane Frank, thanks for that much needed poem. Jane Tucker and Alexa Foley, thank you for your tender attention to the original manuscript, I am still grateful.

Jan Francisco, now also a grandmother, your photos are taken straight from the heart. Your hands caught Zion. Your love has rescued me many times over. Marcia Barnett-Lopez, your drawings give these words wings.

Thanks to Rebecca, Scott, Surreal, and Inti for sharing your beautiful photograph used on the cover.

Jan Tritten and Alice Evans of *Midwifery Today,* you lift me up every time I call for help.

Ashisha and Peggy O'Mara of *Mothering*, thanks for mothering the writer in me.

North American Registry of Midwives, especially Ida Daragh and Sandra Morningstar, who helped me earn those flying papers. Midwives Alliance of North America, who has given me a big community of midwives with whom to hold hands.

Special blessings to the Pan Pacific and South East Asia Women's Association, your support has helped tremendously.

Many men have helped me too: they include the late Theodore Sturgeon, who taught me that writing is a craft of love; Malik Cotter, D.O.C., a brother in the healing arts; Dr. Stephen Chang, always helpful, generous, and inspiring; John Briley, M.D. (still my saint), the man who teaches that "Mother Nature and Father Time are the greatest healers"; Joel Garnier, "go-fer," volunteer, and research assistant; Scott MacDonald, who provided an excellent example of fatherly support for his expectant family while fueling the fire of ideas for my family; Pradheep Chhalliyil, for sharing his beautiful family with me and for biochemical knowledge of human nutrition; Nathan Zenack, ever supporting the women with a smile and a story; beloved Sam Shapiro, for marrying into the *keluarga*; and Lance Sims, who contributed the *After the Baby's Birth* logo, which has become so dear to so many hearts. Special appreciation goes out to the "Yayasan" officers of Healthy Mother—Healthy Baby Foundation in Bali, especially the late Wayan Budiasa, Wayan Windia, and Dr. Made Jawe.

To Tanya Martel and Lakota Hemmerle, who typed for me and made me laugh. I also thank Zhòu Lee for research assistance.

The folks at Celestial Arts: The late David Hinds who made this book possible, I feel your blessings even now; Cynthia Harris enlivened the first edition; Annie Nelson, thanks for production and enthusiasm every step of the way; Kirsty Melville, who provided leadership; Courtnay Perry and Nancy Austin, who created amazing designs; Jean M. Bloomquist, who tackled the copyediting; and Brook Barnum...for so darn much, I am grateful.

To the village of Nyuh Kuning, Bali, Indonesia; the town of Fairfield, Iowa; Haiku, Maui, Hawaii, and Baguio City, Philippine Islands...my homes...*Terima Kasih, Maraming Salamat, Tanks eh!*

My gratitude to Mata Amritanandamayi, the embodiment of unconditional love.

To Wil, my husband, my musical muse. He cooked, cleaned, shuffled the children to violin lessons, copyedited, home-schooled, handled all the financial worries while singing and loving us. Thank you for always dreaming of our lives with me.

And to my astonishing children: Déjà, Noël, Zhòu, Lakota, Zion, Thoreau, and Hanoman. Along with my granddaughter, "Chu-chu," they are my gurus.

Preface to the New Edition

In 1991, when the first edition of *After the Baby's Birth…A Woman's Way to Wellness* came out, I was forced to reinvent myself. That same year my little sister Christine; my midwife, Sunny; and my dear friend Brenda died. Their passing taught me to live only for love. My devotion to my family blossomed, and my commitment to mothers, babies, and their families deepened.

In 1992, I gave up my life as the single mother of four, married Wil, and gained two more children in the bargain. Together we moved to Bali, Indonesia. Early in 1993, our seventh child, Hanoman, was born at home in the Balinese village of Nyuh Kuning. During my pregnancy, two baby owls fell from their nest in a coconut tree and were brought to us to raise. We later learned that to hear an owl's call while pregnant was a good omen. Because two owls came to live with us, the women of our village decided I would be their new *dukin bayi*, or receiver of babies.

When Wil, as my "mid-husband"—received his son at home, people became convinced that the owls had chosen wisely. In the middle of rainy Indonesian nights, I found myself called to births in Balinese homes. And so began my intensive independent study of the art and science of midwifery. Medical protocols from the West had been imported to Asia with questionable results. Hemorrhage after childbirth, mainly due to poor nutrition, was still a leading cause of death on the island. Modern agricultural practices—the use of herbicides, fungicides, pesticides, and "green revolution" rice—put childbearing women at grave risk. Naturally, the women were afraid.

June Whitson, a British nurse-midwife, certified both in the United States and the United Kingdom, came to live with us to train me and guide my hand in the most gentle, culturally appropriate way to welcome babies. Mangku Liyar read me the Lontars, ancient holy books, concerning conscious conception, sacred birth, and enlightened parenting. I volunteered at Indonesian hospitals, where some nights four to six babies were born an hour. Through the North American Registry of Midwives, I became a Certified Professional Midwife. However, it was the families—of Nyuh Kuning, our home village, and across the river in Singa Kerta beyond the Monkey Forest in Ubud, and up the dusty road in Pengo Sekan—who made me a midwife. The needless death of a young birthing mother in Singa Kerta called me to action.

In the postpartum time, I observed that the Asian women I served had excellent care from their own families. This is their culture—to worship children who are closer to God, to elevate women who have become new mothers, and to serve them as they grow strong after childbirth. Sadly, I came to see more clearly how my sisters in the West could expect little or no postpartum care or support, either from health-care providers or from friends and family. The modern lifestyle embraced by the West, sought after and imitated all over the world, has so fractured families that postpartum women today accept and expect to be isolated. I wonder at a culture that decades ago put men on the moon, yet chooses to ignore the most significant life passage of women. In Asia, it is a quite commonly held belief that life becomes richer once one has achieved parenthood. In the West, I often see how my women friends are somehow made to feel diminished when they have a baby.

I grew up between worlds, with an Asian mother and an American father, and so I have looked on both sides of the shadow-puppet screen. I am convinced that a culture is defined by its gentleness with life—the way it protects and nourishes pregnant women, prepares for childbirth, develops rituals surrounding birth (be they spiritual or medical), cares for postpartum women, and nurtures children and the elderly.

It is an exciting time to become a mother. Research has shone bright lights on what women have always known: Dynamic systems are sensitive to start-up conditions. Thus, a gentle birth is life enhancing for the human organism. We know that breastfeeding has tremendous benefits: physical, spiritual, psychological, intellectual, and societal. Our Earth, exploited to the brink of an ecological nightmare, is in grave danger. Jeannine Parvati Baker, the pioneer in perinatal psychology, has said, "Healing birth heals our Earth." So you see, the prevention of birth trauma and the support of breastfeeding open the way for the most amazing humans possible to arrive Earth-side. In this way, loving families are healing our planet, one individual at a time.

History will mark this millennium as the age in which we reinvent ourselves. Who better to teach the world this than postpartum women? Yes, this is, in my opinion, each new mother's exalted role: healer and teacher. And each of you postpartum women reading this can trust that nature has given you the knowledge and the tools to do a splendid job. Your hearth, your very lap, and knee is your classroom.

I once said, "You're pregnant for nine months, you're postpartum for the rest of your life." I meant it. Today I pray for blessings to rain down on every one of you, because we need you so desperately, because I have a granddaughter, and I want her to grow up in an Earthly garden. My work as a midwife and advocate for "the possible family" is devoted to this planet's healing. In these pages I have enfolded what many wise women in many countries have taught me. I have included Natural Family Planning in the hope it will answer one of the questions you most frequently ask: "We've had a baby, what shall we do now?"

Over the years, since *After the Baby's Birth* was first released, I have loved your letters. I have cried with joy when you told me you got stronger or happier or let yourselves be more open to the hearts of your children. I'm not an expert, but I am a mother, a grandmother, a foolish poet, a servant of women as midwife. Because of this, I offer this revision of my first-born book as my prayer for peace.

OM Shanti—ROBIN LIM, MAY 2001

PART I

Now That You and the Baby Have Met

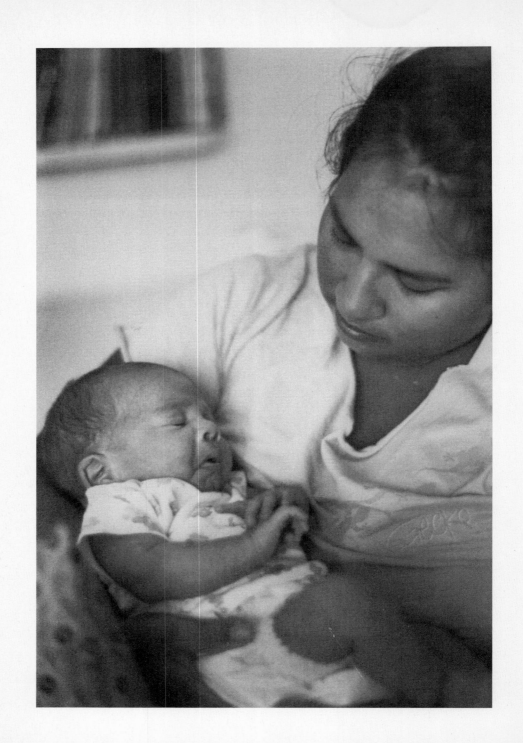

CHAPTER 1

Postpartum:

Unfolding as a Mother

Postpartum begins with the birth of your baby. For the first few days after birthing, it is as if you are between worlds. Both your body and spirit are wide open. If this is your first child, you may be astonished at the powerful bond between you and your baby. For most women, giving birth is their most significant life event.

Depending upon your cultural and religious background, your awareness of God or the greatness of spirit is heightened by the experience of participating so intimately in creation itself by putting a child on our planet. Birthing is the most profound initiation to spirituality a woman can have. In my work as a mother, midwife, and author, I meet and share stories, experiences, and knowledge with hundreds of mothers from many cultures. All of them, even those who prior to giving birth felt no connection to God, Mother Nature, or refined levels of consciousness, are deeply spiritual. It is as if in the process of becoming a mother the heart and mind of the woman get hardwired together. What she does in the world reflects her well of deep feeling. As a mother the woman begins to walk a sacred path. Look in the mirror—you'll see spirit reflected there in your own eyes.

Unfortunately, with our extremely pragmatic twenty-first-century lifestyles, pregnancy, birthing, and postpartum have been deemed merely physical, clinical events. This has forced women to suppress their spiritual natures that unfold in the context of becoming new mothers. A wave of spiritual awakening is pulsing in many hearts around the world and has thrown open the doors for mothers to embrace their innate wisdom and express it openly. Birth is a cause for celebration, and most likely you feel a broad spectrum of emotions from tears to extreme bliss.

Postpartum is a time when you are very conscious of straddling the worlds of the spiritual and the physical. This book was written to help you integrate them. With so much change occurring within your body, heart, and soul, you begin to realize just how intimately one is connected to the others. Keep in mind that, even though some chapters seem to focus on bodily health, the physical cannot be separated from the spiritual, nor the spiritual from the physical.

Your hormones, which enter your bloodstream in minute amounts, have a profound effect on your entire being. I would not be surprised if hormones were someday discovered to be the bridge between matter and spirit. The hormonal fluctuation that occurs during pregnancy, birth, and postpartum certainly contributes to the emotional richness of becoming a mother.

During the last weeks of your pregnancy, your placenta provided relatively enormous amounts of estrogen and progesterone. Your metabolism was stepped up, and the circulation and volume of your blood increased. Your pituitary and many other glands throughout your body were at their peak of hormone production. Labor and delivery, even at its best, is challenging work. At the actual time of birth, oxytocin, the hormone of love, works hand in hand with vasopressin and adrenaline. These powerful hormones employ the uterus to expel the baby and along with endorphins cause you to fall hopelessly in love. This magical bonding enfolds the birth mother, her baby, her most significant other, and her family. Within twenty-four hours after delivery, with the loss of your placenta, hormone levels plunge to a tiny fraction of what they had been. Your blood supply, circulation, and pituitary activity drop tremendously within hours of birthing. The physical and emotional changes are rapid and dramatic.

This is the time to lean on your family and friends. It's your time to delegate rather than to do. In many countries, families do not live far apart, and it is not uncommon for couples to raise their own families as close to their parents as possible. This provides generational support for new mothers.

In America, we've developed a do-it-all-by-yourself attitude. Relatively few women have their mothers' help when they most need it. Many women who have been displaced from their childhood homes are isolated from their immediate family during the postpartum period. Their postpartum care is left to professionals, doctors and nurses who are too busy to give them adequate attention. All too often, the only postpartum care an American woman can count on is one fifteen-minute appointment with her doctor, six weeks after she has given birth. This six-week marker ends an arbitrary period within which she is supposed to have worked out most postpartum questions for herself. This neglect of postpartum women is not just poor health care, it is abusive—particularly to women suffering

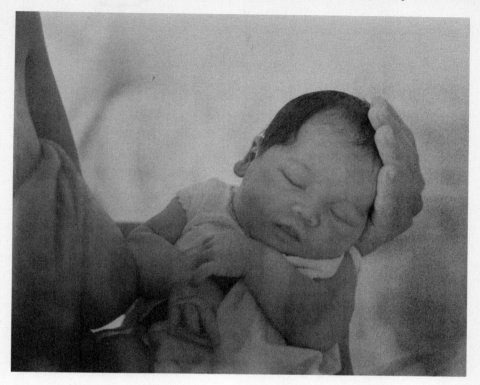

from painful physical and/or psychological disorders following childbirth. It is evident that postpartum care is not a priority for most obstetrician/gynecologists.

Fortunately the vast majority of postpartum women do not need professional care. They need meals cooked for them. They need volunteer baby-sitters if they have other children. They need help with housekeeping. They need juices and herbal teas served to them. They need reassurance and love. Any neighbor, relative, or friend can do these things. Yet for too many American women, postpartum is a lonely time. If friends and family do not care for new mothers, they experience social isolation in addition to medical neglect.

Do You Have the Support You Need?

As a new mother, you need a support network. Do you have someone other than your partner who will do anything for you? When I had my last baby, my friend Jan made helping me a priority in her busy life. When I would thank her, she'd say, "How often do you get to have a baby anyway?" I got my chance to be a postpartum support person when Jan had her fifth baby, my little goddaughter, Ahni. I never dreamed it could be so fulfilling!

Jan always says, "You get what you give." The way to develop friendships that grow to be lifelong support systems is to be of service yourself. As women, we are constantly teaching one another how to live wisely and well. By giving loving postpartum support to a sister or friend, you are laying the foundation for your own future support. Our daughters' daughters will harvest the fruits of this practice as it grows into a postpartum tradition.

Midwives and doctors can help by encouraging pregnant women to network. A bulletin board in the waiting room is a wonderful start. By posting information there, expectant mothers can make contact with women who have similar interests and live nearby.

A person must possess the special talent of skillful loving to be a doula. *Doula,* the Greek word for "servant," has come to mean one who serves or mothers a new mother. A professional doula is someone whose job is to care for pregnant, birthing, and postpartum women and their families. Doulas have special training: this knowledge enables them to restore the age-old tradition of healing birth and postpartum wellness. In this day and age, doulas have become the essential guardians of normal birth. I strongly advise expectant families to hire a professional doula. Just by being available, a friend can give additional postpartum support, like a volunteer doula. When it comes time for you to serve, drop by for a short visit and do a load of laundry for a new mother. Take her family a meal and do the dishes. You can offer to baby-sit. Listen to her; she needs to tell her birth story. Someday someone will be happy to do the same for you. We can all be wise women.

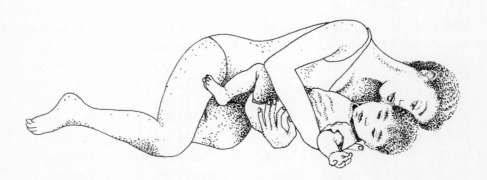

A POSTPARTUM MEAL TREE

After the arrival of the new baby, the mother's friends and family can activate this postpartum meal tree. It is simple to ask people to sign up at the blessingway or baby shower, before the actual birth. However, "the tree" may be organized at anytime, even after the happy event.

Meals should be prepared with the purest possible ingredients. Organic foods are always best. Spices should be minimal. Remember, what is consumed by the mother goes into her milk. Onions, garlic, cabbage, broccoli, and cauliflower tend to upset nursing baby's tummies when eaten by their mothers. Don't forget to take into consideration any food preferences or allergies. Is the family vegetarian? Are they allergic to wheat or dairy? Make enough to feed the entire family, and then some. Have the meal delivered at noontime. What is not entirely eaten at lunch will make wonderful leftover snacks or dinner. The casserole dishes, plates, bowls, and so on can be picked up later.

Activating the meal tree: At the top of the list should be the new mother's best friend. She will get a call when the baby is Earth-side. Meanwhile she has organized a list of friends, who in turn get calls from her. This serves two purposes: to announce the baby's arrival and activate the meal tree. Each volunteer cook chooses a day or two, prepares, and then delivers her contribution. This gives her or him (it may well be a male friend), a chance to peek in on the mother and baby. Remind the cooks not to stay too long and wear out the mother. They can fold a load of laundry while they visit and let the family know that they don't expect serving dishes to be washed when they quietly pick them up the following day. What a wonderful way to build community while selflessly serving a postpartum woman and her family!

Postpartum: The Breakthrough Phases

Many women seem to follow a pattern of breakthrough phases after having a baby. Some women describe the first three days as a time of euphoria. Elizabeth Davis, in her book *Energetic Pregnancy* (Berkeley, CA: Celestial Arts, 1988), calls postpartum days one through three "taking in." She describes the mother in this phase as a passive receiver, with a profound need for sleep and food. She also recognizes the new mother's need to review the details of her birth. Dr. James Hamilton, a pioneer in the study of postpartum depression, calls the first three days and sometimes longer a "latent interval," during which psychiatric symptoms like postpartum blues and more severe postpartum depression do not surface.

Around the third day, your awareness of the real world begins to come back. By this time, your home needs a good cleaning (and you should by no means be the one to do this). If you have other children, they need your attention and want to spend time with the new baby. If you have a partner, he may be returning to work after having taken a few days off for the birth. All this activity springs up around you—just when what you really need is rest and orderliness. The significance of this tender phase, when you are unfolding as a mother, is too

Postpartum Practices around the World

In India, Ayurvedic tradition encourages a new mother to stay at home and be pampered for the first twenty-two days postpartum. Her role as an exalted one is honored. This time of rest helps strengthen the infant-mother bond. In this precious lying-in time, breastfeeding becomes smooth. Rest and protection of both mother's and baby's delicate nervous systems are priorities. Few visitors are allowed. Mother and baby stay out of the wind and weather, decreasing the possibility of exposure to disease. Specially prepared foods are served to the mother.

Immediately after the birth of a child in Bali, a ritual for the placenta, called the *Ari-Ari* (little brother or sister), is held. The men wash and bury the placenta with offerings, giving thanks for the support of new life, establishing the home of the new mother as a place of sanctity. Every day at sunrise and sunset, an elder man runs through the family compound with an armload of burning palm leaves, while another man bangs on a big hollow bamboo. This scares away demons and protects the mother and baby. A Balinese woman does not enter her kitchen nor does she wash her hair until after the baby's cord stump has dried and fallen off; this ensures her rest. On the twelfth day postpartum, the elder women of the family go to a seer priest or priestess with offerings for the mother and child. They read the *Lontars*, Bali's ancient holy books, to discover what this child needs to guide her life. For the first 105 days of life, the child never touches the ground. She is held in arms continuously, floating like an angel from one loving person to another until her *Nyabmutan*, when she touches the Mother Earth for the first time and is officially welcomed to the human family. *

often minimized in our workday society. It is very important to reenter daily activities slowly. By the beginning of this phase, a mother's milk has "come in" and so have the "blues," a natural emotional reaction to childbirth and becoming a mother that 50 to 80 percent of new mothers experience.

Maternity blues, characterized by tearfulness and exhaustion, usually last a few hours to a few days. Your focus should be on breastfeeding and caring for yourself and the baby. The arrival of your milk and the blues at about the same

Most Indonesian women do not go out of the family compound (traditionally a cluster of homes for extended family, set among lovely gardens) or resume their regular responsibilities until the baby is forty-two days old. On the forty-second day, the baby is named, the village participates in the beautiful ritual, and a feast is held.

Some American physicians advise their patients to refrain from "everything" for the first six weeks postpartum. Perhaps this was adopted from the Talmud, which states: "A Woman who has just borne a child should not lie with her husband for forty days." This Jewish practice is shared by many traditional cultures all over our planet. Among the Christian/Animist Igarot peoples of the Northern Philippine mountains, there is also a six-week-long lying-in. I found people of the Muslim faith honoring a forty-two day period of abstinence. For the first three nights postpartum, an Indonesian Muslim father must not sleep; he must guard his wife and baby.

The majority of births in Holland take place at home. Excellent in-home postpartum care is provided by women called *Kraamverpleegsters* (professional maternity nurse). They arrive at 8 A.M. and leave at 5 P.M., for eight days. These angels take care of laundry, cooking, shopping, child care, act as hostess for visitors, and do postpartum checkups as well. They have daily contact with the midwife or doctor who attended the birth, reporting all progress of the mother and baby to her. Infant care is provided, parenting skills are taught, and breastfeeding is supported.

Throughout this book I use the pronouns he and she interchangeably for two reasons: first, to use our language in a nonsexist fashion, and second, to give you, the mother of a girl or a boy, the opportunity to envision your own baby as you read these pages.

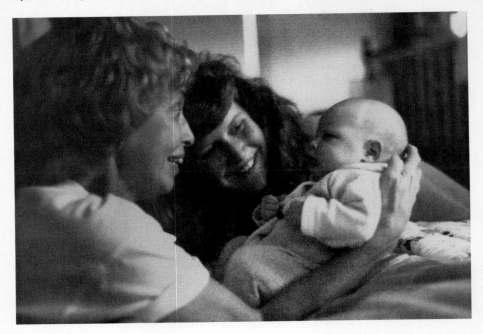

time inspires the wise-women saying "Letting loose the tears helps the milk flow," which should shed a positive light on the common experience of postpartum blues. When your milk comes in, your power also arrives. Some women feel that the arrival of their milk after their firstborn signaled the beginning of their true strength. You become an initiator, a producer. According to Davis, you begin to remaster your own care, to direct your family, and to organize your baby's care. This is a tall order, and without adequate rest, nutrition, and nurturing, you will become exhausted. Many postpartum problems may develop in this whirlwind time. Depression, physical exhaustion, increased uterine bleeding from overexertion, uterine prolapse, breast infections, engorged breasts, and illness can take hold if you do not take it easy.

Be aware that many women report that day five postpartum is a particularly tearful day. I call it "gratitude day." The new mother becomes poignantly aware of the profundity of the passage her birth experience was. She needs to connect, if not in person, at least by phone, with her birth team. She needs to cry and laugh on her midwife's shoulder. Often I've seen wives thank their husbands for the miracle of the baby. He too often cries grateful tears on day five. Remember that neither of you has had normal sleep, and you will naturally feel tender. If the birth was particularly challenging or disappointing, the flowing tears will help initiate the process of healing.

"Taking hold," the next phase, can begin soon after "gratitude day" and lasts through about day ten. In this time, mother and baby are establishing their breastfeeding routine and mother's blues are wearing off. This is the time you will be tempted to get up and put in a load of laundry. Stop yourself. Make yourself stay centered in the beautiful bubble of light created by your birth. The bed and the rocking chair are your domain, and should remain so for as long as possible. Even entertaining too many visitors can cause problems. Many a new mother notices she's running a slight fever and developing soreness and heat in a breast after turning too much of her attention outward. Remember, even if you feel wonderful, you are newly postpartum and must respect your time of lying-in.

From about day eleven and up to week six, the new mother is in her "taking charge" phase, during which she may become exhausted and hypercritical of herself, wondering: Am I a good mother? Why aren't I feeling 100 percent back to normal? Why can't I seem to get much done? Usually she is not getting the help and emotional support she needs because the excitement of her birth has worn off, and friends and family have left her to fend for herself. Obviously a mother must eventually "take charge" of her life and home. However, in traditional cultures this is not expected of a postpartum woman for many weeks. "Take charge" in "baby steps" and the transition will be smoother.

Postpartum depression, which 3 to 20 percent of new mothers suffer from and which can be quite debilitating, can set in any time after delivery. Severe postpartum psychosis is rare, only about 1 per 1,000 new mothers suffers from it. Onset of postpartum psychosis is usually between day three and one month postpartum. (See the Postpartum Emotions chart that shows how to distinguish the blues from moderate or severe postpartum depression, and the treatment appropriate for each. Chapter 16, Issues of the Heart, covers postpartum depression in detail.)

Sometime between the second and fourth month postpartum, most women feel "settled" and less vulnerable. This coincides with the settling of the baby who becomes more present and comfortable in the body. Loneliness and exhaustion are still issues in a new mother's life, especially if she has other children and must maintain a high level of activity to meet her family's needs. Exhaustion becomes even more of an issue if you are returning to work after six to eight weeks, the customary period for maternity leave. If possible, try to put off returning for as long as possible so you can recuperate more fully and enjoy your baby. When you do return to work, you will have the challenge of juggling the life of a mother with the life of a professional. (See page 254 for more on returning to work.) Your coworkers cannot begin to understand how vulnerable you are and how tender your emotions can be unless they have also returned to work after a short maternity leave. It is not unusual for a new mother to find herself crying on her coffee break. Don't criticize yourself for being softhearted; you have plenty of reason to be. Look for emotional support and practical advice from friends who returned to work when their babies were young. Whatever you do in these early weeks

POSTPARTUM EMOTIONS

	% Affected	Onset/Duration
Postpartum Blues	Approximately 50%–80%; 500–800 postpartum women per 1,000	Begins about day 1–3 postpartum; lasts from a few hours to several days
Postpartum Depression (PPD)	Approximately 3%–20%; 30–200 postpartum women per 1,000; reoccurrence rate for women who previously had PPD = approximately 10%–35%	Can set in any time after delivery; may last for a few weeks to several months. For 4% of women suffering from PPD, symptoms persist for as long as one year.
Postpartum Psychosis	Approximately .1%; 1 per 1,000 postpartum women	Onset is severe and sudden; usually begins within the first month postpartum; 80% of the cases set in within 3–14 days postpartum; duration varies and recovery is gradual, but averages 3 months once treatment begins

NOTE: *This simple chart is included with the hope that people can see at a glance when help is needed. Please read chapter 16, pages 259–70 for more information about this important postpartum issue.*

postpartum, make sure you allow for enough rest and for good nutrition. If you neglect yourself, you will put yourself in extreme physical and emotional risk.

By about the eighth or ninth month postpartum, babies enter a phase of increased physical independence from the mother. Babies at this age may be crawling, sitting up, and eating solid foods. Most have one or more teeth. Some

Symptoms May Include	How To Treat
Tearfulness; exhaustion; worry; irritability; cravings or loss of appetite; lack of confidence; sadness	Review the story of your baby's birth with a beloved friend; rest, eat well, and cry (see chapter 16 for more remedies and coping suggestions)
Headaches; numbness; chest pains; heart palpitations; hyperventilating; despondency or feelings of despair; feelings of inadequacy; inability to cope; hopelessness; helplessness; impaired concentration or memory; loss of normal interests; thoughts of suicide; bizarre or strange thoughts; panic attacks; hostile behavior; new fears or phobias; intrusive thoughts; nightmares; exaggerated guilt; fear of not bonding with baby; overconcern for baby; feeling out of control; no joy; feeling like you are "going crazy" *(Symptoms' frequency and severity vary from woman to woman. A woman may experience some or all of these symptoms.)*	Get additional loving support from understanding friends and family; seek professional guidance; if your doctor prescribes medication and/or psychotherapy, make sure you get emotional support as well; take a good look at your diet—you must eat well to be well; take small steps toward feeling good: brush your hair, go for walks. PLEASE: The family must help get professional guidance for the woman suffering from PPD.
Refusal to eat; agitation; fatigue; inability to stop activity; frantic excessive energy; hyperactivity; extreme confusion; delusions; feelings of hopelessness and shame; loss of memory; failure to identify familiar people; incoherence; rapid speech; bizarre hallucinations; hearing voices; suspiciousness; irrational statements; alteration in mood; preoccupation with trivia; distorted thinking	Immediately the family must intervene and get the woman suffering from symptoms of postpartum psychosis *experienced professional help;* the safety and well-being of both the mother and the baby is at risk! This is a medical emergency that requires immediate hospitalization and medication; psychotherapy and nonjudgmental love and support are essential.

babies are taking their first steps and making their first attempts to verbalize. Yet at the same time, the baby's psychological attachment to the mother has grown profound. The baby is anxious and will cry when mother leaves the room. Whereas younger infants will accept the breast of any woman, most babies will not breastfeed with other women by the time they reach this age, unless they have grown accustomed to being breastfed by aunties or a friend. I often witnessed this custom of women sharing the responsibility of breastfeeding, while living in Asia. It is becoming more and more acceptable in the United States.

By the ninth month, the mother has been postpartum about as long as she was pregnant. Some women feel this is a good time to wean, but because the baby is anxiously attached psychologically, it is in fact a difficult time. During the baby's "dependent/independent" phase, some mothers become impatient with the physical condition of their bodies. A mother may think, "I was pregnant only nine months, why should it take me longer than nine months to get back my old shape?" This is a good time to start a dance or yoga class, preferably one that other mothers are attending and that allows you to bring your baby along. Because many aerobic exercise classes are quite competitive and physically straining, I don't recommend them for new mothers. Dance classes (especially those with a tribal drumbeat focus if you can find one) are generally less competitive and more for having fun as you condition your body. If during a dance class you feel exhausted or sore, stop and rest. Remember, it is never good to overwork your body.

Unfortunately I've observed an extraordinary large number of couples separating and divorcing between the eighth month and first year after the birth of a baby. Is it because most women have begun to return to fertility by this time? The risk of another pregnancy may increase anxiety for couples who feel they already have more than they can handle. With the emergence of the baby's independence, does the father somehow feel that he is no longer needed?

Of course, in reality, he is needed very badly. At about the time of the baby's first birthday, the "stress and mess" phase begins. With increased mobility, a baby contributes more mess to the home and adds considerably to household chores.

The "stress and mess" phase is a long one. You are making the gradual ascent to full strength. You may feel great one day, only to suffer a setback brought about by several sleepless nights when you were caring for a cranky, teething baby. On the bright side, this period is peppered with joy. You can get out more with your baby. Slowly you will find time to spend on creative endeavors. Though at times your baby will be as brash as a bull in a china shop, at others he will be as gentle as the laughing Buddha.

Year two postpartum is more fun. Even women who have had a difficult first year seem to enjoy their role as mother more in the second year, despite the fact that their baby is in the terrific twos! Toward the end of the second year, women wishing to have more children begin to seriously consider getting pregnant again. If you have a choice, spacing children four or more years apart is easier on your body. In addition, a lower incidence of sibling rivalry has been observed when children are spaced at least four years apart. However, for some families spacing children closely works out wonderfully.

Year three is spent in companionship with your child. In general by this time, Mom feels very good, very active, and her child is delightful to her. Three-year-olds are quite civilized compared to two-year-olds. They like outings and travel well. If all other aspects of life are good, a mother will share wonderful times with her little sidekick.

A big breakthrough comes in year four. Physically all of a woman's systems are go. Even those who have had physical or emotional postpartum difficulties usually feel whole by now. This is not to say that body, mind, heart, and soul are just as they were before the baby. You will never be the same. You are better!

Whatever you do, do not view postpartum as merely pregnancy's "fourth trimester." That attitude implies that you should have achieved total physical recovery and that your life is back to "normal" within three short months. The most profound physical changes a woman ever undergoes *do* take place during the first few days after giving birth, but far-reaching changes in body, lifestyle, emotions, attitudes, and spiritual experience continue to unfold for as long as you live. You were pregnant for nine months; you are postpartum for the rest of your life.

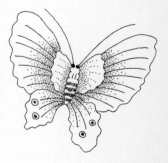

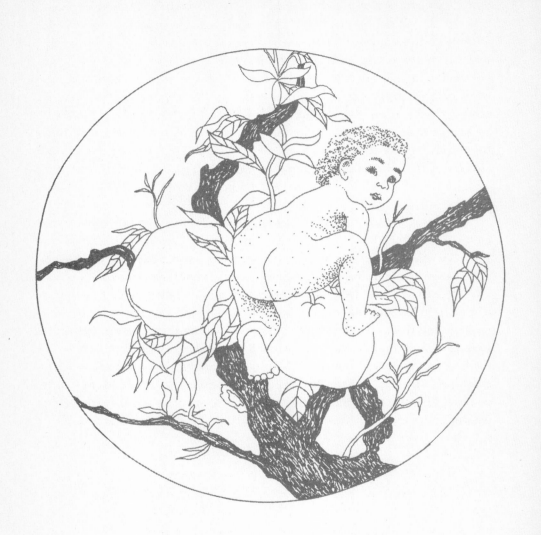

CHAPTER 2

Write about Giving Birth

Use these pages to write about giving birth to your baby. Breathe deeply as you remember all the details. What was your first signal that labor had begun? What did you feel as this profound reality sunk in? Who was there for you? What disappointments did you have?

What is your most joyful birthing memory? Describe your first impressions of your baby. What did your body experience while birthing and afterward? How do you feel spiritually and emotionally? How would you like your postpartum to unfold?

Processing the details of your birth is an essential part of your postpartum recovery. While writing down the story, you will most likely feel compelled to talk about the birth. It would be wise to find a friend who will listen. You may wish to ask your baby's father about his perceptions of your birth if you were anesthetized or if you lost consciousness at any time during labor. If he was not there, find out what he was doing and feeling. If you have other children, where were they and what did they feel? Even knowing what happened in the world news that day will be significant as you incorporate your birth history into your life.

Do not hold back if you feel yourself laughing or crying. This is the story of your most significant life passage, the most profound experience of your life-the birth of your child, and your own rebirth from maidenhood into motherhood.

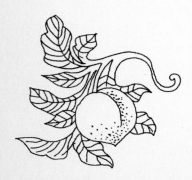

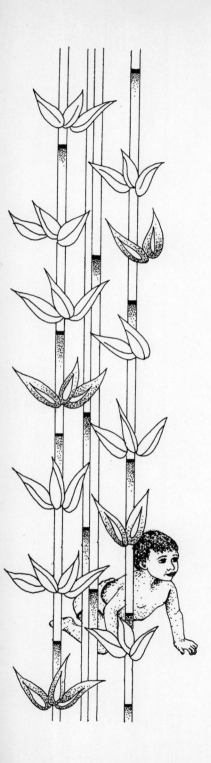

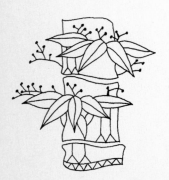

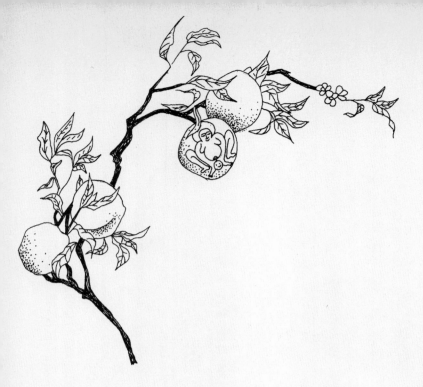

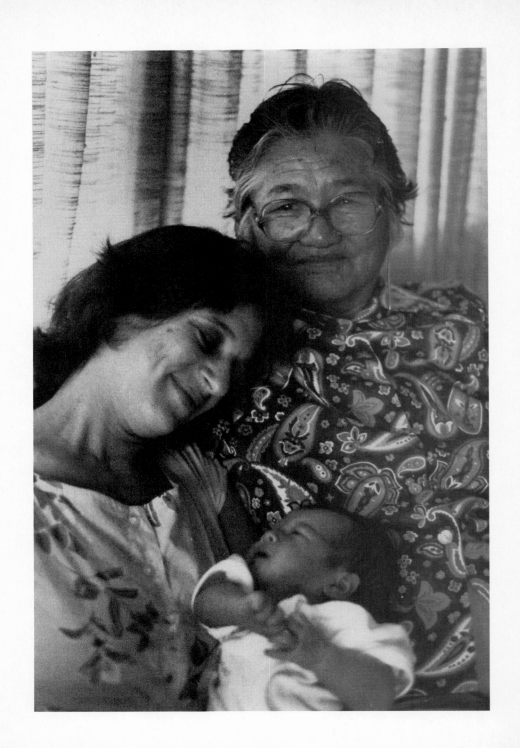

CHAPTER 3

The First Days Postpartum:

A Delicate Passage

Nature arranged the best possible preparation for motherhood: the experience of pregnancy and childbirth. In the long months of pregnancy, you watched your body, and indeed, your baby grow. You waited for, nurtured, loved, and clung to this precious life harbored in your womb. Then the day came when you were compelled by the force of your own body and the baby to let go. You gave birth. This letting go is like no other human experience. Another life issued from your body. In this letting go, you became a mother, and now the relentless giving and joyful receiving begins.

During their first pregnancy, most women have many thoughts and wishes about the baby but few about their new role as a mother. Over the short period of time from the onset of labor to the actual birth, some of the most profound physiological changes that the body can undergo take place. The development of your body during pregnancy took nine months; the changes during birth took only hours. Following the birth, you are not only in a totally transformed body; you are also in a completely new role, which is wonderful and challenging. Not only are you getting to know your new baby, but also in the process of giving birth, a new you was born. If you did not think extensively about what being a mother would entail, you are not alone. Many women experience a fair amount of surprise at the demands and joys of being a mother. Loving support for yourself from your heart, and from others, is essential as you may feel that not one aspect of your former life is intact. If all of your friends are childless, you may feel alienated from them. But given time, they too will fall in love with your baby and accept your new life as a mother. They may be curious to find out what having a child is like and may be willing to help out in any way they can. Include your friends in your new life and you will remain a part of theirs.

In the first days after birth, your every move is guided by what many call instinct, something that some women feel is a part of their ancient heritage. Your emotions will have an intensity you may have never felt before. All that you see, taste, touch, hear, smell, and feel will seem exaggerated. Some days will be too much. One moment you may feel deeply saddened by the profound emptiness of your womb. The next moment your heart will soar with joy at the fullness of your arms as you hold your child. These days are a time of healing and recovery. Soon you'll be remembering this time of your life tenderly, holding it in your heart forever.

Because both you and your baby are emotionally and physically vulnerable, you will be wise to follow certain guidelines. No matter where or how you had your baby, a long period of postpartum nurturing is essential. If you gave birth in the hospital, the details of eating, resting, and caring for your baby may be orchestrated by the staff for the first few days. Let yourself feel like a pampered queen; you deserve to be given good care. Don't hesitate to ask for whatever you desire. Let the hospital staff know your baby's needs and your own needs and desires. Hold firm to the fact that your baby needs you. It was your body that held her as she grew from embryo to fetus to baby. Your waters cradled her. Your voice soothed. Your every step was baby's dance. Separation, even if your baby is just down the hall, is frightening and painful for her. Try, from the moment of birth on, to be inseparable from your child. You, as mother, know much better than anyone that baby needs you.

Some women because of medical necessity experience prolonged hospitalization, but the choice of many families today is early discharge from the hospital or birth center. Home birth is also a viable alternative. This later choice means that family and friends will have full responsibility for the mother and newborn immediately after birth.

Before taking leave of you, the doctor or midwife should examine both you and your baby thoroughly to make sure all is well. If there is any indication that further medical attention is needed, you should not be left unattended. If you have any questions, even a shadow of a doubt, now or later, ask your doctor or midwife.

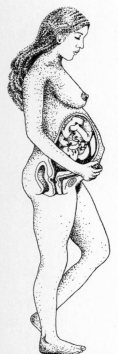

Pregnant,
full term

Getting Help

Birth is a rite of passage, the journey into parenthood. You may be anxious or amazed at your self-reliance. In either case, for the first few days it is important

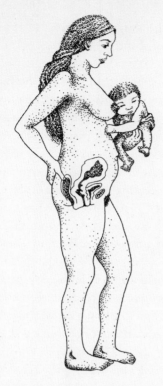

Immediately following the birth, before involution (from the outside, the mother may
appear to be 5–6 months pregnant).

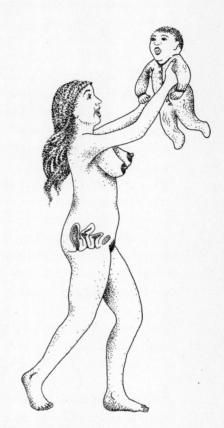

About six weeks postpartum the uterus has
nearly regained its pre-pregnancy shape,
size, and position.

that you reach out for the support of those around you who love you. In many societies the world over, postpartum care is assured. In North America, we are only beginning to recognize the bedrock importance of mothers and babies. A well-nurtured infant grows up to be a caring adult who in turn raises children who can live harmoniously with others and contribute to society's well-being. Spending these early days showering your child with love and attention is impor-tant, not just on the level of the individual or her family, but for the entire planet's future. A well-nurtured individual grows up to respect his or her fellow humans, the plant and animal kingdoms, and the fragile ecology of the Earth. Mothering is our world's most essential occupation. For this reason, I beg families to protect the new mother.

If you are not in a hospital for the first forty-eight hours following the birth, someone should be, must be, around to help with your needs and the care of your baby. This can be the baby's father, but if he, too, is tired and disoriented from his own passage into parenthood, a doula or labor coach, a close friend, a relative, or a neighbor should be called upon to help. The people chosen need to be alert to and intent upon your needs. Let them know you are counting on them.

You are being bombarded with physical and emotional stimuli and deserve the best care. Too many visitors may wear you out. Naturally your attention is focused on your newborn, and you need much rest. Friends and family will understand if you ask them to postpone visits for a few weeks. By then, you will appreciate the company.

Get those who do visit in the early days to help out. Let family and friends know that you won't entertain them. The support and love of those close to you will be the greatest gifts they can give. Ask someone to bring a camera over and take pictures for you. You may wish to post a note on the door that says:

Glad you are thinking of us. Baby and mom are resting peacefully right now. We sure would love a helping hand with…
    ❏ *housework*   ❏ *errands*   ❏ *the kids*   ❏ *meals*   ❏ *other*

Recently in Iowa, I received a baby during a week of wicked winter weather. Inside the glow and warmth of this home, a child was being born. Just outside, someone had anonymously come in the night to shovel the driveway and sidewalks. This sweet gesture will never be forgotten by the family, nor will they ever know who did it.

Your partner will be feeling tender in these first few days. It is likely he was shaken by the power and wonder of your child's birth. He is probably eager to help. It may seem like he's avoiding you when, in fact, he fears he'll tread on the delicate aura surrounding you and his newborn child. Include him by asking for back rubs, nice meals, and special nurturing. Get him to hold the baby. Tell him that you, too, are just getting to know this little stranger. Invite him to share in the intimacy of this bonding period.

If at all possible, follow the ancient tradition of many cultures and stay home with the baby for a prolonged lying-in period after the birth. The Ayurvedic tradition, practiced in India, suggests that mothers and babies spend the first twenty-two days postpartum quietly at home. Don't be too eager to break the bubble of peace that surrounds you and your baby. These days are precious.

Newborn Care

Although the focus of this book is you, the new mother, your focus is also very much on your baby. Because you may have many questions about newborn care, especially if this is your first baby, I've included a brief overview here. Your best sources for help and advice concerning your newborn, however, are other mothers, midwives, and wise women. You may want to read some of the new books or contact organizations listed in Reading and Resources at the back of this book.

Caring for the newborn means giving him or her love, as well as observing your baby's breathing, temperature, heart rate, and ability to eat and eliminate. How your baby looks and acts to you is usually the best indicator of how well he's doing. The following information will help you understand and monitor your baby's wellness in the first weeks after birth.

TEMPERATURE
Your health-care giver will probably check your baby's temperature regularly during the first days. She or he may take the baby's temperature under the newborn's

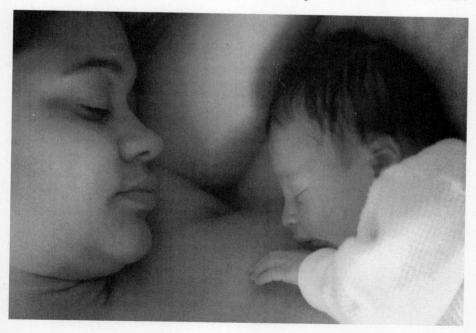

arm. (It is not necessary to take the temperature by mouth or rectum, but add one degree to the reading you obtain from under the arm.) An under-the-arm reading of 97.6° is normal for a newborn, with the actual temperature being 98.6° (from 97.5 to 99.5° is considered normal for newborns). If your baby feels too warm to your touch or looks too cold (blue hands, feet, or lips), take a temperature reading carefully; otherwise it is not necessary to take baby's temperature unless so advised by your health-care giver.

HEART RATE

At rest, a full-term neonate's heart rate should be between 80 and 160 beats per minute. (Occasionally a healthy newborn in deep sleep will have a heart rate as low as 70 beats per minute.) If your baby was born prematurely, his or her mean heart rate may be slightly higher than that of a term newborn. Some irregularity can be normal. Sleep cycles such as dreaming can affect the heart rate. To take

Postpartum Practices around the World

Sweden encourages mothers to stay home with their babies by giving them two years of maternity leave with full pay. This time off from work to nurture the baby may be used entirely by the mother or split with the baby's father.

On the island of Maui, in Hawaii, women who choose to give birth at home can depend on three to four postpartum visits by their midwives in the first week. The midwives like to arrange an in-home professional massage for the new mother on about day four postpartum. The midwife visits again at two weeks postpartum and at six weeks. On Maui, and in other family-centered communities in the United States, mothers are networking to improve their postpartum experiences. Friends often bring food and volunteer to do the housecleaning. Once mother and baby have become settled and are ready to reenter the world (about six weeks after birth), they gather at the beach with other mothers who have babies of about the same age. Groups of mothers and children, and often entire families, get together for films and potlucks. This experience your baby's pulse, place two fingers over her heart and count for thirty seconds, then multiply that number by two.

BREATHING

Your baby's breathing should not seem to take any effort. In the first day of life, the normal respiration range is forty to sixty breaths per minute, with wide variations. Unless your baby's breathing is labored, he is gasping, or his chest is retracting when he inhales, there is usually no reason to worry over his respiration. To determine his rate of respiration while he is quiet, count the number of breaths he takes for one full minute. A new baby's breathing can be irregular. Do not be alarmed if your baby seems to be breathing deeply and then suddenly takes a few quick gulps of air.

If your baby's breathing is noisy, she probably has a bit of mucus in her nose or throat. Usually the swallowing required to breastfeed will clear this. You can suction out the mucus with a bulb syringe, which can be purchased at any drugstore. *Be sure to ask your health-care giver to show you how to do this correctly.* Before inserting a bulb syringe into a baby's mouth, make sure all the air has been squeezed out of it, and go gently.

UMBILICAL CORD STUMP CARE

Your baby's umbilical cord stump normally needs no special care. Some mothers like to dab it with a cotton swab dipped in rubbing alcohol or hydrogen peroxide to keep it clean. I do not recommend alcohol or hydrogen peroxide as they are harsh and may cause the baby to feel painful burning. They also tend to reopen the healing wound. An old Native American tradition was to sprinkle the ash from a volcanic eruption on the healing cord stump. In Indonesia and the Philippines, the crushed antiseptic leaf of the bitter cucumber vine is often applied to cord stumps.

No matter what you do, your baby's cord stump will have a fleshy smell before it dries up and falls off. If you do clean around it, be very gentle. (Even before the cord stump has fallen away, you may bathe baby in warm water, using no soap, and pat her dry.) In approximately one to three weeks, the stump will fall off. Keep the area uncovered by folding diapers back so urine does not seep into it. After the stump has fallen away, your baby may still have a slightly open umbilicus for a few days. Continue to keep it dry and uncovered until it heals completely. Call your doctor or midwife if the area around the cord becomes red or hot or pussy.

Lotus Birth…Care of the Placenta

Cutting of the umbilical cord after the birth of a baby is a medical ritual. It is not practiced in all indigenous cultures. It is in fact not necessary. If you choose to avoid all violence, by keeping the cord intact, you are making the beautiful choice to give your baby a "lotus birth." Any birth in which cord cutting is delayed until after the placenta is born is indeed a lotus birth. A full lotus birth entails no cutting at all, and allows the cord to fall off in its own time.

Having helped many families with this gentle choice, I am in awe of its significance. I urge expectant families to consider this completely natural option.

Sometime after the birth, when mother and baby are stable, bring a warm bath of water to the baby and his or her still-connected placenta. Gently wash as much of the blood from the placenta as you can. It is the blood that quickly begins to smell decayed. By washing the placenta, you slow that process down. Next rub the placenta with ground dried rosemary or fragrant herbs of your choice. This will help speed the drying process and eliminate most of the odor. Wrap the placenta in a cloth diaper and place it in a small basket, beside baby and mother.

The presence of the placenta, called the "little brother" or "little sister" in many cultures, has a protective quality. The family will stay more centered, quiet, and reverent around the new mother and child, until the baby himself either pulls off or kicks away the placenta. This process of respecting the baby's timing is so beautiful. I have seen babies grasp their umbilical cord as it changes and dries, so tenderly, integrating the changes in this, his most familiar companion in the womb. Siblings often will not leave the home, even to go outside and play, until the cord has fallen away in its own time. This is not a rule but a subconscious guardianship within the family that can spontaneously take place when patience and faith are present.

Leaving the newborn baby connected to the placenta will greatly limit the amount of moving around the mother and child do. Some folks find this inconvenient. However, as a midwife, I greatly appreciate the depth of rest my lotus birth families are able to enjoy during the few days of transition before the cord and placenta fall away. I've seen it take three days, an average of five, and as many as eight days for the cord to fall off. All members of the family will experience the depth of the mystery of life and death as this gentle process unfolds. One lotus birth father, Scott, had vivid dreams. He and his wife, Rebecca, both spontaneously woke on the third night when their new son, Inti, kicked free of his cord and placenta.

In Bali, the Hindu Dharma people believe the placenta, called Ari-Ari, is the physical body of the baby's guardian angel. Science has taught us that the placenta is the advocate for the baby during pregnancy. Knowing this, may we in our culture learn to respect the astonishing placenta.

For more information on lotus birth, look for the book Lotus Birth *by Shivam Rachana and order the Lotus Birth Information Packet by Jeannine Parvati Baker. (See Reading and Resources in this book for addresses.)*

SKIN CARE

Your newborn has a unique smell. Don't be quick to wash away this lovely scent, for it will be gone all too soon.

Even before the baby's cord stump has healed, you may bathe her in warm water (make sure the water is not too hot or cold by testing it on the inside of your forearm). Avoiding soaps is best, but if you do wish to use soap, choose a mild product that contains no chemical additives. Always pat baby dry thoroughly. Keep her out of drafts.

You may give your baby a daily massage with a pure grade of olive, sesame, or coconut oil. If baby's skin is dry, peeling, or cracking, the oil massage will quickly help soothe the delicate newborn skin.

Remember the baby is accustomed to the warm wet skin-friendly environment of the womb. Even soft clothing may feel abrasive to newborn skin. All your baby's clothing should be washed and double rinsed before she wears them. Buy an odor-free natural laundry soap; avoid harsh detergents. Some newborns are so sensitive that I ask families and visitors to stop wearing perfumes (essential oils are natural and generally okay), even antiperspirants. Any strong odor will feel harsh to the newborn senses of smell and touch.

Cotton cloth diapers are kinder to our newborn's skin than the single-use throwaway kind. They are also kinder to our environment (as well as your pocketbook). Please consider using them.

CARE OF THE PENIS

Expectant families must do much reading, research, and heart searching before making the decision to circumcise. It is an irreversible, painful procedure. Please, please, if you have not circumcised your newborn son, do not do it. He is made perfectly and need not be surgically altered.[1] There is a wealth of information available to support your decision to keep the baby intact. Visit the NOCIRC Web site listed at the back of this book, or call NOCIRC ; they are willing to help.

If you had a boy and had him circumcised, you will need to take very good care of his healing penis. Be sure to get thorough care instructions from your doctor at the time the circumcision is done. It is extremely important to ensure that no infection sets in. Though leaving diapers off all newborns is best, it is especially important for boys who have been circumcised. Let him lie without pants, and place a diaper under him to catch waste. Rubberized puddle pads (available in most baby shops), placed under the open diaper, help keep the bedding dry. If you suspect that your baby's penis is getting infected, *get medical care immediately.*

Uncircumcised baby boys need no special attention or cleaning. *Do not pull back your baby's foreskin.* This is painful and unnecessary. If you take your baby to see a pediatrician, make certain he or she knows you do not want the baby's intact foreskin retracted. Be firm. This could cause scarring between the foreskin and penis. In time, your son will retract his own foreskin, gently, without pain or harm.

See Reading and Resources in this book for NOCIRC contact and Web site information.

EYE CARE

If drops to prevent infection were placed in your baby's eyes, they may become red and swollen. Most states still require the use of drops. The hospital may give you a choice between silver nitrate or antibiotic ointment, the latter being less invasive. If you birthed at home and decide not to apply drops, you may put a drop or two of colostrum, the first milk your breasts produce, in baby's eyes during the first few days of life. This rich, yellow secretion carries your antibodies and serves as natural "insurance" against infection.

When cleaning baby's eyes, wipe from the inner portion of the eyelid to the outer. Use clean, wet cotton balls, a fresh one for each eye.

If the discharge from the eyes becomes green or yellow, tell your health-care giver. Minor eye irritations can usually be healed by squirting a bit of your breast milk in the baby's eyes. Breast milk cannot hurt your baby's eyes and has been known to work wonders. Note that it takes at least a few days and up to a few weeks for baby's tear ducts to mature and work properly, so don't worry if her eyes look a bit goopy or get stuck shut.

JAUNDICE

About half of the world's healthy newborn babies become a little yellow or jaundiced. Physiologic, or newborn, jaundice is caused by the buildup of bilirubin, or bile pigment, in the blood, which the newborn's liver is not yet able to process.

If your baby seems jaundiced—has yellow skin or yellowed whites of the eyes, or is irritable or seems too sleepy—call your midwife; she will want to check the baby. Most mildly jaundiced babies are fine, and three or four minutes' exposure to direct sunlight (weather permitting) or up to twenty minutes of indirect sunlight through a window a couple of times a day clears up the condition. Do not overexpose your baby to the sun as his skin is tender and burns easily. Always protect baby's eyes by covering them, and never leave your newborn alone outside or by a sunny window.

In white and African American babies with physiologic jaundice, there is a decline of the unconjugated bilirubin level about five days after birth. This will be seen as a clearing up of the yellow skin color. In Asian and Native American newborns, this takes seven to ten days.

Jaundice Prevention Tips

- Breastfeeding often is the best way to resolve jaundice.
- You can put vitamin E directly on your nipples. This soothes sore nipples and helps resolve jaundice as the baby nurses.
- You can drink freshly squeezed citrus juices daily. This enriches your milk with vitamin C, which the baby will get when he nurses. Vitamin C reduces jaundice.
- Consult a homeopathic practitioner about a remedy for jaundice.
- If your baby's jaundice lasts longer than seven to ten days, please have her checked for pathologic jaundice. This condition is rare, but requires medical treatment.

FEEDING

Babies should be fed when they are hungry. This means anywhere from eight to twelve good feeds, and sometimes a few "snacks," a day. You need not wake up your baby for feedings to be sure he or she is getting enough nourishment. However, if your baby seems overly sleepy and is not wetting six or more cloth diapers per day, you must wake her up every four hours for a good feed. Look at your baby's fontanel, or soft spot; if it is deeply depressed, your baby may be dehydrated. It is imperative the baby stay well hydrated, preferably by breast milk. (Don't give the new baby water. Breast milk only is recommended by the WHO, La Leche League International, and most health-care givers.) Just be sure she takes your breast with enthusiasm, is sucking and swallowing well, or gets enough commercial formula and digests it well.

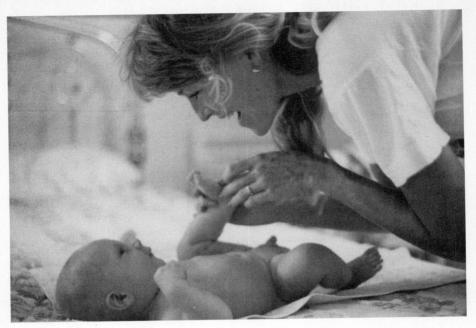

You will want to discuss feeding with your health-care giver and experienced mothers to be reassured that your baby is eating well. If you decide not to breast-feed, watch for allergies or negative reactions to formulas. If your baby seems unable to digest her formula, or shows symptoms of allergic reaction like skin rashes, you will need to change formula until you find one that is compatible with your infant. Breast milk, being the perfect new baby food, will not present the same nutritional concerns as formula (see chapter 5, Breastfeeding, Bottle-Feeding, and Breast Care).

Not all of your baby's cries mean "feed me." However, in the early days when feeding is getting established, this is often what they mean. As your baby grows, you will soon know exactly what your little one is trying to say.

Spitting up is normal; however, if your baby suffers from projectile vomiting (i.e., the vomit seems to shoot quite a distance, out of baby with little or no warning), see your health-care giver so she or he can determine if medical attention is needed.

ELIMINATION

Your baby should have at least one bowel movement and urinate at least once in the first twenty-four hours after birth. For about the first three days or so, your baby's stools will be tarlike, almost black and sticky, and will stain clothing and diapers. This is meconium, the contents of your baby's bowels before he was born. As your milk comes in, his bowel movements change to a yellow, curdlike stool. Once breastfeeding is established, or the baby is taking formula, he will have at least six, and probably many more, wet diapers a day. If you feel that your baby eliminates very frequently or very infrequently, be sure to ask your health-care giver about it. They can put your mind at ease by helping you discover the normal rate of elimination for your baby.

YOUR MOTHERLY INTUITION

Learn to trust your mothering instincts. It may take time, but be assured your instincts for knowing how to care for your baby will develop. As you get to know her, you will become sensitive to her unique needs. Ask your health-care giver about your baby's temperature, pulse, elimination, breathing, or anything else you think of to help you gain confidence. They can help you learn how to determine the baby's well-being. Watch just how keenly aware of your baby and her needs you become as you learn to trust your intuition.

Don't hesitate to call upon more experienced mothers in your community for help in developing your own mothering skills. The early days postpartum is a perfect time to rekindle a special closeness with your own mother. Even by phone or e-mail, her wise words will soothe and reassure you.

On her third day postpartum my daughter said, "Now I know how much you love me."

The Mother's Special Needs

In the first precious days following birth, your awareness is so intent on the baby that you may neglect your own needs. You will heal faster and be equipped to be an even better mother if you get enough rest, eat nutritious food often, drink plenty of healthful fluids, and get lots of help. Your moods may swing; one moment you will be elated, the next down. You have a great need for sleep. You struggle to find balance with your body image as you go from bulging with life, to birthing, to breastfeeding.

You may feel the strong urge to talk about your birth. (Later, if you have not already done so, you will want to write down this story, using the blank pages in chapter 2.) This is not only natural, it is essential that you go over every detail. A good friend or family member will love to listen to you recount your birth story. You may want to keep a pen and paper by your bedside; your notes and observations of your child's first days will be precious stories to tell as he or she grows.

You may feel full of energy, but don't overextend yourself. This is mainly emotional energy. Physically you are tired, especially if you had a long labor and difficult birth. Doing too much in the first few days and weeks postpartum may cause you to have a longer overall recovery period. Keep in mind that doing too much may mean simply being on your feet too long. It is especially easy to push beyond your physical limit if you have other children and need to keep up the home.

YOUR PLACENTA

If you have a chance, take a close look at the placenta. It weighs only about one pound. On the baby's side, the umbilical cord is attached with its main vessels radiating outward. It looks like a tree of life and is smooth and glossy. On the maternal side the surface is irregular and spongy. Remember, this side was once attached to your uterine wall and has now been torn away.

During the baby's development, your placenta provided for his or her nutritional needs, respiration, and excretion of waste products, and acted as barrier to protect the unborn child from harmful bacteria and most foreign molecules. The placenta also served you and baby as an organ of synthesis. Hormones (estrogen, progesterone, gonadotrophin) as well as certain foodstuffs and local enzymes were synthesized and employed by your placenta.

After the birth, your uterus is empty. Not only is the baby gone, but your placenta is no longer with you. It is no wonder a profound feeling of loss is experienced after having a baby. The placenta, which sustained your baby, also provided you with a level of hormonal activity to which you have grown accustomed.

The drug and cosmetic industries have long known the valuable properties of human placenta. Doctors of Chinese medicine can dry your placenta so you can put the powder in capsules to take like vitamins. For centuries, women in China have preserved part of their placentas in this way. Later in life, they can take the dried placenta as a remedy for symptoms of menopause.

Animals eat their placentas. Distasteful as it may sound, human mothers would benefit if the practice of eating the placenta after giving birth became commonplace once again. Traditionally in many cultures, mothers chewed a piece if the placenta after birth to prevent or stop hemorrhage. By ingesting the placenta, you take back some of the nutrients and hormones you've lost in birthing. Many women who have been reluctant to try this are surprised to discover the artfully cooked placenta is delicious. It is interesting to note that placenta is the only meat that is not obtained by killing an animal.

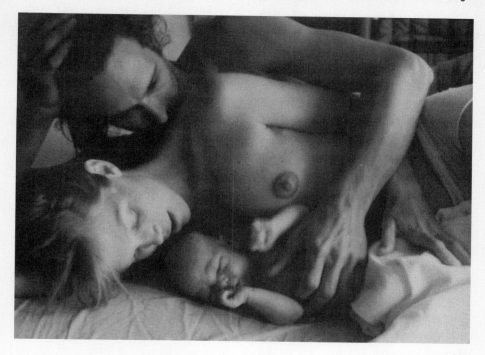

Even if you choose not to eat your placenta, remember it belongs to you and need not be treated like garbage. Ask the hospital or your midwife, ahead of time, to save it for you, but don't depend on them to do so. Have your birthing partner bring a sturdy plastic bag or two-quart bowl with a lid that seals tightly along to birth. Then the placenta can be taken home and frozen until you decide what kind of tree you would like to plant with it. Many women experience a feeling of loss after birthing, and rituals, like planting a placenta tree, may lessen the sorrow. A growing child will marvel at the peach tree that derived its strength from the same organ that sustained him before birth.

ELIMINATION

It is important to urinate soon after you give birth. An over-full bladder can cause excessive postpartum bleeding. Your midwife probably will not leave until you have had at least one urination after birthing. Small abrasions, tears, and/or stitches in the perineum will hurt when you urinate for a few days. However, do not let this discourage you; you must pee. Very concentrated urine is more uncomfortable to pass, and you need to be well hydrated to heal well and establish a good milk supply. Please, drink plenty of fluids. If you've had stitches, don't be concerned, urine is sterile when it first comes out. Pat dry gently, rather than wiping.

Using a clean squirt bottle filled with warm water, irrigate your vaginal area as you urinate. The warm water helps prevent stinging; it is even more soothing if you irrigate with warm comfrey tea.

By drinking lots of fluids, you dilute the urine and reduce burning caused by urine coming into contact with tender vaginal tissue. Your urethra may be traumatized from the birth, making it difficult to urinate. If this is the case, sit patiently on the toilet when you feel the urge, giving your body a chance to relax and do its job. Once things get going, you may find you urinate frequently and perspire more than usual because of your increased breast size, any extra weight you may be carrying, and hormonal changes.

In the first days following birth, your bowels may be sluggish, almost afraid to move, especially if you had an episiotomy or tear and are afraid of damaging the stitches. It is important for you to eliminate, but it is equally important not to strain. Try to relax on the toilet. Take slow deep breaths, and don't hurry or push. You may apply pressure, using a gauze pad, to your perineum to protect your stitches while having a bowel movement. Get plenty of liquids and eat fresh foods that are nonconstipating (see page 115). If you don't have a bowel movement within the first couple of days, tell your health-care giver.

Hemorrhoids are a common postpartum complaint (see page 112). The pressure of childbearing on the pelvic floor and the increased blood volume from pregnancy can cause swollen veins to protrude from the anus. This is extremely painful. If you are suffering from hemorrhoids, it is very important that you avoid constipation and never strain on the toilet. Warm, shallow baths offer some relief, and Tucks, an over-the-counter hemorrhoid care product, can make you more comfortable, but building your ability to heal by resting is the best medicine.

Both the sitz bath below and/or the herbal pack will help soothe the pain of skids (those painful hot spots or abrasions) and tears, the discomfort of stitches, and hemorrhoids while promoting healing. All women, even if they don't tear, experience some discomfort in the pelvic floor after having a baby. Herbal packs and sitz baths feel so good and really do help.

BLEEDING

Following the birth, you will bleed. This discharge is called *lochia*. For several days, it will be red and similar to a heavy menstrual flow. Then it becomes brownish and lasts for a couple of weeks or more. If your lochia turns bright red

Bev's Herbal Postpartum Sitz Bath

½ oz. comfrey leaf and or root (promotes cell growth and healing)

½ oz. rosemary (antiseptic, reduces swelling)

½ oz. urva ursi leaf (heals the urinary tract)

½ oz. shepherd's purse (promotes clotting)

½ cup sea salt (for healing properties of saline)

TO MAKE: Add herbs to boiling water with salt; let steep. Strain through a clean piece of cloth, or a diaper in a colander, into the bathtub. Sit in this warm shallow bath (you may add water as you please) 1 to 2 times a day for the first few days to one week postpartum.

---

after it has been brown, you are probably exerting yourself too much. Lie down with your feet elevated for the remainder of the day. Staying off your feet, as much as possible for at least your first five days postpartum, will help prevent excessive bleeding.

If your lochia smells foul, or if your bleeding becomes heavy (soaking two large pads with blood in less than half an hour after the first twenty-four hours following the birth), call your health-care giver. Another cause for concern is persistently passing a clot larger than a golf ball. Your bleeding should not be excessive; if you suddenly gush blood, call your health-care giver immediately.

For the first two to three days postpartum, deeply massage your lower abdomen with your fingers, about every half hour or when you wake up from sleep. Your uterus should respond by remaining contracted; it should stay hard and about the size of a grapefruit. If it becomes soft and does not respond to massage by remaining contracted, call your health-care giver. Suckling your baby inspires the presence of oxytocin, a hormone that helps keep your uterus firm, preventing excessive bleeding.

Afterbirth contractions or afterpains are normal (see page 107). After your second or subsequent birth, they are sometimes quite severe, and you may need to use relaxation and breathing techniques like those used during labor to get through them. It helps to remember that the pains are beneficial, assisting your uterus to return to its pre-pregnancy state.

When to Be Concerned

If you faint, get severe headaches, have pain anywhere, bleed heavily, feel frightened about your physical or mental health, are worried about your baby, or feel you cannot cope, don't hesitate to talk to your health-care giver. Perhaps the most serious physical postpartum condition that could develop and remain undetected unless the symptoms are known is uterine infection, referred to in the past as "childbed fever." The pain associated with uterine infection may not be severe enough to cause you to contact your health-care giver, but these infections can result in death, so you must be aware of and watch for the symptoms, which are

- Tender uterus
- Lower back pain
- Foul-smelling discharge
- Elevated temperature (over 101°)
- Elevated pulse
- Cold sweats

If you have any of these symptoms, you should call your health-care giver immediately.

SORENESS

Your perineum may be sore from stitches, slight tearing, skid marks, or stretching. In the first few hours following birth, you may use an ice pack for relief of swelling and pain. I've found that the best ice pack for this purpose is a condom, filled with approximately 1½ cups water. Freeze this before you go into labor, then it will be on hand if you need it. Later, a warm, shallow bath will speed the healing process. A squirt bottle of warm water while you urinate will help with the stinging and serves also to clean the area. When you are sore, there's nothing like sitting on a little pillow. You may wish to try sitting on two pillows, spaced a few inches apart, with one buttock on each.

Your entire body may be quite sore from labor and delivery. You may wish to get a thorough postpartum massage from an experienced masseuse within a few days after the birth.

The herbal compress or pack described below is my favorite first aid for postpartum soreness in the perineum, the scary area.

Melody's Herbal Yoni* Pack

Very handy, soothing and promotes healing. It's best to obtain these herbs before the birth, or send someone out to buy them for you.

A generous pinch of each of these herbs: comfrey root or leaf, slippery elm, and goldenseal powder.

Open a sterile gauze pad. Sprinkle the herbs into the center. Fold into a shape like a pad or flat cigar, making sure to tuck the ends in, so the herbs don't escape. Lay in a bowl and pour approximately two ounces of boiling water over the pack, let steep five minutes. When it is cooled off, but still pleasantly warm, pick up the ends and twist to squeeze some of the excess water out. Place the pack right in your underpants, close to your yoni, with a maternity pad beneath to hold it in place. Wear twenty to sixty minutes. Remove and dry area thoroughly. Your yoni needs to be dry most of the time to heal well.

BREASTS

Your breasts will become full when your milk comes in, within thirty-six to seventy-two hours after you give birth. Prior to this, your breasts provide colostrum for your baby. This thick yellow substance contains your antibodies to disease, which are essential to your infant's optimal health. Just before the onset of the flow of your "true milk," a low-grade fever (below 101°) known as "milk fever" often sets in. This fever lasts about twenty-four hours and is alleviated once the milk begins to flow.

If you will not be breastfeeding, please do not take prescription medication to dry up your breast milk. There is a controversial drug called bromocriptine (Parlodel), the use of which may cause vomiting, diarrhea, fainting, loss of appetite, seizures, and stroke. As far back as 1989, an FDA advisory group recommended the agency withdraw approval for drugs and hormones prescribed for the suppression of lactation. The FDA did ask the manufactures of bromocriptine to stop labeling the drug for use as a lactation supressant for new mothers. Sandoz, the maker of this drug commonly called Parlodel, declined to follow the FDA recommendation. Lactation suppression drugs are prescribed to an estimated 700,000 women each year; they are only marginally effective.

To naturally suppress lactation, bind your breasts but not too tightly. Avoid eating alfalfa sprouts for a couple of weeks, as alfalfa increases milk supply. Drinking sage tea can also suppress lactation. Your breasts may still become engorged or overly full (see page 88), but do not hand-express milk unless you

---

*In this chapter and throughout the book I will use the Sanskrit word for vagina, yoni. To me the word yoni honors this sacred part of the female anatomy.

are told to do so by your health-care giver, as removing milk encourages its production.

Do not be alarmed by the drawing and tingling feeling in your breasts. This sensation, which can be powerful, is called the *letdown reflex*. It signals the presence of milk and lets you know all is well. Letdown is experienced at various times. Sometimes it occurs at the thought, smell, or sight of your infant. The sound of your baby crying or smacking her lips can cause it. Even a smile from your partner, a giggle from your four-year-old, all can activate your oxytocin, the hormone of love and the hormone that causes the letdown reflex. Usually once breastfeeding is established, letdown happens after the baby's first few sucks.

During the feed, make sure the baby is well on the breast, not just sucking your nipple but taking a good amount of breast tissue into her mouth. Sit comfortably or side-lie, positioning yourself and baby belly to belly. You will notice that when mother and baby are belly to belly, the baby need not twist her neck to reach the nipple. If you notice baby twisting her neck to reach your breast, gently turn her body toward you. Poor breastfeeding positioning can cause sore nipples, numerous breast problems, and difficulty establishing breastfeeding.

Between feedings, keep your nipples clean and dry. Don't use soaps or creams, except for lanolin ointment, which is especially made for breastfeeding mothers. Vitamin E, right from the capsule, can be applied to nipples after feedings to prevent soreness or cracking. Do not wear a tight bra. Hot packs or hot compresses made with freshly grated gingerroot help relieve the discomfort or engorgement. (See page 90 of chapter 5 for details on preparing a ginger compress.) Frequent feeding and remembering to feed from both sides each time will help relieve engorgement and ensure an adequate milk supply.

If you notice changes in your breasts or experience pain with breastfeeding, discuss your condition with your health-care giver. Painful, feverish breasts can lead to serious infection if not treated quickly. If your breasts become red, hard, or painful, or if you run a fever *over* 101°, see your health-care giver. (A temperature up to 101° is normal about day three when your milk is coming in.)

If you have difficulty getting started or experience discomfort during breastfeeding, don't become discouraged. Ask for help and support from mothers who have nursed babies. Organizations like International Lactation Consultants Association (ILAC) and La Leche League may be found online. (See Reading and Resources in this book.) They can answer questions, give support, or help you find a professional lactation consultant if you need one. Mothers of premature babies or babies who are hospitalized for any reason may still breastfeed, but it will take determination (see Premature Babies, page 273). Chapter 5 (Breastfeeding, Bottle-

Feeding, and Breast Care) provides details and expands on the information provided here.

NUTRITION

This is not time to diet. As a postpartum woman, you need almost as much protein and more vitamins and minerals than you did when you were pregnant. If you are breastfeeding, your nutritional needs are increased further because the baby receives approximately 1,000 calories each day from your milk. If you diet while you are breastfeeding, you compromise your baby's nutritional needs as well as your own. Even if you are not breastfeeding, poor nutrition will leave you susceptible to colds and other infections. It can also cause you to be irritable because your nerves are raw and you feel exhausted. To avoid getting run-down, it is essential that you eat several well-balanced meals a day. Don't forget to eat a complete protein with each meal. This need not be a meat protein; many vegetarian women have breastfed their babies successfully.

Postpartum Belly Pack

Just look at the size of your beautiful baby. He or she plus the placenta and the amniotic fluid all fit neatly into your belly such a short time ago. Now your organs are finding their original placement in your abdominal region. These organs and your intestines were slowly displaced over many moons. Now all of a sudden, they are looking for their once familiar places. This process can be greatly aided, plus general healing of your entire body will be enhanced, by applying the following postpartum belly pack. You may do this daily for the first week. I've seen improvement in muscle tone and the mother's general feeling of well-being even if the belly pack is applied only one time.

Ask a friend or family member to help you.

1. Fill a hot-water bottle with very hot water.
2. Rub your belly with a generous amount of odor-free castor oil.
3. Lay a clean cotton diaper over your belly to protect you.
4. Place the hot water bottle on your belly on top of the diaper.
5. Rest for at least twenty minutes.
6. You may wish to rewarm the water bottle now and again.

Cesarean Birth

If you had a cesarean birth, you have more to cope with afterward. You have undergone major surgery and must heal. You must also care for your baby. Women have many strong feelings after birthing. As a cesarean mother, you must process the emotional and physical strain of surgery, as well as make the adjustments to mothering a newborn. If you have other children at home, the demands made upon you are huge.

With so much emphasis on naturalizing birth, you may feel let down and angry because you didn't deliver vaginally. This is natural. You may feel that your experience was not ideal, yet you cannot change what occurred. International Cesarean Awareness Network (ICAN) is a very good support organization available to help mothers deal with both the physical aspects of and their emotional responses to cesarean birth. You can write or call their national headquarters and request their list of publications that deal with cesarean birth and recovery as well as information on preventing future cesarean deliveries. They can also refer you to cesarean support groups in your community. If ICAN does not have a group near you, they will refer you to the local chapters of related organizations that do. (See Reading and Resources for address and phone number.) *Mothering* magazine has been a very supportive publication for cesarean mothers. You may wish to write and ask them for reprints of *Cesarean Poems* and the Cesarean Special Issue (see address in Reading and Resources).

As a cesarean mother, you may have had greater blood loss than a woman who delivered vaginally. The folk remedies for iron-related anemia are getting lots of rest, eating leafy green vegetables, and snacking on raisins. The best herbal tonic for treating or preventing anemia is yellow dock root. You can find it in tincture form at health-food and herb stores. A good liquid iron supplement is recommended for all cesarean mothers and women who have hemorrhaged after childbirth. You may also want to ask your doctor about iron tablets (though I prefer the liquid iron supplements over the tablet form) to supplement your diet if he or she doesn't prescribe them, because a change in diet alone is sometimes not enough to treat severe anemia. One consequence of obtaining iron from supplements is that it can cause constipation (iron-rich foods usually don't have this effect), and postpartum cesarean women often tend to have sluggish elimination already. To counteract the irregularity the iron supplements may cause, increase your intake of liquids and roughage (see Constipation, page 114). Walking also helps get a sluggish system moving. If you increase your exercise and adjust your diet and still find that your stools are very hard, dark, and difficult to pass, you

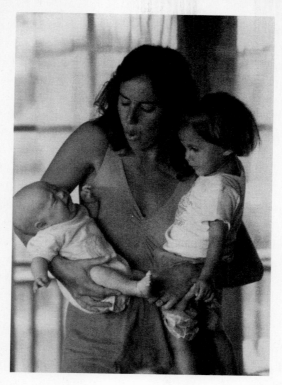

may want to discontinue the supplements for a couple of days and favor leafy green vegetables and make sure you get plenty of rest.

Most women who deliver by cesarean section stay in the hospital for a minimum of four days and up to a week. By day two or three postpartum, the incision should look well sealed from the outside; however, this does not mean you should be running laps or doing sit-ups. The commonly prescribed painkillers have been known to work so well that there have been reports of women being unaware that they reopened their incisions when they jumped back into strenuous activity too quickly. Straining or reopening the incision sets back the healing process, increases the risk of infection, and causes more scar tissue to form. Support your incision with your hand or a pillow before coughing, sneezing, or laughing. *Absolutely do not lift anything heavier than your baby for a minimum of three weeks and preferably longer.* This means you must ask for help when you need it. Try to arrange for your mate, a friend, or a family member to be at home with you for at least the first two weeks you are home from the hospital. You will need the support. If you are home alone, let the chores go. Don't be tempted to "go ahead and get a few things done." Wait until someone is there to help out.

After you leave the hospital, it is safe to shower daily. However, do not scrub your incision site, and follow the instructions your physician gives you. Many women experience itching around the incision. Itching is a good sign; it means you are healing. After the tapes have been removed after four to seven days depending on how quickly you heal and your doctor's opinion, you may gently apply vitamin E to the area. Some women report that vitamin E helps reduce itching and decreases scaring.

If you are breastfeeding, experiment with nursing positions to find those that are most comfortable for you. Often cesarean mothers prefer to breastfeed while lying on their sides.

Severe gas pains are a problem for some women when recovering from a cesarean birth. The herb valerian has helped many women who suffer from gas and can also reduce pain from the incision. (Comfrey is another herb especially beneficial for cesarean mothers as it promotes healing. See chapter 11, Herbs for the Postpartum Woman, which tells how to prepare these herbs and others you may wish to take.) Elizabeth Noble's book *Essential Exercises for the Childbearing Years* (Boston: Houghton Mifflin, 1988) has excellent suggestions for cesarean mothers who experience postoperative gas pains. Sometimes taking deep, cleansing breaths, as if you are filling the entire body with oxygen and then blowing it out, helps with gas pains. You can breathe deeply while tightening and contracting the abdominal muscles at the first twinge of a gas pain. Your breath is one of your strongest rehabilitation tools. By blowing, hissing, huffing, and panting, you use your full lung capacity, inspiring better circulation and providing oxygen to your healing tissue. In addition, breathing deeply is important following general anesthesia when respiration is slowed down and the lungs tend to collect mucus. To prevent the stagnation of this mucus in your lungs' base, you must ventilate fully.

A Note about Vitamin and Mineral Supplements...

If you were fortunate enough to have taken a quality well-balanced multivitamin and mineral prenatal supplement during your pregnancy, please continue to do so for as long as you breastfeed. If you suffer from anemia, remember that a multivitamin/mineral supplement is a better value than buying iron tablets separately, as your body needs a balance of all the nutrients.

Walking is very helpful for mothers recovering from cesarean and all births. In the hospital, you were asked to walk to decrease the amount of time it took for the anesthesia to wear off and to ensure that the body's systems such as circulation, respiration, and elimination did not atrophy. Now that you are home, walking speeds the healing process by improving circulation. Weather permitting, you can take short walks outdoors immediately after you return from the hospital. Walk, but do not strain.

Three exercises from chapter 8, Toning What's Inside, that are safe and beneficial for cesarean mothers during the first two weeks after surgery are Constructive Rest Position, Yoni Exercises, and the Belly Squeeze. After two weeks, all exercises in Toning What's Inside are safe for you to do them. *Essential Exercises for the Childbearing Years* contains an entire section devoted to exercises and early recovery for cesarean mothers.

"Once a cesarean, always a cesarean" was common medical practice until about fifteen years ago. Physicians feared that the stress of labor on the scar would cause problems with delivery. But vaginal birth after cesarean (VBAC) is becoming more common and, in most cases, is considered safer than repeat cesarean births. If you are planning to have more children, discuss this option with your health-care giver. You may need to change health-care givers if your desire to have a VBAC is strong, and he or she does not consider VBAC as a option for any woman. Find a health-care giver who has experience with VBACs and will encourage and support you. To prepare for a VBAC, stay in good health. This means get some form of gentle exercise daily and eat a well-balanced diet. For good news about VBACs, read *Artemis Speaks* (see Reading and Resources for address) by Nan Koehler. Koehler's book is an excellent guide for mothers who wish to have a VBAC. Keep a positive attitude and plan for a VBAC, but don't be too hard on yourself if it doesn't work out.

In the future, you may choose a "trial vaginal birth," which means you have had a cesarean in the past but want to try to deliver vaginally. You and the baby will be monitored carefully. If either of you becomes "distressed" during the labor, you may be given a cesarean section.

You may decide that your next birth will be a "prepared cesarean birth." Mothers who have placenta previa (the placenta laying over the cervix) are likely candidates. If there is any possibility you may have a cesarean, prepare yourself. Many hospitals offer classes and allow fathers who take the classes with their mates to be present at the birth.

HOW DO I KNOW WHEN I'VE DONE TOO MUCH?

- If your bleeding or lochia has become brown, then returns to bright red, you've done too much and must return to resting.
- If you begin to run a fever and or get a sore or red (hot) spot on your breast, that is a sure sign you've overdone it and must rest.
- If you are finding it hard to cope with the needs of your baby, you need more help and more rest.

Twins and Multiple Births

As a mother of more than one newborn, you will feel blessed and bombshelled. One baby alone is a lot of work. You will get less sleep and the demands made on you will be far greater than on the average new mother.

Breastfeeding may leave you feeling more like a dairy than a mother. If you are concerned about having enough milk for more than one baby, remember that in the past, wet nurses provided milk for up to six infants. You must, however, *try* to get plenty of rest and you *must* eat extremely well to

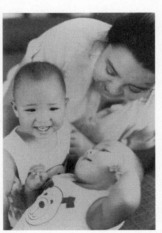

ensure sufficient milk supply. Try as you might to put your babies in a breastfeeding and sleeping routine, they will have their own ideas.

Asking for help is essential. After the first few days when the novelty has worn off and friends and family no longer remember to bring over casseroles, remind them of your need for continued support. With all the caring you must provide for your babies, don't forget that you are postpartum and need to be cared for too! A wonderful gift you might ask a friend to give you is the opportunity to nap.

PAMPER YOURSELF

Pregnancy was a physical test. Birth was hard work. This is your time to rest and recuperate.

You are the center of your new baby's world. Taking good care of yourself is good for your baby. Pamper yourself and let others pamper you. You've given the world a treasure, a child.

Get someone who loves you to come and take over your babies and your home. Unplug the telephone and lock yourself in your bedroom for two hours. (This is especially wonderful if it can happen regularly!)

Because of the stress on your uterus from having had more than one baby, you may have bled more than average. Also, your afterbirth contractions may be stronger and last longer than those experienced by mothers who birthed a single baby. Take it extra easy, follow the guidelines for all mothers in this chapter, and pamper yourself even more. I encourage you to read Elizabeth Nobel's book, *Having Twins: A Parents' Guide to Pregnancy, Birth and Early Childhood* (Boston: Houghton Mifflin, 1991). Also, subscribe to *Double Talk,* a newsletter for parents of twins. Talk with mothers of twins who are older. It may comfort you to know how they were able to cope with taking care of more than one baby while keeping up with the day-to-day chores of running a home. Find out what they did on those days when coping seemed impossible.

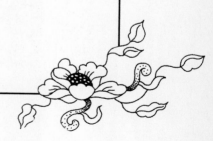

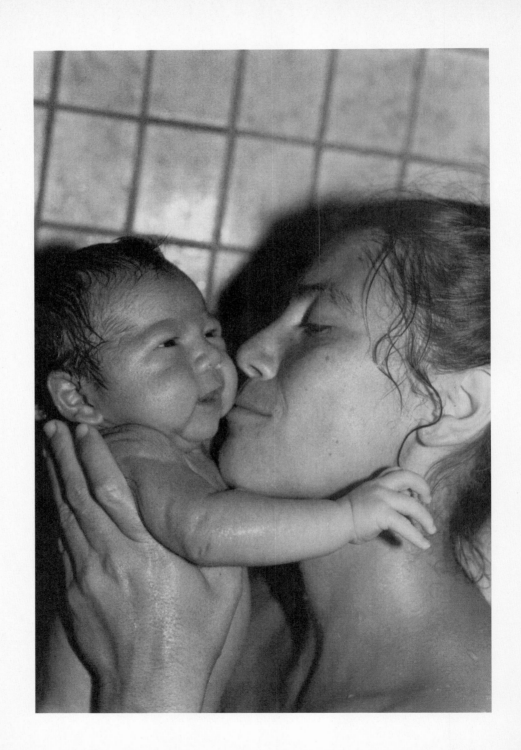

CHAPTER 4

Postpartum Primer:
Taking Care of Yourself and Your Baby

As a mother, your attention will be focused on your baby. This is natural and appropriate because your baby has great need of you. Almost no other mammal on earth is born as helpless as humans. Our offspring remain unable to survive on their own for years. The miracle of maternal bonding, the intense psychological and psychic connection a mother feels for her child, is essential for the baby's survival (see page 240). Bonding creates devotion on the part of the parent and trust on the part of the baby, both of which are life supporting.

Each day is important to your growing baby. To a ten-day-old baby, one day represents one-tenth of her life experience outside your womb. For adults, one day represents only a small part of their lives. So you see, each and every hour of every day is important to your baby. Realizing this makes it easier to set your priorities. Taking care of yourself and your baby are at the very top of the list.

It is important for you to understand that taking good care of yourself *is* taking care of your baby. You are, after all, the baby's primary caretaker. If you are sick or sad or hurt, the baby suffers. If you go without, your baby goes without. Your positive attitude and thoughts glow like light around you and your baby. This is a good time to sculpt your environment and experiences: Choose to be surrounded by uplifting music, supportive people, beautiful settings, healthy and delicious foods, and fresh air.

The postpartum period is also a good time to practice loving-kindness toward yourself. As you unfold in your role of mother, you will see your own strength and beauty as well as your inadequacies. Loving and taking care of yourself when

51

Postpartum Practices around the World

On the island of Palau, new mothers are honored in a celebration called "Ngasech." After four to ten days of ritual cleansing, the "Ngasech" ritual elevates the postpartum woman to her exalted role of mother with chanting, feasting, and flowers.

you have so many other demands on your energy is no easy task. You may not be getting enough sleep. You may feel overwhelmed by the round-the-clock job of being a mother, so taking care of yourself is a tall order.

In the early stages of motherhood, we evolve in the mundane, everyday world. The dishes in the sink, the laundry that needs folding are our testing places. On some days, they feel like battlegrounds. Learning to live graciously among the ordinary chores of family life is a great and, too often, unsung accomplishment in our culture. This chapter outlines some ways in which you can consciously take care of yourself from day to day.

Some days won't be easy. Just as you step into the shower, the baby will cry. You may get so busy that you forget to eat. Mothering takes patience at the very times you feel you have none left. Sometimes you just won't get everything accomplished that you were certain had to be done in that day; even so, find a little time for yourself. Ask friends and family for help so you can take a leisurely bath, sit under a tree, go buy yourself something lovely, or simply brush and floss your teeth and brush your hair.

Taking care of yourself does not mean neglecting the baby. You will become a wizard at responding to the needs of your baby, your mate, and your other children. Soon you will carry your baby while preparing a meal, but in the first weeks after giving birth do not try to take on everything. Breastfeeding and recovering from birth require a tremendous amount of energy. Don't be upset with yourself because you tire easily. The time will come when you will have the energy to accomplish anything you wish to do.

For right now, go easy and go one step at a time. Pace yourself. Do the things you really want to do first so when you run out of steam, the less important tasks are the ones left undone. Don't schedule activities that you know will be impossible to manage with a baby. If you do, you may end up feeling disappointed and defeated.

Labor pushed you to your limits and beyond, demonstrating just how much inner strength you have. Eventually you will use this reserve of strength in your creative endeavors. It takes several months for your strength to return. In fact, your full strength can take a year or more to come back. For every baby I had, it was not until the fourth year postpartum that I said, "Yes, I've really got my stamina back in full." If you rest and take it easy, you won't suffer energy setbacks. In time, you may feel that being a mother makes you more vivacious and energetic than you ever were. Many women claim that their children have kept them young.

In the meantime, give yourself a bit of private time each day. Call it an hour, or one half of an hour, of prayer or meditation, play, or rest. Just set aside some time to sit and play your favorite song on the guitar, to stretch and do the body toners in this book, to read or daydream. This time is essential food for your spirit. It renews you. Without this refreshment, how can you be the well from which your child draws love? The Chinese philosopher Chuang Tsu believed that "Easy is good." So take it easy, and take good care of *you*.

Appearance

It is imperative that you do not neglect yourself after giving birth. New mothers all too often focus so much attention on the baby that they forget to brush their teeth and wash their hair.

You feel better when you look better. Shower daily, or more if you like. Water often washes away much more than dirt. It can wash away stress and loosen any stuck tears you need to cry in these tender days when you don't even need to have a reason to cry.

Warm shallow baths help soothe episiotomy and hemorrhoid soreness. Deep baths are usually not recommended until the vagina and surrounding area are well healed. Do not douche. Douching, which is seldom helpful at other times, would disturb the healing process now.

The gifts that friends give to new mothers can be very personal—a new hairbrush, a bottle of massage oil, a nice package of herb tea, a book of poetry, a tape of soft or rockin' music, a massage, or a nightgown. The baby will get plenty of gifts, so a thoughtfully chosen gift for the mother may lift her spirits, making it easier for her to feel better and to care for her baby.

Breath

Your breath brings life-giving oxygen to every cell in your body. Let it be deep and full. Allow yourself to be nourished by your breath. Remember how vital your breath was while you were birthing? Even now, each inhalation feeds your cells. Each exhalation takes waste from your body. When someone is under stress we say, "Take a deep breath." There is wisdom in that advice.

As a breastfeeding mother, you wish to provide optimal milk for your baby. If your breath is shallow and inadequate, your milk will not be as good or as abundant. The entire body is involved in making milk because all of your body's systems are interdependent. Oxygen is a vital element for feeding this system. Cows that are allowed to graze and breathe fresh air produce more and better quality milk than cows confined to crowded cattle lots. I've observed the same result with women. When I see women who are having difficulty breastfeeding, I've found very often they are shallow breathers.

So take some deep breaths. Take this wonderful gift to every part of your body. Feel it in your toes and fingers. Feel it in your entire body, telling your breasts to make excellent milk.

Clothing

Hardly any woman fits into her pre-pregnancy clothing immediately after delivery, but most women never want to see their old maternity clothes again. Plan ahead. Pull out or purchase some loose-fitting yet flattering garments to wear in the first weeks postpartum.

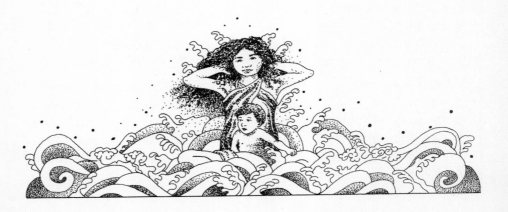

Give away your old maternity clothes. Keep only the ones that are especially beautiful, ones that you will want to wear during future pregnancies. If you're shy about your postbirth weight, remember that you won't hide anything under oversized clothing. Well-fitted, comfortable clothing makes you look best.

When you plan your postpartum wardrobe, remember that with a new baby, tops and pants or skirts and blouses work better than one-piece outfits. Whether or not you are breastfeeding, your baby needs access to your breast for skin-to-skin contact. The beat of your heart is a tonic to your baby. Most dresses are impossible as you cannot put the baby to your breast modestly. Some ready-made nursing garments are available, and pattern companies are beginning to offer designs for the nursing mother too.

Dress in something fresh and clean every day. During your first week postpartum, you may wish to wear only your pajamas to emphasize that this time is for rest and recovery. If you must stay in bed for some time after delivery, change into fresh pajamas often to make yourself feel better.

Beautiful colors make you feel more vital. Babies love to look at you when you wear bright colors.

"I'll never forget the look of awe on the face of our two-day-old son when he saw his father in a yellow shirt. His little lips pursed. His big eyes grew bigger. We soon discovered that yellow was his favorite color."

Lisa

Jewelry must be worn carefully as babies will pull on pendants and earrings, get poked with pins, and grab your gems.

Colic

"As a colic survivor I want to share this: Not only did my baby survive, he grew up 'normal,' happy and well adjusted. It may be a comfort to know, in a time when you are wondering if your child will be permanently scarred by all the crying, not only did my baby survive, he thrived."

Alesia

Almost every baby gets an occasional tummy ache. You can comfort him. Hold him, rock him, gently massage his tummy, and eventually the pain will go away and he will sleep. Burping is often all that is needed. Sometimes simple tummy aches will be remedied by a slight change in a breastfeeding mother's diet. Onions, garlic, chocolate, broccoli, cauliflower, and beans, to name a few

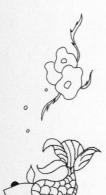

foods, have been known to upset a baby's stomach through the breast milk. You may drink fennel tea to make your milk more soothing to baby. If your baby is formula-fed, changing the formula sometimes solves the problem.

Some unfortunate babies have "true colic" or "evening colic." Beginning in the first three weeks after birth, the baby with "evening colic" screams when he has finished, or soon after finishing, his evening feeding. This screaming is much more intense than his cries at other times. He may draw up his legs because of the acute tummy ache.

Nothing you do may seem to help. Holding, cuddling, stroking, putting gentle pressure on his tummy, and nursing all seem to comfort the baby for a few moments. Then the crying resumes. Your baby can be screaming in pain one moment, and shaking and sobbing the next. Both you and the baby are miserable.

Check and double-check to be sure the baby is as comfortable as he can be under the circumstances. Hold your suffering baby. Don't leave him in a closed room to "cry it out." Your instincts will tell you to comfort your child, even when it's tough. If you do not extend your care, you will feel even worse.

The colic episodes can last a few minutes or up to three hours. When you think you've come to the end of your rope, look at the clock. You will see that the episode will end soon. Ask your mate or a friend to help you. Take turns comforting the baby. No one likes the sound of a suffering baby. Don't blame. It is not your fault, nor your mate's. Don't take it out on each other. Colic is never a reaction to breast milk. Over the ages, doctors, midwives, and parents have searched for the cause of colic. It develops mysteriously and usually disappears suddenly, by the time the baby is three months old. It will soon run its course. Other parents and their babies have survived colic, and you will too.

"Before 'colic time,' I would try to get in a nap or a foot rub or a quick-paced walk. This would give me the courage to face what was surely ahead, two hours of constant crying. Sometimes when my baby was crying, it helped to let go and cry some too. I got into the habit of taking a long relaxing bath after my baby was finally asleep. I got through it this way."

Elizabeth

The best advice veteran "colic parents" have passed on is *accept*. Just knowing your baby will cry every day at about the same time and that the crying will stop can help you prepare for it. Don't plan outings or activities during "colic time."

Check your pediatrician to ensure that the baby is healthy. Almost always, colicky babies are physically perfect. A visit with your baby's health-care giver will put your mind at ease, which helps you to live with colic until it goes away.

Diapers and All That Laundry

Each year in the United States alone an estimated eighteen million "disposable" diapers diminish our natural resources and pollute our environment. If you were to rely on disposable diapers alone, your baby would use between eight thousand and ten thousand of them before he or she is potty trained. The cost to you would be about $10 to $15 per week for approximately two and a half years.[1]

While the risks to our environment and your budget are obvious, the health risks to your baby are not yet clear. Single-use diaper manufacturers are not required to list the chemicals they use to increase absorbency and to deodorize. These chemicals are in contact with up to one-third of your baby's total body surface and in direct contact with the baby's genitals. Add the universal solvent, water, which is the main component of urine and the chemicals are easily absorbed into the baby's skin. Would you feed your baby vegetables soaked in unknown chemicals? Why, then, would you wrap and let your baby soak in them? The outer plastic wrapping serves to warm it up and ensure that the urine and other substances stay right against your baby.

Cloth diapers mean more laundry. Plus there are environmental issues of using detergent and water for washing. Please use an earth-friendly laundry product; it will be kinder, to both baby's skin and the environment. Newborn babies go through a lot of diapers every day. Older babies use fewer, but their waste is more unpleasant than a newborn's. The very thought of cloth diapers can be staggering when merely having a new family member already increases your laundry load. However, cloth diapers are more personal. They are your baby's very own. Several brands of wool and cotton diaper wraps or covers are available now, so you don't have to rely on those binding plastic pants. Most wraps feature Velcro closures, eliminating the need for pins. (Once your baby is toddling, you may wish to pin the wraps anyway to make sure he doesn't take them off.)

Diaper services, which pick up and deliver to your home, are quite inexpensive and make using cloth diapers as convenient as using disposables. The cost averages about $15 per week.

When doing your laundry, use a mild soap and rinse twice. This keeps clothing from accumulating soap residue, which can be irritating to your baby's skin.

A good way to beat the laundry doldrums is to do your folding when friends come to visit. This way you get plenty of help, and it feels less like work and more like fun.

Dreams

You may notice as do many mothers, that your dreams have become more vivid during postpartum. This may happen because you wake up several times in the night with your baby, and when you wake at night you tend to remember more dreams and in greater detail.

Dreams serve several functions. Some simply release tension and stress. Nightmares typically fall into this category. A nightmare is a result of the process of letting go of scary things, worries, or concerns from your awareness. It helps not to dwell on nightmares.

Prophetic dreams are another type. Perhaps you dreamed of your baby while you were pregnant, and he or she is indeed the same baby you saw in your dreams. Some people see future events clearly in dreams. The experience of prophetic dreams brings a feeling of deep peace.

New mothers often have wisdom dreams. In a wisdom dream, you envision something of universal significance. Wisdom dreams are enriching. You feel you can share what you've learned with others. Sometimes members of a family or group of friends will have the same wisdom dream. Tasks, such as baking bread as a healing process or gathering women for a sewing circle, a prayer circle, or a yoga or exercise group, may be revealed to you during wisdom dreams.

Meredith's Wisdom Dream

"I am taken throughout the world by a being dressed in a white sadra. We see hundreds of thousands of people from many walks of life. Each one has a white circle around his or her head. The circles are made of white light, pierced through with circles of hearts. The wise being points out this light that surrounds each person and says, 'Do you see she has a white circle? Do you see he has a white circle?', as if he wishes to be sure I don't miss this. I acknowledge. Yes, I see each individual has a white circle. And then he says to me: 'This is the light of God, that no one lives without. Until you look at everyone and see this, you will not really see.'"

Meredith

Going Out

In the first six weeks after giving birth, it is best for both you and your baby to stick pretty close to home. In some parts of India, twenty-two days of rest after birth is the common practice. In Bali, new babies and their mothers stay home in the family compound for a minimum of forty-two days. On the forty-second day of life, the baby gets his or her full name, along with elaborate rituals of welcome. In these lovely cultures, women are served and treated like queens during this rest-and-recovery period. Mothers heal faster and babies are more settled when they are at home. It also provides a quiet, peaceful span of time for bonding to occur.

Even if you are bored at home and feel certain that you can brave the world right away, be aware of the acute sensitivity of your baby's brand-new nervous system. She is imprinting everything that goes on around. It is up to you to soften the first impression she has of this world. Avoid loud sounds, polluted air, extremes of temperature, and any sort of environmental stress. This is your very special time to savor with the entire family. Your baby will never be a neonate again.

After the six-week rest period is over, break back into the world slowly. If you cannot accomplish a six-week period of lying-in, please try to stay home for a minimum of three weeks. Plan your first ventures out. Make them short. Make sure your partner or a friend comes along for support. Don't go out on several consecutive days. Space your outings, giving yourself and your baby a chance to resettle at home.

Hair Loss

During pregnancy, you may have noticed that your hair became thicker and more beautiful. The larger amounts of hormones present in your system during pregnancy can make your hair healthier. After giving birth, those hormones are reduced, and breastfeeding taxes you nutritionally. This combination causes hair loss in some women. Don't panic. Ask your health-care giver to suggest vitamin- and mineral-rich foods and/or supplements. I recommend that women eat seaweeds, and hijiki in particular. This and other seaweeds are available in health-food stores. In the early morning in Hawaii, one can find it on leeward beaches. Also make sure that you eat lots of leafy green vegetables and that you rest, rest, rest. If you were fortunate enough to have taken a quality prenatal vitamin during your pregnancy, don't stop now. I advise women to continue taking their prenatal vitamins for the entire time they breastfeed. Vitamin deficiency can also contribute to hair loss. Your hair will stop falling out as your hormone levels stabilize.

Postnatal hair loss usually starts the third or fourth month of postpartum. It diminishes gradually and should stop about the sixth month postpartum.

Housework

Your housework may pile up during the first few weeks after you have the baby. Visitors will practically parade through your home to see the newest member of the family. Don't be surprised when your Aunt Norma, whom you haven't seen in years, appears at your door with a basket of gifts and flowers, and plans to spend the whole afternoon with you and the baby. The bad news is you'll have to tell her just how little energy you and your baby have for visitors right now. It's up to you to put a time limit on visitors to avoid getting burned out. If your baby does not feed well while you have visitors, you have even more reason to lay down the law.

The good news is Aunt Norma won't expect your house to be clean. She may even offer to help. Let her. You need to rest as much as you can. Save your energy for the important job of caring for your baby and yourself. The two of you should never be compromised because the living room needs dusting.

If you are feeling physically strong after the first six weeks or so but out of control emotionally, cleaning your house or just one room may help you regain a sense of orderliness. When not taken too seriously, cleaning can be good therapy.

Women in Bali are not permitted to go into their kitchens until the baby's cord stump has dried up and fallen off. This absolutely keeps the new mother from cooking or doing dishes. Even after she is welcomed back into the kitchen, other women in her extended family cook and clean for her for at least forty-two days.

If Illness Comes Around

Mothers are often spared when a flu or a cold goes around. Though mothers are always on the go, many times not getting enough rest, they are resilient to disease. Perhaps it's a bit of magic, the strength of mother's love.

If you have the misfortune of falling ill, you must rest as much as possible so you can recover quickly and completely. Your family will rally around you. Meals will get cooked and the dishes will get washed. Your baby will be cared for by family and friends. If you are married or living with a mate, ask him to take off

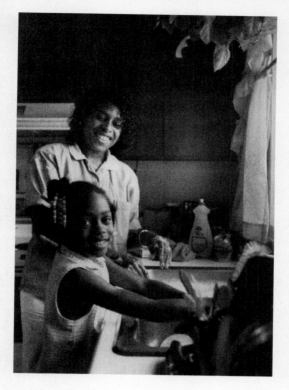

from his normal routine to take care of you and his family. Do not hesitate to ask friends for help. You would do the same for them.

Breastfeeding need not be interrupted by illness. If your doctor prescribes medication, tell him or her that you are breastfeeding. To be certain the drugs will not have a negative effect on your nursing infant, call a pediatrician. He or she will know what medications are safe for breastfeeding mothers and their infants.

Drink extra liquids to avert the danger of dehydration. Even if you cannot eat, take plenty of warm fluids. Warm is better for your body than cold. Fresh orange juice, honey, and hot water make a good healing drink. Above all, drink good old-fashioned H_2O.

Rest

It's true, I keep bringing up the issue of rest. This is because the importance of getting plenty of rest in the postpartum period cannot be stressed enough. Nap when your baby naps; you'll need it. Fatigue undermines recovery and healing.

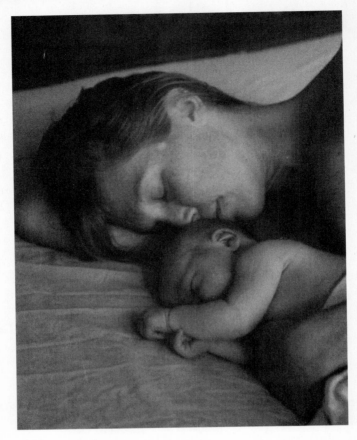

Lack of rest will make your first weeks as a mother frustrating rather than joyful. You owe it to yourself and your baby to enjoy this precious time. Don't allow fatigue to rob you of a beautiful postpartum. Lay in the Constructive Rest Position (see page 130). It is terrific when you need to get the maximum amount of rest in a short period of time.

Meditation techniques can help you attain a wonderful state of deep rest. This "restful alertness" is very beneficial for mothers as well as for people in all walks of life. One technique is transcendental meditation, or T.M. For more information, call a local T.M. center, located in most cities in the United States and in many cities throughout the world. Prayer or creative visualization are wonderful methods of getting rest too. Settle into a comfortable fetal position and gently pray, or visualize the world as you would love to see it. Let yourself slowly fall asleep. While you are meditating, as with any other form of rest, there will be occasions when your baby or older children interrupt. Because meditation has a mystique about it, you may feel that interruptions at this time are especially bad. But they are fine. Whatever program of relaxation you choose, your baby is your most powerful guide along the path to your heart and to unity with your God or Spirit. Don't be upset if your toddler drives a little truck over your face while you are visualizing.

Mata Amritanandamayi is a teacher of great compassion, also known as "Ammachi." Nearly every summer she makes a tour of the United States. If she comes to your area, it is worth going to see her. You may request a "Japa" mantra from her, which she will give you free of charge. This Japa mantra may be done while nursing the baby, folding laundry, washing the dishes, or walking. It is a wonderful way of reducing stress while keeping in constant contact with your higher self. Japa meditation may be enjoyed by people of all faiths as it does not interfere with one's personal religion.

Skin

Pregnancy may have caused increased skin pigmentation (cholasma, sometimes called the "mask of pregnancy") or extra hair growth on your face. These will diminish gradually and may go away entirely now that the pregnancy is over. Some Native American tribes recommend using the baby's first bowel movement, like a cream, as a cure for "mask of pregnancy."

It is important for your well-being that you look your best. Cleanse your face thoroughly and use a light natural moisturizer every day. You should use makeup lightly, if at all. Heavy makeup distorts one's facial features, providing the baby with an artificial image of you to bond with. Makeup's texture and perfumes also put a barrier to intimacy between you and your baby.

Sleeping Arrangements

Some people believe strongly that babies should sleep in cribs well away from the parents. Others advocate the family bed. Sleeping with an infant is not a new idea by any means. Throughout history, parents all over the world have shared beds with their children. In more recent times, particularly in the United States, sharing a bed with the children has become almost taboo. But in nature, no mammal, except humans, sleeps separated from their newborn.

Babies thrive on the physical closeness a family bed affords, and sleeping with your baby makes it easier to hear her and respond to her needs in the night.

Keeping your baby with you in the family bed is a very personal choice; make it without the "help" of anyone who might be critical of your decision.

If you sleep with your child, you will need a bigger bed. Little people take a lot of room. Care should be taken that the family bed is safe for your baby. Regular beds are often dangerous because babies fall off of them. Babies have also been hurt when they scoot between the wall and the bed. A cotton futon placed on or very near the floor works well and is also very comfortable. Soon the baby will crawl on and off easily.

Stretch Marks

Just about all mothers have stretch marks. Even if you buttered yourself with special oils every day of your pregnancy, chances are you still have them somewhere. The abdomen, breasts, and thighs are stretch marks' favorite spots. They may be small and of little concern, but some women have very large ones. The skin's elasticity, which varies from one woman to the next, determines just how much it can stretch before thinning and leaving marks. Greasing up during pregnancy helps only a little (it certainly can't hurt, especially if the oil is applied lovingly). Having surveyed many people on the subject, I found that most don't find stretch marks unsightly in the least.

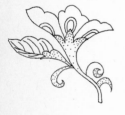

"A woman should be proud to be marked by her childbearing experience. It's like having a sign on your body that says, 'Hey look, I had a baby!' I think they're really neat."

Lee, a father

Sweat

Try to do something every day that causes you to perspire for about five to ten minutes. If a brisk walk does not accomplish this, soak in the bathtub. (Remember to wait until your lochia has stopped flowing and your stitches are well healed before sitting in a tub of deep water.) While soaking, massage your body. This helps break up cellulite. In *The Tao of Balanced Diet* (San Francisco: Tao Publishing, 1987), Dr. Stephan T. Chang recommends that you not perspire for more than ten minutes daily because you will lose too many nutrients through the skin.

Because of increased breast size and additional water weight carried during pregnancy and postpartum, you may find you sweat more now than you are accustomed to. This is healthy and cleansing and will normalize over time. Some new mothers experience night sweats so profuse they must get up and change the sheets. Aside from the inconvenience, they need not be alarmed unless other symptoms of illness are present. Postpartum is a time when the body rebalances itself, and night sweats are one of its quick methods of adjusting.

Teeth

Your teeth and gums are important. Brush and floss every day. If you put off seeing a dentist during your pregnancy to avoid X rays that would be harmful to the fetus, make an appointment soon after you've reentered the world, because pregnancy may have taxed your calcium supply and introduced cavities. In many countries, it is not uncommon for a woman to lose at least one tooth for every child she bears. If you are breastfeeding, tell your dentist so he or she does not use anesthesia or other drugs that would pass through your breast milk and affect your baby. Your health-care giver may prescribe calcium supplements while you are breastfeeding to help you maintain your dental health. For the sake of your teeth and the rest of your body, it's a good idea to continue taking a well-balanced prenatal vitamin and mineral supplement for the entire time you breastfeed.

Vitamins

Your nutritional needs during pregnancy and postpartum are greater than before childbearing (see chapter 12, Making Friends with Food). If you are breastfeeding, your need for additional vitamins and minerals increases greatly. If your health-care giver recommended prenatal vitamins, don't stop taking them now. Continue at least as long as you are breastfeeding. Always check with your doctor or midwife before adding or changing your supplements. Common sense should be used where vitamins are concerned; too much can be more hazardous than too little.

Keep your vitamins hidden and well out of your children's reach. Vitamin overdose is the leading cause of poisoning of children in the United States. The toll-free number of the poison control center in your area is listed in the front of your local phone directory. The people who answer are trained to give you immediate instructions for treating your child.

Walking

Going for a stroll with your new baby is one of the finest experiences there is. As the first few days postpartum pass, you will probably feel the need to get out of the house. A nice walk, not a hike, is perfect for mother and baby. The whole family can come along. If you take your partner along with you and your baby, a sunset walk is perfect time to renew the bond of love.

In earlier cultures, people walked. Daily life required people to be physically active. Exercise and fresh air were an integral part of life. In our culture, we tend to drive just about everywhere. We get in the car, and go from *inside* our house *into* the store. Weeks can go by before we find ourselves spending time outside. Don't allow this to happen to you or your baby. Take a walk. It's terrific exercise, and you will return home feeling exhilarated.

Holding the baby in your arms is the simplest, most natural way to walk with him. A baby pack that fits on the front of your body and is comfortable for both you and the baby works great. Backpacks designed for carrying babies are dangerous as the baby can climb out and fall.

Babies love the intimacy of being held in your arms or carried in a frontpack. You will probably feel best holding your baby close, as opposed to having him ride in a stroller where you can't see him. Also, strollers are not recommended for newborns unless they can be adjusted so the baby can lie flat. The sitting position of most strollers can strain a newborn's spine.

When your baby is bigger and you do begin to use the stroller, be careful not to slouch while pushing it. Good posture and long, enthusiastic strides make walking very enjoyable and healthful.

Avoid taking your baby for walks on very windy days. According to Ayurvedic and Chinese medicine, the wind tends to cause physiologic imbalances that can make the babies as well as adults restless and unable to sleep.

Weight

Healthy is your goal, not skinny. To meet her nutritional needs, a breastfeeding mother requires between 1,000 and 3,500 calories per day more than at other times in her life. The number of additional calories varies from woman to woman, and from day to day, depending on body type and activity level. Eat a well-balanced diet and eat when you're hungry. Drink plenty of water or other healthful fluids whenever you are thirsty to avoid dehydration.

Breastfeeding mothers must not diet, even if you are considerably overweight after your baby's birth. Postpartum is a good time to incorporate commonsense eating habits and a regular movement and exercise routine into your life. (See chapter 12, Making Friends with Food, and chapters 8 through 10.) The ultimate beauty goal is a happy heart and good health.

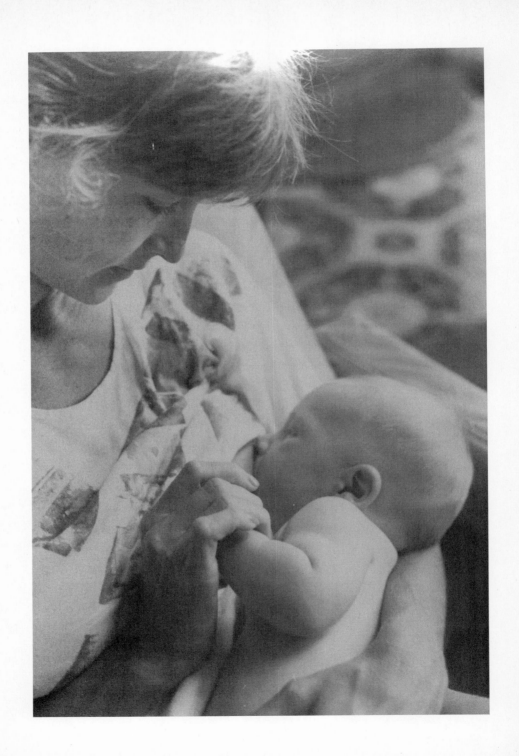

CHAPTER 5

Breastfeeding, Bottle-Feeding, and Breast Care

For a woman in the childbearing years, the breasts are of primary concern. In one woman's words, "They are a hot spot."

When my own daughter was expecting her baby, I took her to a La Leche League meeting. Each pregnant woman there was asked why she wished to breastfeed her baby. Everyone of them gave the health benefits of breastfeeding as the main reason they were for it. When it was Déjà's turn to speak, my daughter said, "I know breastfeeding is healthier, but that's not the reason I want to do it. I can still remember the happiness I felt while feeding at my mother's breasts. That is the feeling I wish to share with my baby." Generation after generation, breasts have nourished and nurtured human beings. It is my belief that babies receive more than their essential food from the breasts of mother. That *more* is the very culture, the essence of the baby's people.

With the onset of pregnancy, the breasts change. They increase in size and the nipples become larger and change color, from rosy pink to brown or deep eggplant. When lactating, the breasts change even more. This chapter examines the physical, emotional, and practical aspects of breastfeeding and postpartum breast care.

The American Academy of Pediatrics says:

"Human milk is the preferred feeding for all infants, including premature and sick newborns, with rare exceptions."[1]

The Physiology of Lactation

The human female's breast contains fat, mammary glands, and ducts. Each consists of fifteen to twenty lobes that are separated by fibrous tissue and embedded in fat. Each lobe has its own ductule, emptying into milk ducts that deliver milk first to milk pools, located concentrically behind the areola, with openings at the nipples. After conception, tremendous hormonal activity turns the breast into a "dairy."

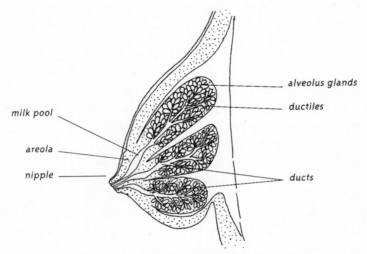

Structure of a lactating breast

At about the fifth month of your pregnancy, your placenta began to produce a hormone called "human placental lactogen." The presence of this hormone initiated the development of milk sacs. These internal changes caused changes in the appearance and color of the areolae, the dark area surrounding the nipples, as well as the arrival of colostrum, or "first milk." You may have seen colostrum, which is thick, sticky, and slightly yellowish, emitting from your breasts toward the end of your pregnancy.

Once you give birth, colostrum is expelled before your true milk comes in. Your true milk arrives anywhere from as early as twelve hours to four days after the birth. Colostrum contains the mother's antibodies against disease and provides a baby with protection from infection. In addition, the baby's suckling at this early stage stimulates the nerves in your breasts, signaling the hypothalamus and pituitary gland to start the flow of the true milk.

Prolactin, a hormone produced by the anterior pituitary gland, triggers the production of breast milk. This hormone is ever-present in the pituitary, but until you deliver a baby, its secretion is inhibited by substances secreted by the hypothalamus. Prolactin is released for as long as your baby is suckling. More sucking equals the release of more prolactin, which equals more milk.

Milk is produced in the lobes of the breasts. Meanwhile, back in the posterior lobe of the pituitary gland another hormone, oxytocin, is released. It causes the muscle cells in the milk lobes to contract. The contractions force the milk into the milk ducts. This process is called the "letdown reflex," and the perfect formula, at the perfect temperature, is delivered to your infant. Breast milk can be quite white, creamy, or sometimes it will appear clear, bluish, or thin. You may have heard of the myth that "blue" milk will starve the baby, but this is not true at all. Human milk, which is more unctuous (oily) and sweeter than cow's milk, is somewhat like warm ice cream!

Your body is beautifully designed to nourish a baby. Your baby's crying, or even the sight or mere thought of your child, causes the release of oxytocin into your bloodstream. The suckling baby causes the further release of oxytocin. In addition to triggering letdown, oxytocin also causes the uterus to contract. In the first few days postpartum, this may be felt as mild to painful cramping. Each contraction hastens the recovery of the uterus to its pre-pregnancy condition.

Stores of fat accumulated during pregnancy are used for milk production and mothers who breastfeed return to their normal weight more quickly than those who don't. This is not to say your normal weight will be exactly the same as before you had your baby. Full breasts weigh more than inactive tissue. What is a stable weight for you while you are breastfeeding will probably be a few pounds more than before you were pregnant.

Is Breastfeeding Best for Women?

Clearly breastfeeding is best for babies. Is it really best for the mothers? According to the American Academy of Pediatrics, "Extensive research in recent years documents diverse and compelling advantages to infants, mothers, families and society from breastfeeding and the use of human milk for infant feeding."[2] Here are some of the ways in which breastfeeding is best for women:

• Involution, the return of one's uterus to its pre-pregnancy state is completed more quickly, due to uterine contractions inspired by the presence of oxytocin. It is the baby's sucking that causes the mother's pituitary to provide her with this essential and wonderful hormone. This means less blood loss for the mom.[3]

- Oxytocin, the hormone that is responsible for the letdown of one's breast milk, is also responsible for that warm, wonderful feeling one gets when one is loved and in love. It facilitates bonding with baby and helps the new mother feel closer to her circle of loved ones. The hormones oxytocin and prolactin have a calming effect on the breastfeeding woman.
- A fully breastfeeding woman is less likely to become pregnant again soon after her birth. This natural child spacing is due to the suppression of ovulation.[4] (See chapter 18.)
- Prolonged lactation causes women's bodies to be more efficient. This means they become fit and trim more readily after childbirth and return to their pre-pregnant weight earlier.[5]
- Breastfeeding women enjoy improved remineralization, which prevents osteoporosis later in life.[6] This also means reduced risk of hip fractures in elderly women (postmenopausal) who have breastfed. [7]
- Breastfeeding mothers enjoy a reduced risk of ovarian cancer[8] and premenopausal breast cancer.[9]
- Mother's who breastfeed are spared the economic strain of paying for costly infant formula.[10]
- A breastfeeding mother does not need to sterilize bottles and artificial nipples, mix and warm formula, or carry around all the gear necessary to bottle-feed. Breastfeeding is clearly more convenient.

"As a breastfeeding mother, I know that I am providing my baby with something wonderful. Breast milk is truly a wonder food. It affects almost every aspect of my baby's health in a positive way. When I breastfeed I feel powerful and wise; I am the source of this wonderful fluid that provides my baby with all she needs."

Ivana Kurtz, mother of Antonia and Alex

Nursing: Getting Started

"Mothers need to ask that their baby be given to them right after delivery, even before the cord is cut. It is during the first one to two hours of extra-uterine life that a newborn is exquisitely ready to bond and breastfeed."

Mary Kroeger, CNM

The sooner your baby starts suckling, the faster your milk will come in. Research has shown that the sooner a newborn goes to the mother, skin to skin, and initiates breastfeeding, the more successful overall is the breastfeeding experience. A mother needs to know just how essential it is not to be separated from her baby after delivery. Stay close, don't let anyone take the baby from you. Swedish research has shown that a normal newborn left completely undisturbed on her mother's abdomen will, on her own, crawl and wriggle up to her mother's breast, find the nipple, and latch on.[11] The average time for this miracle to occur is between twenty and fifty minutes. The researchers urge that delivery room routines like weighing, bathing, administering medications, and so on be postponed until this kind of natural initiating of breastfeeding has occurred. The WHO/UNICEF joint statement on maternity services, "Ten Steps to Successful Breastfeeding" (see below) includes this practice along with nine others that are based on evidence, known to protect, promote, and support breastfeeding. These steps address the need to support new mothers, even if they had a cesarean birth, or if mom or baby has special needs. The mother who has had epidural anesthesia will need extra help from her caregivers to initiate successful breastfeeding. The "Ten Steps" are designed to help initiate the first breastfeeding as early after birth as possible, anywhere and everywhere in the world.

TEN STEPS TO SUCCESSFUL BREASTFEEDING
—A joint statement from WHO/ UNICEF
Every facility providing maternity services and care for newborn infants should:
- Have a written breastfeeding policy that is routinely communicated to all health care staff.
- Train all health care staff in skills necessary to implement this policy.
- Inform all pregnant women about the benefits and management of breast-feeding.
- Help mothers initiate breastfeeding within a half-hour of birth.
- Show mothers how to breastfeed, and how to maintain lactation even if they should be separated from their infants.
- Give newborn infants no food or drink other than breast milk, unless *medically* indicated.
- Practice rooming-in—allow mothers and infants to remain together—twenty-four hours a day.
- Encourage breastfeeding on demand.
- Give no artificial teats or pacifiers (also called dummies or soothers) to breast-feeding infants.
- Foster the establishment of breastfeeding support groups and refer mothers to them on discharge from the hospital or clinic.

A Dream for the Future of Breastfeeding...

The first step toward successful breastfeeding should be to provide women with "mother-friendly" prenatal care and gentle labor and delivery practices.[12] Throughout history, midwives have been the protectors, promoters, and supporters of breastfeeding. The advent of modern technological doctor-managed births has done grave damage to the mother-baby bond that must be intact for breastfeeding to again be universally successful.

PACIFIERS, DUMMIES, SOOTHERS, BINKEYS, PLUGS, GUCKERS...

Whatever you wish to call an artificial teat, designed to soothe baby and give mom a break, can cause breastfeeding problems. Using these will also cause you to return to fertility earlier—they are best avoided altogether. [13]

COLOSTRUM

For the first two or three days, your milk will be sticky, thick, and slightly yellow. This is colostrum, or first milk, which is high in protein and very nutritious. Colostrum contains antibodies and provides your baby with protection against infection. It also encourages the baby to have bowel movements. To give you an idea of how important colostrum is to new life, kids of dairy goats not fed their mothers' colostrum are not expected to survive. Colostrum is extremely beneficial to human babies too, though most infants will live even if they don't receive it. Because colostrum is so important to a baby's well-being, I have advised mothers who had decided not to breastfeed to allow their babies to nurse for the first few days just to give them the precious colostrum. In every case, the mother began to enjoy breastfeeding and continued to breastfeed for a year or more!

TO PREPARE OR NOT TO PREPARE YOUR NIPPLES

Your nipples may be sore for the first few days. Current research shows that little or no difference exists between the amount of soreness felt by women who "prepared" their nipples by pulling and rolling and women who have not. No special nipple preparation for breastfeeding is necessary during pregnancy as oil glands (Montgomery tubercules) prepare us automatically as pregnancy progresses.

The very best way to prevent nipple soreness in the early days of breastfeeding is to make sure the baby attaches well to the breast and is well positioned from the very first feed, and for every feed. If you have flat or inverted nipples, see page 81.

The Importance of the First Two Weeks

The first two weeks postpartum is the critical period of establishing a nursing relationship. A nursing mother needs physical, emotional, and practical support. The issue of feeding—whether to breastfeed or bottle-feed—is highly charged. Both sides have strong opinions. A tremendous amount of pressure may be put on a new mother to bottle-feed her baby. Many people may tell her that she and the baby would be better off using commercial formula. Studies have proven that breast milk is the superior food. Not only is it nourishing, but it also provides effective protection from illness and allergies. The American Academy of Pediatrics and the Canadian Paediatric Society strongly recommend breastfeeding.

La Leche League, a network of caring mothers who are ready to help you nurse your baby, can provide you with support and practical advice you need. They are breastfeeding experts. What to you may seem like a giant problem actually may be a tiny obstacle. Through La Leche League's mother-to-mother work, the lost art of breastfeeding is back. Visit their Web site at http://www.laleche-league.org/LLLIlang.html.

Other very important helpful organizations are The Nursing Mother's Council and the International Lactation Consultant's Association. (See Reading and Resources for information on contacting NMC and ILCA.)

Learning the Art of Breastfeeding with Your Baby

SIX MAIN START-UP POINTS
1. Hold baby close to you.
2. Make sure she's well supported.
3. Turn her toward you.
4. Make sure her mouth is even with or just below your nipple.
5. Baby's head, neck, and back must be in a straight line.
6. Make sure baby's hands and arms are not in her way as she latches on.

Breastfeeding is an art, and like any art it must be learned both by mother and baby.[14] Getting the baby on the breast correctly is of primary importance. Sit up straight. Do not lean forward or back. **Bring the baby close to your breast.** Do this by holding your baby very close and securely, turning his body toward you. **You and baby should be tummy to tummy,** so baby's neck is not twisted to one side. (See pages 79–80 for more information on breastfeeding posture.) **Make sure baby's whole body, from head to bottom, is well supported in your arms;** pillows also may be used for this purpose. **Baby's mouth and your nipple must be at the same level** when he feeds; it is all right if he is *just below* your nipple as you bring him toward your breast. In order for your baby to be easily able to swallow your milk, **his head, neck, and back should be in a straight line,** not twisted.

The nearness of you causes her to *root,* the natural reflex of searching with an open mouth for your nipple. If she roots in the wrong direction, simply stroke the cheek nearest to your breast.

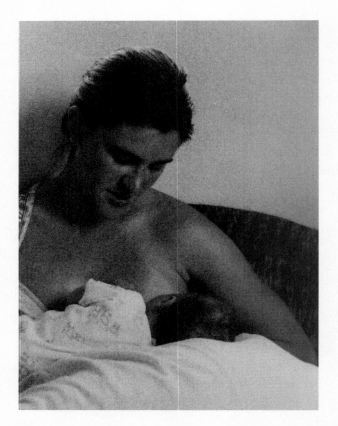

The baby's mouth should open wide to take in not only the nipple but much of the areola and some breast tissue. Nursing babies manipulate the areola and sinuses around the areola with their tongues.

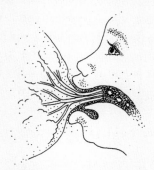

A baby well on the breast takes much of the areola
as well as the nipple into his or her mouth.

If your baby's hands and arms are in his way, he can become frustrated. Help him by carefully positioning his hands and arms where they won't block his efforts to latch on. This does not mean, however, that baby's hands need to be pinned to his side. Comfort is essential for both mother and baby.

You need not force your breast into your baby's mouth. The baby will *take* you. Try tickling his lips with your nipple; **when he opens wide, bring him close, and he'll latch on.** Bring the baby close to you, as leaning toward him does not work as well and may strain your shoulders. Adequate back support lets you sit up straight and *relax* while nursing. Most breastfeeding start-up difficulties are resolved once a mother learns how to offer her breast and baby becomes practiced at receiving it.

Some mothers may wish to be sure the baby has a clear airway to his nose. This is almost never a real concern; however, if your breasts are very engorged or the baby is positioned incorrectly, his nostrils may be blocked. Cupping your hand under your breast changes its shape so your baby's breathing is not so muffled. Do not, however, scissors-pinch your nipple with your index and third finger. This can cause plugged ducts and other problems.

Each time you nurse, make sure that your baby's mouth is centered over the areola. Sucking off to one side can cause painful clogged milk ducts (see page 91). Also, be sure your nipple is drawn deep into your baby's mouth. Sucking just the tip is very inefficient and can make you sore.

Sometimes when a healthy mother and baby have trouble starting to nurse, the letdown reflex is not occurring. This has nothing to do with milk production. Tension is the biggest obstacle to letdown. Relaxing will help.

Many women can feel their milk let down. You may experience it as a pulling or tingling in the breasts. Don't be alarmed if you cannot feel letdown. **If you listen closely, you can hear the baby swallow your milk when your milk lets down.** This can be so reassuring. Another indicator that your baby is swallowing milk is observing her ear or jaw move. If your baby is a gentle sucker, he will take longer to stimulate your letdown. Be patient with him and all will be well.

Is My Baby Gaining Enough Weight?

Bottle-fed babies sometimes gain weight more rapidly than breastfed babies.[15] A breastfeeding mother and baby can be doing just fine and some one will say the baby should be gaining more. Do not wean your baby onto formula just so he'll gain weight more quickly. If your baby is truly underweight, you may need help with breastfeeding. Consult a pediatrician who believes avidly in breastfeeding, or call your chapter of any breastfeeding support group such as La Leche League, Nursing Mothers Council, International Lactation Consultants Association, or a knowledgeable supportive woman in your neighborhood. I have seen breastfed babies fill out to the point where they surpass "chubby." This is baby fat at its best; when a "rapid grower" baby becomes an active toddler, he will slim down naturally.

Some small or premature babies are simply not strong suckers; try leaving the baby on your breasts for longer periods of time. An avid sucker brings down milk faster and need not nurse as long. Some babies just prefer to take their time, and it is common for babies to pause midfeed to smile or simply enjoy the comfort they derive from breastfeeding.

In the beginning, it is important to breastfeed your baby often, even as frequently as every hour. Let your baby tell you how often and how long she wants to feed. Feeding often keeps the breasts from becoming too full and can prevent engorgement (see page 88). It also is better for a newborn baby whose body is adjusting to receiving milk, just as your body is adjusting to producing it. In the days of breastfeeding start-up, supply and demand establishes your milk supply.

To reassure yourself that your infant is getting enough breast milk, check the number of wet diapers. If she is really wetting six to eight cloth diapers per day (five to six disposable diapers), then you can feel certain that she is well fed. Another sure sign that baby is getting plenty to eat is frequent bowel movements.

IS MOTHER'S MILK SAFE?

Environmental contaminants do find their way into human milk. Rest assured that mother's milk is still the safest way to nourish your baby. Cow's milk and soybeans used to make the breast milk "substitutes" are not toxin free. Cows eat grass, grain, and hay that is sprayed with pesticides. Formulas containing soy contain much more aluminum, lead, cadmium, and manganese than breast milk. Several brands (Neocare, Isomil, Ross Lab's, Similac, Carnation's Alsoy, and Mead Johnson's ProSoBee) test positive for genetically engineered corn and/or soy. Additional concerns arise when one considers whether or not the water used in the formulas is pure.[16]

Tips for Lowering the Levels of Environmental Pollutants in Your Milk
- Drink only purified water and lots of it; tap water is always questionable.
- Choose to eat organic foods.
- Wash and peel your fruits and vegetables.
- Reduce your intake of red meat (vegetarian mothers have fewer toxins in their milk).
- Remove fat and skin from chicken.
- Avoid fish from places known to be polluted.
- Ingest fewer dairy products.
- Do not smoke or drink alcohol.
- Don't pump your own gas. (Some always seems to get on your skin when you do.)
- Avoid pesticides and hazardous chemicals in cosmetics and housecleaning products.

BREASTFEEDING POSITIONS

It is a good idea to vary the position in which you breastfeed your baby. Nursing your baby in different positions makes use of all of your milk ducts and helps prevent plugged ducts (see page 91). The cradle position, in which the baby lies across your lap with pillows on your forearm, is comfortable for most women and babies. Also try nursing while you are lying down on your side on the floor or bed (a small pillow placed under your rib cage will make you more comfortable). The baby can lie beside you, or on top, lying across your body. Another position is to hold the baby tucked under your arm like a football. In this position your baby's body will be beside you, rather than on your lap.

Breastfeeding "experts" vary in opinion on the "feeding the baby on both breasts every time" issue. Some women are more comfortable if they feed their baby from both breasts at each feeding. Your baby does not need to feed for a set amount of time on a particular breast to get the "hind milk," or higher fat-content milk. The best way to know that your baby is getting the hind milk is by the *feel* of your breast: It will feel softer when this has occurred. At that point, you may wish to switch to the second breast.

In the early days of breastfeeding start-up, some mothers put a safety pin on their bra strap to remind them on which side the baby began the previous feed. They then start the next feed on the opposite breast. This ensures that each breast is used to begin feedings half of the time—when the baby's strongest suckling occurs. Don't worry, your breasts don't really ever get empty. Sometimes they are firm and fuller, other times they are softer and the milk supply is replenishing.

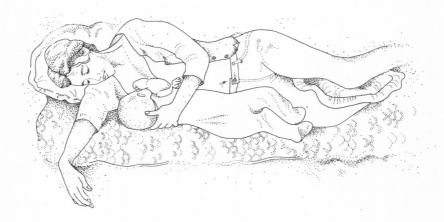

LEAKING

Your breasts will leak some milk. Don't be alarmed if you wake up some night in a puddle of milk; it only means that your milk let down in your sleep. Letdown is powerful and can happen at home, in the grocery store, or wherever you happen to be. Even when your baby is not near, just thinking of her can trigger your milk to let down. Because your milk is the same temperature as your body, it is possible to leak and not notice that your blouse is wet for quite a while. Many women find that with practice they can control letdown. When you first begin to feel the tingling sensation of letting down, think, "Oh, this is not necessary now," and the flow will diminish or stop. Another trick that will help stop the flow is to gently press upward, with your hand in a loose fist, against your nipple area. If you are shy to do this in public, you can pretend you are covering your mouth for a yawn…and press firmly with your inner forearms simultaneously.

Nursing pads are available at many drugstores. They keep the milk from seeping into your clothing but can be hot and uncomfortable. I advise wearing pads only if you really need them, because infections and cracked nipples have been caused by overusing them. It is important to avoid buying pads that have a layer of plastic in them; these pads cause the most problems. While nursing the baby, nothing works quite as well as putting a cotton diaper over the unused breast. In cold climates, wool nursing pads are wonderful for preventing clogged ducts caused by the wetness of leaking breast milk (making one's breasts cold when one goes out in the weather).

INVERTED NIPPLES

The size and shape of your nipples should not affect your ability to nurse. Some women's nipples (or it can be just one) are either flat or inverted, turned in. A woman whose nipples do not protrude can still breastfeed successfully. You will need perseverance, and in some cases help, but you can do it.

I am a big fan of "breast shields," also called "breast shells," which are plastic devices available through La Leche League International. These cups, with reservoirs for catching leaks, are designed to be worn under the bra, next to the skin. They train flat or inverted nipples to protrude. I have seen them work very well for mothers who were frustrated and on the verge of giving up. A study published in the *British Medical Journal* warns that the use of breast shields or Hoffman's exercises to make nipples protrude should not be so stressed that the mother becomes nervous.[17] Nervousness is counterproductive to breastfeeding.

Having the newborn initiate breastfeeding, right away after birth, is especially important for the mother with flat or inverted nipples. In the first hours of life, the baby (born to an undrugged mother) is awake and highly motivated to suck strongly. Also, the breasts are still soft, so the nipple can be more easily pulled by the baby's sucking into a teat. If there is a delay in initiating breastfeeding until the mother's milk has come in, things become more difficult. The mother and baby may then have flat nipples *and* engorgement to contend with. Even if this happens, don't lose hope. Get someone to provide you with a pair of nipple cups and get some support. Don't give up. Have patience with yourself and your baby.

BREAST SIZE

Your breasts will be considerably larger than usual while you're nursing. You may have one breast a good deal larger than the other. Try to notice whether the baby favors the larger breast. Sucking determines the milk supply. If the baby sucks more on one side, that breast will be larger. If this is the case, make a conscious effort to put the baby to the less-used breast more frequently. After weaning, when both breasts diminish in size, they will again appear equal. Keep in mind, though, that hardly a woman in the world has breasts that match in size exactly. If before your pregnancy you had very small breasts, it does not mean you will have difficulty providing adequate milk for your baby. You may enjoy having larger, fuller breasts for the period you are breastfeeding.

WHAT ABOUT SAGGING?

This question is often asked by new mothers. Some mothers are concerned that breastfeeding will cause breasts to sag. Since milk-filled breasts are heavier than dry breasts, and sagging is caused primarily by the pull of gravity over time, nursing can speed the process. The increased weight can cause ligaments that support your breasts to stretch, but with the help of a good bra and good posture, a nursing mother's breasts will not change substantially from their pre-pregnant appearance. During feedings, keep a pillow snugly under the baby to support his head. This reduces pulling on the breasts.

It is important to note that women without children also have slack breasts in their later years. Aging causes most of the change in breast shape. The breasts' fibrous tissue slackens over time. Since the breasts have no muscle tissue of their own, no amount of exercise will reverse the effects of gravity. Working the pectoral muscles, which surround the breasts, can make the breasts appear a bit more pert.

To some extent, sagging breasts are hereditary. Daughters of large-breasted women are generally large breasted themselves. Larger breasts weigh more and respond more quickly to the pull of gravity. Short of surgery, wearing a good bra to help prevent sagging is about the only way to combat it. It is silly to think that if one avoids breastfeeding her breasts won't ever sag. The greatest changes in breast size occur during pregnancy, before delivery. Poor posture exaggerates a little droop, so stand tall, and breastfeed your baby.

BRAS

Nursing mothers may wish to wear a bra within a day or two after delivery. When your milk comes in, it really comes in. A bra that fits well can lessen the pain of engorgement and prevent some stretch marks on the breasts. If your bra is binding, it may cause soreness and clogged ducts that could lead to infection. Ask a salesperson for help if you are uncertain of the fit. It is difficult to achieve proper fit for a nursing bra, unless you buy it after your milk comes in. However, I do not want new mothers out shopping for bras in the early days postpartum. I

Breastfeeding and Mothers with Special Health Concerns

Diabetes: If you are a diabetic, it is still possible for you to breastfeed. Your midwife or doctor will help you make adjustments to your diet and it is probable that you will be taking less insulin. If you had a cesarean birth, or even if you require special treatment in the hospital, you can still nurse your baby.

Cancer: Even if your family has a history of breast cancer, you can still breastfeed. There is no increased risk to you or your baby's health. Consult your midwife or doctor about breastfeeding and cancer. There are studies that indicate that breastfeeding benefits for the mother include possible reduced risk of ovarian and premenopausal breast cancer.[18]

Breast Surgery: Women who have had breast surgery may have some difficulty breastfeeding. However, take heart: There is a lot of good news on this topic. Removal of cysts or benign lumps normally leaves little scarring and usually causes no problems.

A woman who has had a breast removed can fully breastfeed a baby from her remaining breast. The miracle of supply and demand will cause one breast to produce as much as the two would have.

Usually breasts that have been enlarged through surgery and implants will still work fine if the milk-carrying ducts and nerves that innervate them have not been cut. This system must be intact to allow the milk to reach the nipples. If the breasts have been made smaller by the removal of tissue, it is more likely that the ducts and nerves were cut to reposition the nipples. Successful breastfeeding after surgery will greatly depend upon the type of surgery one has had. La Leche League is soon to publish a book about this very topic. Visit the author's (Diane West) Web site at www.bfar.com for information about breastfeeding after breast surgery.

solved this problem by buying a high-quality organic cotton sports bra, in a size larger than what I wore during pregnancy.

A mother who decides not to nurse may wish to wear a bra that fits firmly if she becomes engorged. This lessens the distension of the breasts and may reduce discomfort.

Special nursing bras can be purchased at department stores, mother-baby specialty shops, or by mail order. These bras have front flaps that give you easier access to the breasts. There are many styles of nursing bras, so you should try on several and choose the style that you can manage most easily. The flap closures on some can be opened with one hand, which you will find essential when juggling a baby. With practice you will become adept at getting your breast in and out of the bra quickly and discreetly.

Cotton bras breathe better and prevent rashes that synthetic materials promote. The comfort of cotton is especially important while breastfeeding, as your full breasts generate more heat.

If you live in a cold climate, wool breast pads are a must. Running in and out of doors can cause breast milk that has leaked to get very cold. This cold wetness can cause plugged milk ducts. Wool remains warm, even when it's wet. So, for those cold leaky days, wool breast pads.

On warm days, cotton breast pads are great. However, do not leave wet pads on for long periods of time. Your breasts need to stay dry to prevent clogged milk ducts and cracks.

Choosing Not to Breastfeed

Although just about all women can breastfeed, not every new mother does. Because more emphasis has been put on breastfeeding in recent years, the mother who feels she cannot or does not wish to breastfeed is too often left feeling guilty. Your baby can be nourished with commercial formula. Babies thrive on love, the most important thing you can give whether you breastfeed or bottle-feed. Mothers who bottle-feed love their babies as dearly as breastfeeding mothers.

According to Mary Renfrew, Chloe Fisher, and Suzanne Arms, authors of *Bestfeeding: Getting Breastfeeding Right for You* (Berkeley, CA: Celestial Arts, 1990, updated in 2000), most women make their choices about whether to breastfeed long before the baby's birth. If you are not breastfeeding, you may have one or more of the following reasons:

- Breastfeeding may be distasteful to you.
- It seems inconvenient.
- You are returning to work soon after the birth and cannot see a way to coordinate breastfeeding and working.
- You may have had problems with breastfeeding in the past.
- You lack skilled support.

Loving Bottle-Feeding

For mothers who choose not to breastfeed:

- Choose the formula that is most compatible with your baby. Experiment until you find the right one.
- Prepare your baby's bottles with love. Your feelings will go into the formula you are preparing. Think about the meals you enjoy making and how they seem to taste better than those you do not like to make.
- Always hold or ask someone to hold your baby while she is bottle-feeding. Do not simply prop up the bottle. Nothing you could be doing is more important than holding your baby while she eats.

CHECK IT OUT www.4woman.gov

If you have any doubt regarding the health benefits of breastfeeding, the surgeon general has launched a National Breastfeeding Initiative. The U.S. Department of Health and Human Services' "Blueprint for Action on Breastfeeding" is a collaborative effort by fourteen federal agencies and twenty-three health-care professional organizations, including the American Academy of Pediatrics and the American Academy of Family Physicians.

Societal attitudes of the past may have influenced your decision about breastfeeding. In our culture only a generation ago, breastfeeding was considered old-fashioned, even primitive, by many. Perhaps this opinion can be traced to two sources: our country's puritan roots and industrialization. Over time puritanical laws, which were put into practice initially to regulate married couples' sexuality, filtered through the entire culture to affect how we touch, or don't touch, our babies. Intimacy in any form was discouraged and a "touch not" tradition prevailed. Industrialization advocates efficiency and standardization. Breastfeeding fell to the wayside as it was considered too time consuming to be a good value. In a society that values the precision of measurement that comes with standardization, breastfeeding may be viewed as inferior because mothers and doctors cannot monitor the exact amount of milk the baby receives at each feeding as they can with bottle-feeding. The supply-and-demand system (the more a baby suckles, the more milk a mother produces) that has worked beautifully for mothers and babies throughout human existence came to be distrusted. Also, both industrialization and puritanical ethics are preoccupied with cleanliness; perhaps breastfeeding came to be seen as too earthy.

Hearing one or another myths about breastfeeding may have made you decide not to breastfeed. Two common, and untrue, beliefs about breastfeeding are some mothers' milk is "too thin" or "not rich enough" to nourish a baby and breast-feeding can cause jaundice.

"When I had my first baby in 1956, the military doctors told me breastfeeding was not done in America. Though I had assumed I would breastfeed, like all mothers did in the Philippines, I followed my doctor's advice and believed I was making a better choice for my children. I had five babies, all bottle-fed. Years later, when I saw my oldest daughter breastfeeding her baby, I began to have regrets. I know I missed something."

Crescenia

A good health-care giver will understand your desire to breastfeed and help you fulfill it. The surgeon general's National Breastfeeding Initiative states that health-care workers should be taught how to encourage their patients to breast-feed. It also recommends that "[w]omen who return to work after childbirth should have access to childcare facilities or private rooms on-site to accommodate breastfeeding."

Make sure you are eating well and supplement your diet with more leafy green vegetables, root vegetables like beets, and alfalfa sprouts (see chapter 12, Making Friends with Food). You should also drink plenty of pure water. If your nutrition is adequate and your milk is letting down, there is no reason to feed your baby formula. Breastfed babies normally gain weight at a slower rate than bottle-fed infants.[19]

The standardized growth curves for babies were based on the weight gain of bottle-fed infants. The growth of breastfed babies may differ from the standard-ized weight-gain charts. Weight loss is normal during the first three to four days after birth. A weight loss of up to 7 percent is considered normal. Within two to three weeks most infants regain their birth weight.[20]

If you are concerned about your baby's growth and weight gain, consult a La Leche League leader, a lactation consultant, and/or a pediatrician who is support-ive of breastfeeding. A knowledgeable support person will individually evaluate your baby's breastfeeding positioning and attachment as well as the baby's weight and size.

BREASTFEEDING AND JAUNDICE

Breastfed babies do develop more jaundice that bottle-fed babies, but this jaun-dice is not harmful. Many healthy babies develop a yellowish cast to their skin during the first few days after birth, especially around the second or third day. This happens because infants are breaking down excess fetal red blood cells that were produced before they were born and began breathing oxygen. Excess bilirubin, which is yellow and causes the baby to appear yellow, is a by-product of fetal red blood cells breaking down. The high level of bilirubin in the baby's bloodstream will make her appear yellow.

Breastfeeding soon after the birth, frequently and in positions that allow for good milk to flow, is often the best prevention and cure for jaundice. Colostrum works as a laxative to help the baby pass meconium (the first stool), which is high in bilirubin. The rarest form of jaundice, which some doctors believe is due to the baby's reaction to breast milk, has been referred to as "breast milk jaundice" and develops after the first week of life. Though the baby retains a yellowish cast, it is almost never dangerous and it is not necessary to discontinue nursing. Continued breastfeeding and exposure to sunlight (see pages 32–33) will gradually disperse it over a period of several weeks. It is not necessary to give a jaundiced baby water. This used to be common advice, but in fact this practice interferes with breastfeeding and does not clear the bilirubin any faster. Breastfeeding makes for more stools, accelerates the passing of bilirubin, thus decreasing the jaundice.

Should jaundice persist, your pediatrician should assist in monitoring your baby, and advise you if he or she feels that the baby needs phototherapy to reduce the level of bilirubin in his bloodstream. Much headway has been made in the last ten years regarding the treatment of newborn jaundice. Some babies may even go home with "wallaby lights" strapped to their torsos. This allows for phototherapy at home, which does not disrupt breastfeeding as much as a hospital stay.

HOW STRESS EFFECTS YOUR LETDOWN REFLEX

The most common situation in which a mother feels she cannot breastfeed is when her milk will not let down. This usually happens when a woman is under a great deal of stress, either physical or emotional. She may be faced with the following scenario: She produces plenty of milk, but the milk is not delivered from her milk sacs to her waiting baby. Anxiety causes adrenaline to be present in the body, and adrenaline suppresses oxytocin, the hormone responsible for milk letdown. Many discouraged women put their babies on formula because they "did not have enough milk," yet they then become engorged.

When a woman reduces the number of feedings by supplementing with formula, her body begins to produce less milk. She becomes more upset and a cycle of frustration for mother and baby sets in. In this case, a better solution than partial or total weaning is to take a good look at the mother's life and to find ways to reduce her anxiety. When some of the stress is eliminated, her body may allow her milk to let down.

HOW TO SUPPRESS LACTATION

If your baby dies, is given up for adoption, or if you choose not to breastfeed, you will need to suppress lactation because your breasts will have colostrum initially and then fill with true milk about day two or three postpartum. The best advice for keeping yourself more comfortable is to bind your breasts before your milk comes in. Do this by wearing a well-fitted cotton bra—cotton because it breathes and will lessen discomfort. If you become engorged, express your milk only enough to keep comfortable, gradually cutting back. Remember, expressing will stimulate milk production, so do it conservatively. Talk to a La Leche League leader, midwife, or health provider for help in this matter. In the past, physicians prescribed hormones to inhibit lactation, but this was found to be detrimental. (See chapter 3, page 41.) Sage suppresses lactation and can be taken alone or with other postpartum herbs in tea (see chapter 11, Herbs for the Postpartum Woman), or use sage generously to flavor your food.

To reduce pain from engorgement, apply ice packs for ten minutes on/ten minutes off until discomfort is reduced. Mild pain relievers like acetaminophen (Tylenol) may be taken under the guidance of your health-care giver. Engorgement usually subsides in two or three days and nearly disappears within a week.

Postpartum Breast Care and Problems That Might Occur

ENGORGEMENT

Just when you think you've felt it all—pregnancy, contractions, the birth itself, stitches, or skid marks—and you figure it's easy from here on out, you wake up in the morning, eager to cuddle your two- or three-day-old baby, and you feel as if a two-ton truck is sitting on your chest. You may also be running a low-grade fever.

You are engorged. Overnight a tremendous amount of hormonal activity caused your milk to come in. My milk actually drops in, like a lead doughnut. All humor aside, sometimes it hurts. This early stage of motherhood is painful for some women, while others experience no discomfort at all. Some women have different experiences with different babies.

At the first sign of engorgement, go to bed with your baby. Mother Nature is letting you know that you need to rest and stay centered.

If you are breastfeeding and experience a lot of pain, it does not mean you are failing at breastfeeding. It does mean that you will need extra encouragement to persevere.

The best remedy for engorgement is prevention. Prevention is best accomplished by early initiation of breastfeeding and frequent feeds. Because it was once hospital policy to separate mother and baby after the birth, and babies were given supplemental feedings of infant formula in the nurseries, engorgement was thought to be normal. One is less likely to become painfully engorged if separation from baby never occurs, if the baby is breastfeed frequently and on demand, and if the mother learns to position the baby correctly while feeding.

If you do get engorged, you must persevere in letting the baby feed at your breasts. Your baby is the best possible cure. If you have pain, when you put your little one to your rock-hard breast, it hurts even more. But you must nurse often and from both breasts to relieve engorgement. Do not avoid nursing your baby on the side that hurts the most; this will make it worse. Even the areolae around your nipples can be swollen. If the baby can't get well attached to your overly full breasts to take out enough milk to bring you relief, don't give up. Your partner can gently suck out the milk. If you are not breastfeeding, do not remove milk as you will encourage milk production and extend the process of drying up your breasts (see How to Suppress Lactation, page 88).

Warm showers are helpful when the breasts become hard and painful. Let the milk flow in the shower to relieve the pressure. Then feed, taking a deep cleansing breath before the baby "latches on."

Following a dairy farmer's trick, especially if you have had painful engorgement with previous births, may help to lessen your discomfort: Farmers give new mother goats no alfalfa on days two and three postpartum. This is because alfalfa increases milk production tremendously. So on day two to three, eat no alfalfa sprouts.

An effective homeopathic remedy for engorged breasts is Phytolacca 30X, which is prepared pokeweed root. This remedy may be purchased without a prescription at drugstores, some health-food stores, and herb shops. At the first sign of hot, swollen breasts and/or painful breasts, take according to package directions or follow the advice of your homeopathic health-care giver.

Engorged breasts are very sensitive. Centering your nipple in baby's mouth reduces the pain. If you experience severe pain while nursing, you may consider taking acetaminophen (Tylenol—aspirin is not advised for new mothers due to its anticoagulant effect) twenty to thirty minutes before feeding. Consult your health-care giver before taking this or any other over-the-counter products.

Instant Relief...

A compress of strong gingerroot tea or applying mashed gingerroot to the breasts has helped many mothers. Grate the gingerroot and pour a small amount of boiling water over it. Make a compress by soaking a clean cotton diaper in the tea, or just place the warm, grated ginger mash directly on your breasts. Applying cold cabbage leaves directly on breasts has been scientifically shown to reduce engorgement.

If these suggestions don't help, keep in mind that the pain goes away within a day or two. Your hormones will decrease the signals sent to your milk-producing glands and things will settle down. If done correctly, breastfeeding will not hurt over the long run. Engorgement can occur at any time during the period you are breastfeeding, but most often it happens when you are first beginning or when you miss feedings, especially when you are weaning your baby and cutting back the number of feedings. Following the advice given here will help whenever engorgement occurs. Someday you will be telling an expectant mother about the joys and trials of early motherhood and may even forget to mention engorgement.

CRACKED OR SORE NIPPLES

To prevent sore nipples when first starting to breastfeed, the most important thing is to help baby to attach well from the very first feed. This involves getting the baby to open his or her mouth very wide before latching on. If the breasts are not over-full, it is easier for baby to open wide and get well attached.

If baby pulls and bites, it is sometimes helpful to start your milk flowing by hand before putting her to your breast. Do this by massaging your breasts, or taking a warm shower. Pulling the baby off too quickly is another cause of nipple injury and soreness. When removing your nipple from baby's mouth, break the suction gently by pressing your breast away from the corner of her mouth with your finger. Leaning forward, toward baby, is a better way to remove her from your breast than pulling forcefully away.

Treat cracked nipples by applying a little bit of your own vitamin-rich colostrum or breast milk. Keep your nipples clean and *dry* between feedings, but don't wash with soap. Soap dries out the nipples, further compounding the problem of cracked nipples—and your baby won't like the taste. Don't forget to problem of cracked nipples—and your baby won't like the taste. Don't forget to nurse on both sides, even if one breast is more sore than the other. Don't apply tea bags to your sore nipples. The pure (pesticide free) Lansinoh (lanolin) Cream is affordable and has been endorsed by La Leche League International. It can be found in many drugstores and is hypoallergenic. It does not need to be washed off before breastfeeding. I would use this only as a last resort, should cracked or sore nipples persist.

PLUGGED DUCTS

If you notice a tender area or a lump in your breast that is sore and may be hot, you probably have a plugged duct. This can happen when your baby decides to sleep through a night. Your breasts may be accustomed to being emptied several times during the night. If baby sucks at the breasts irregularly or inadequately, they can stop up. An overly tight bra can press on a milk duct and clog it. *Lack of rest, however, is what I consider the leading cause of plugged ducts.* Sometimes when they occur, you cannot figure out their cause.

The first thing to do is downsize your stress level. Let any and all unessential responsibilities become someone else's job. Plugged ducts can develop into breast infection (mastitis) if not cared for properly. Don't try to do anything more than be with the baby. Nurse often and long. Also gently massage the hardened area while your baby is nursing. This helps move the stagnant milk along and out. A continual flow of milk will loosen the duct that is plugged. (See page 89 for information on homeopathic Phytolacca 30X.)

BREAST INFECTIONS (MASTITIS)

Inflammation, soreness, redness, or excess heat anywhere on your breast indicates that you have mastitis. *If your breasts become infected, don't stop nursing your baby.* Unfortunately some people are still quick to recommend that mothers with mastitis stop breastfeeding. Because mastitis is often caused by incorrect milk flow, discontinuing is not only unnecessary but makes things worse in most cases. The pain from breast infections can be a throbbing, burning sensation. Fever and a low level of energy often accompany the infection. Plugged ducts, poor diet, lack of rest, emotional stress, or a weakened immune system can all lead to breast infection.

Get help from your health-care giver. If you need to be treated with antibiotics, make sure the medication is safe for your baby. Tell your doctor that you are breastfeeding and that it is imperative you get an antibiotic compatible with breastfeeding. I repeat, do not stop breastfeeding. By continuing to feed your baby, you will recover more quickly, without sacrificing your nursing relationship. If you possibly can, let the baby nurse on the sore side first. The baby's initial sucking is more efficient and will keep the milk flowing in the affected breast. Drink plenty of liquids to help flush toxins from the infection out of your body and to promote healing.

How to Examine Your Breasts

LOOK FOR CHANGES

Stand in front of a mirror with your arms at your sides. Turn slowly from side to side, checking your breasts for

- Changes in size or shape. Nursing mothers have many expected changes occurring in their breasts. Frequent self-examinations will help you learn to distinguish between changes from nursing and unexplained changes.
- Puckering or dimpling of skin.
- Changes in nipple size or position. Compare one nipple to the other.

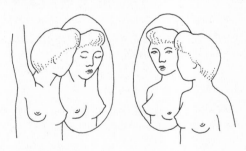

FEEL FOR CHANGES

Examine your breasts in the shower.
Your hands will glide more easily over wet skin. With fingers flat, move your hand gently over every part of each breast. Check for

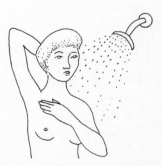

- Lumps
- Hard knots
- Thickening under the skin, either deep in the breast tissue or near the surface.

If an infection develops into an abscess, you need immediate medical attention. Your doctor may need to drain the abscess. You can continue nursing; however, for a few days you may be able to nurse the baby on only your good side and hand-express or pump milk from the infected side. As soon as possible, resume breastfeeding on both sides.

To prevent abscess, immediately upon noticing signs of mastitis: rest, eat well, keep your milk flowing by feeding your baby more often or expressing your milk,

Lie on the floor or bed. To examine your right breast:

- Put a pillow or folded towel under your right shoulder. Place your right hand behind your head (this distributes breast tissue evenly).
- With your left hand, fingers flat, press gently and move in small circular motions around your breast. A ridge of firm tissue in the lower curve of each breast is normal.

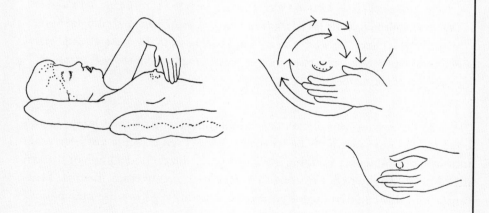

- Move inward an inch at a time and spiral slowly toward your nipple. Examine every part of the breast this way.
- Squeeze your nipples, checking for discharge, either clear or bloody.
- Do the same procedure on your left breast. Put a pillow under your left shoulder and place your left hand behind your head.
- Report any changes to your doctor.

and use a variety of nursing positions to ensure that all of your milk ducts are being used. If a fever should develop, call your health provider immediately.

BREAST LUMPS

Nursing mothers are not immune to breast cancer, though some studies indicate that breastfeeding may decrease the risk of developing this disease. A self-examination should be done weekly so that you become familiar with the normal fluctuations that occur in your breasts throughout your monthly cycle and during breastfeeding. Note any changes in your breasts. Early detection has saved many breasts.

If you have not been doing breast examinations regularly up to this time in your life, the postpartum period is a good time to begin a lifelong routine. Self-examinations are particularly important now because the hormones of pregnancy tend to speed up the growth of preexisting abnormal cells.

"When my baby was seven months old, two things happened. My neighbor died of breast cancer. She was only thirty-five. She had four small children and was still breastfeeding her one-year-old baby when the cancer spread out of control quickly. The second thing that happened was that I developed a breast lump. My doctor could not feel it. I knew it was there, so I went to a surgeon. He did a biopsy. It was uncomfortable for a few days. I did not wean my baby. I did not have cancer. Now I have this scar; it's very small compared to the tremendous peace of mind I gained. If I ever have another breast lump, I definitely will choose to have it checked thoroughly."

Robin

Don't depend on your doctor, or medical provider, to discover lumps in your breasts. You know your body better than anyone. Even if you've just been examined by a doctor, report anything questionable. If you do find a lump or thickening, don't be frightened. Most breast lumps are not cancerous. Because breast cancer is readily cured in the early stages, conducting regular self-examinations is choosing to live.

If you have a lump and you and your health provider feel a biopsy is necessary, you can continue to nurse your baby. Be sure your health-care giver knows you are breastfeeding. Discuss what painkillers will be used, whether you will receive a local or general anesthesia, and what effects the procedure will have on you and your child. The support of your loved ones will be very important now. Express your feelings and ask for extra loving care.

Storing Breast Milk

Mothers who work or are students worry that they will not be able to breastfeed, but many mothers who return to a job or school continue to nurse. You, too, can work this out. What you arrange will depend on your schedule and your baby-sitting arrangements. If you are close enough to where your child is being cared for, you can nurse her during your lunch hour or other breaks. Or you can breastfeed while you're home, express milk from your breasts either by hand or with the aid of a breast pump while you're away, and refrigerate or freeze the milk for the feedings when you won't be home. *Be careful not to go too long without nursing as you may become engorged* (see page 88). Remember, your breasts produce milk on a supply-and-demand basis: if you cut back on feedings, your breasts will soon make less milk; if you add feedings, you will produce more.

When storing breast milk, always take care to ensure that the bottles or plastic bottle liners are sterile. This protects your baby from disease. Bottles can be sterilized in the dishwasher or by being immersed in boiling water for five minutes.

Never heat breast milk by boiling or in a microwave oven. Breast milk has many protective antibacterial properties that are destroyed by heating over 130° F. *Infants have been burned by hot milk.* A bottle heated in the microwave may feel cool to your touch but can contain dangerous "hot pockets." Hot pockets can severely burn your baby. On the other hand, never serve a baby ice-cold milk. You can thaw your milk in its container by holding it under cool and then gradually warm running water and shaking it, until milk is thawed to room temperature. Or move it to the refrigerator to thaw slowly, then run under cool then warm water.

TIMETABLES FOR HUMAN MILK STORAGE [21]
These guidelines apply to mothers who

- Have a healthy, full-term baby
- Are storing their breast milk for home use (as opposed to hospital use)
- Wash their hands before expressing
- Use containers that have been washed in hot soapy water and then rinsed well, or sterilized in the dishwasher (sterile bags may also be used)

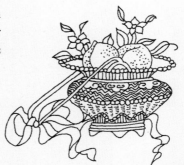

Milk kept at room temperature:
- Colostrum—12 to 24 hours
- Mature milk—6 to 10 hours

Refrigerated milk:
- Mature milk—up to 5 days

Frozen milk:
- Stored in a freezer compartment located inside a refrigerator—2 weeks
- Stored in a self-contained freezer unit of a refrigerator—3 or 4 months
- Stored in a separate deep freeze at a constant 0° F—6 months or longer

Label each container, with the month, day, and year. Use milk in the order in which it was expressed. Remember, if your baby is in a hospital or day-care setting, you must put your name on the label as well.

Never refreeze breast milk.

To prevent waste, store your milk in servings of 2 to 4 ounces.

BREAST PUMPS

According to the La Leche League International's *The Breastfeeding Answer Book,* "A full-size automatic electric breast pump is the fastest, easiest, and most effective way to express milk."

Choose a pump to suit your needs. The mother who is just going to express her milk occasionally may be better off renting a pump, rather than buying it. If you decide to get a hand pump, choose one that can be sterilized. Note that the "bicycle-horn" type pump cannot be sterilized, is quite ineffective, and has been known to cause tissue damage, as the suction cannot be regulated. Some electric pumps come with an option for a double-pump attachment. This allows the mother to pump from both breasts simultaneously. The double-pump attach-

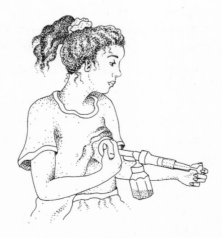

ment will cut pumping time in half and avoids milk loss from leaking, which occurs often when only one breast is being used.

These days the pump manufacturers (see Reading and Resources) provide detailed instructions for all aspects of pumping; follow the instructions provided with your particular brand of pump. Some women feel that it's best to purchase a pump through a lactation consultant or a La Leche League chapter. This way they will get caring personal instruction as well as a pump that is dependable.

> "My baby was born with cleft soft palate, a birth defect which prevents her from being able to form suction in the mouth, and therefore prevents breastfeeding. I chose to feed my baby exclusively on my own breast milk, and so I have spent countless hours pumping the one and a half quarts per day that my baby needs. It has been painful and an incredible challenge, but I am so thankful that my baby has been able to get all of the benefits of my breast milk. My love for her would never allow me to have made any other choice. I know that she is getting the best possible start for her wonderful life!"
>
> *Lonica*

WHAT ABOUT BURPING?

As a midwife in Bali, I was summoned to help a baby crying inconsolably in the middle of the night. Upon arrival, I found the baby in distress, the young mother and entire extended family in a panic. I picked the baby up and burped her. She immediately calmed down and slept.

Don't laugh, I've been called at 3 A.M. to rescue families in the same predicament in the United States. Both bottle-fed and breastfed babies need burping sometimes. Bubbles in the stomach hurt and cause babies a lot of pain and confusion.

Simply place your baby on your shoulder and *gently* pat or rub his back. (Put a clean diaper or small towel over your shoulder to catch any milk that may come up with the burp.) Just holding your baby in an upright position usually will bring up most of the air bubbles. Also lying your baby across your knees while rubbing his back helps him burp. Be sure to support his head while he is still very small.

After a big burp, see if the baby wants to have a little more of your milk. The bubble may have made him feel full, before he was truly satisfied.

rooms. If someone asks you to do this, ask them if they would like to eat their next meal in a bathroom.

It looks like the future will be more accommodating toward breastfeeding mothers. Already many department stores have installed "mothers' rooms" with changing tables and armchairs for nursing.

Many mothers prefer to nurse privately. Some babies do better if they are fed in a quiet, more private spot. Listen to your own inner voice; it will tell you where you and your baby will be most comfortable. In many situations, you will want to nurse discreetly. Do so, but do not let your baby go hungry to make others more comfortable.

"In order to encourage mothers to breastfeed, we must foster a positive environment where they can feel comfortable. This attitude must extend beyond hospitals and homes and into places like the U.S. Capitol building."

American Academy of Pediatrics[22]

How to Breastfeed Modestly in Public

- Don't ask permission to nurse your baby. You are not doing anything unnatural or illegal. By asking, you are inviting criticism.
- Don't wait until your baby is crying to nurse. A crying baby attracts immediate and negative attention. If he begins to fuss while you are enjoying a meal in a restaurant, simply put him in your lap, drape a napkin or a receiving blanket over your breast, and nurse while you eat and converse.
- Good nursing bras allow you to unlatch them with one hand while holding a baby in the other arm. (Look for those that are all or mostly cotton; you'll be cooler and more comfortable. Buy yourself more than one nursing bra. You will need them.)
- Don't worry about people looking at you while you nurse (they usually don't). As more women choose to breastfeed, mothers nursing in public places will become as commonplace as apple pie.

"In order to encourage mothers to breastfeed, we must foster a positive environment where they can feel comfortable. This attitude must extend beyond hospitals and homes and into places like the U.S. Capitol building."

American Academy of Pediatrics [22]

Relactating

If you weaned your baby for some reason or started him out on a bottle and then decided you wanted to breastfeed, it is still possible to nurse, though it will take patience and dedication. Sometimes a mother is convinced that breast milk is not the best thing for her baby. She weans the baby only to find that he has trouble on formula. (Nothing is as easy for a baby to digest as mother's milk.) In some cases diarrhea, diaper rash, and stomach pain are caused by formulas.

Without the baby's sucking, the mother's milk begins to dry up. To reestablish the milk supply, sucking is necessary. As often as possible, put your baby to your breast. At first, there will be little or no milk. Let the baby suckle you while he's voracious, then supplement your milk with bottled milk. The Nursing Supplementer, available from your local La Leche League leader, is a fantastic device that provides supplement to the baby along with whatever milk the mother is producing while nursing at the breast. I've seen it work both in the establishment of milk supply in an adoptive mother and for the reestablishment of a birth mother's milk supply.

Usually by doing this several times a day, the milk comes back within two to six weeks. At first, there will be only a few drops, but eventually it pays off and you're fully breastfeeding. The challenges of relactating are very individual; women have extremely varied experiences. It will take courage, so reach out for assistance and loving knowledgeable support.

"Several months after I weaned my son, he got sick. He was not able to eat solid foods. I wished I could still breastfeed him. He was so hungry, and getting weak. I felt helpless. I wanted to nurture and nourish him. In desperation, I put him to my breast. He nursed! Several times a day he took my breast. He seemed to thrive on what I thought were empty, dry breasts. To my delight, within a couple of days I had milk again."

Annie

To relactate, a mother needs a tremendous amount of support, which La Leche League and Nursing Mothers Council can provide as well as further information.

IF YOUR BABY BITES YOU...

while breastfeeding, it can really hurt. Biting the baby back, which some people recommend, is usually not effective, and it's mean. Biting a baby only teaches biting. The most natural reaction to being bit is to jump (or to scream, or at least squeal). You need not rehearse this, it will happen. When it does, the baby may cry. Calm and comfort her. Stay as calm as possible; do not frighten your baby. Don't pull away forcefully or pop your baby off of your breast; this can cause nipple injury. It is better to lean toward the baby to gently release your nipple. You will soon learn to be on the lookout for times your baby may tend to bite. The two of you will work it out.

Weaning

"Exclusive breastfeeding is ideal nutrition and sufficient to support optimal growth and development for approximately the first 6 months after birth.... It is recommended that breastfeeding continue for at least 12 months, and thereafter for as long as mutually desired."

The American Academy of Pediatrics [23]

Just as you and your baby establish nursing and feel settled into it, someone will ask, "When are you going to wean him?"

When he's ready, your baby will wean himself from your breast. Babies who have gotten teeth do not need to be weaned, but the arrival of teeth signals that the enzyme ptyalin, which helps digest solid foods, is present in the baby's body. Child-led weaning, when the child loses interest in breastfeeding and seemingly magically weans herself, requires surrender on the mother's part. It can mean that you will be nursing as long as three years or more. If an extended period of breastfeeding will not work in your situation, it will be necessary for you to encourage earlier weaning. When other mammals feel irritated while breastfeeding, they encourage their young to eat solid foods. The manatees, however, never do wean. I have seen a mother manatee breastfeeding her baby, while herself nursing on the grandma manatee!

Whenever you decide to wean, it should be done gradually and lovingly. You can encourage the natural process of weaning by introducing appropriate com-

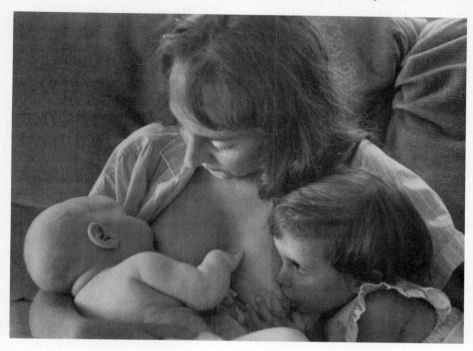

plementary foods at about six months or older. Soft mashed fruits and mashed staple foods like well-cooked rice are good starter foods for baby. Try chewing your baby's food for her, and putting it directly into her mouth.

If you feel that breastfeeding your toddler has become an enormous energy drain, look at *all* aspects of your life. Perhaps it is not the child's demand for breastfeeding that is tiring you. Feel it out; you may need to downsize a less important part of your life, so you have more energy for being a mother.

Sometimes mother's milk becomes a silencer when other forms of loving are more appropriate. Try cuddling or having a little talk or singing a song with your child. Sometimes when she is hungry or thirsty, she may actually want solid food or a drink of water, but she does not know how to distinguish between asking for breast milk and asking for something else. You can help her learn to ask clearly for what she really wants.

If you decide to have another child while you are still breastfeeding, you have some choices to make. Pregnancy changes the breasts, and the amount of milk you produce will decrease and it will taste different. For some children, these changes are enough to cause them to stop nursing on their own. Others rebel and demand to nurse even more often. It is possible to breastfeed throughout pregnancy. Indeed, many women have done so and remain perfectly healthy. Some women who have become pregnant while breastfeeding report an increase in irritability. This may be nature's signal to wean. Other mothers experience no discomfort when breastfeeding while pregnant. With a new baby on the way, it is especially important to wean gently and with love. You want your child to associate the arrival of a little brother or sister with more love, not with loss.

Tandem nursing, breastfeeding a new baby as well as an older child, is also an option. Many mothers say they thoroughly enjoy this shared nursing. Others have become exhausted trying to meet the demands of two nursing children. In many cultures, both contemporary and ancient, it is not uncommon for women to breastfeed more than one child.

Breastfeeding is a wonderful form of giving. Gradual weaning is best not only for your baby but also for your health. Tune into your baby and your own heart. When you do, weaning comes naturally and easily, and when the time is right.

According to a recent study published in the American Academy of Pediatrics,

"The longer infants are breastfed, the more likely they are to have positive cognitive and academic outcomes into early adulthood." [24]

Gradual Weaning Guidelines

- Tune into the messages your body and emotions send. If you feel that both you and your baby (toddler/child) are both really ready, it may be time to begin weaning.

- One at a time, introduce solid foods to your baby in small amounts. In some Asian cultures, a mother chews the food and passes it from her mouth to the baby's. Besides beginning the digestion process and preventing tummy aches for the baby, this also keeps feeding on an intimate level.

- Keep in mind that your baby will miss not only your milk but also your touch. Extra cuddling will reassure her.

- Drop one breastfeeding session every few days until you are down to one feeding a day. By eliminating feedings slowly, over time, your milk supply will taper off gradually, and you can avoid engorgement. You may decide you want to continue with this one very special session for a long while.

- Wearing a T-shirt or nightgown with no buttons in the front will discourage feedings in the middle of the night. Out of sight, out of mouth.

- You will want help. Discuss this with your partner. Ask him to give loving care to the baby when you would normally be breastfeeding. Get him to commit to one or two weeks of helping out at night; this will entail holding, rocking, walking, and generally comforting the baby (and in the case of weaning a very young baby, he will also give the infant bottles). If you are a single mother, ask a friend to spend some nights helping you. Both you and your baby will benefit from the emotional and practical support.

- Watch for signs of swollen or engorged breasts as you cut back on the number of feeding sessions. Massaging the breasts gently, wearing a bra that fits well, and resting may help prevent engorgement, but for some women discomfort is inevitable. Expressing a small amount of milk while in a warm bath or shower relieves the pain and pressure. Ginger compresses (see page 90) also help relieve the pain.

- Take care of yourself and let others pamper you so engorgement does not develop into mastitis. A run-down mother with mastitis risks developing a breast abscess. Get extra rest, drink plenty of water, and eat well.

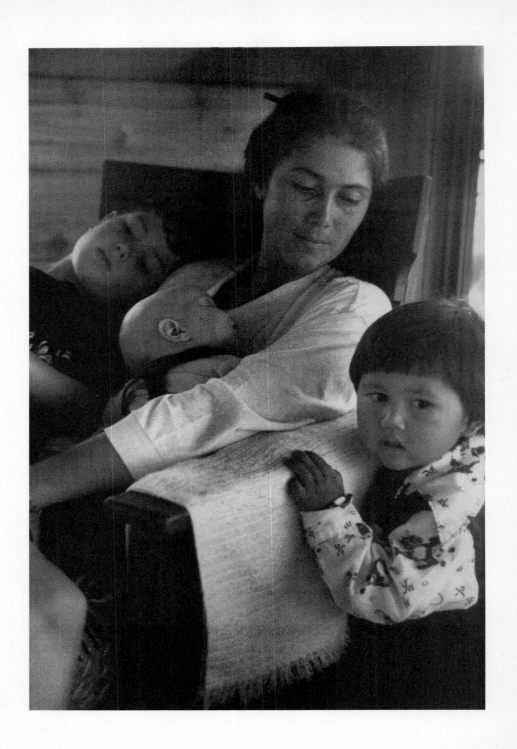

CHAPTER 6

Postpartum Pelvic Health

No one word comes close to describing or dispelling the myths associated with the region of the body that includes the vagina, cervix, uterus, urinary tract, perineum, anus, fallopian tubes, and ovaries. A woman's pelvic region is the focal point of her physical sexual pleasure and during pregnancy the cradle for her developing child. For lack of a better term, at home my children and I mischievously refer to this as the "scary area."

After childbirth, it is very important to become comfortable, even friendly, with your "private parts." This euphemism reflects the attitude predominant in our culture: Some aspects of life and the body are not to be shared. In our society women are not encouraged to ask questions or seek and share information regarding their reproductive anatomy. The result is that they often don't receive the knowledge necessary to ensure adequate postpartum health care, and confusion regarding sexual concerns may also arise. Fortunately, in Hawaii where my family lived, the ancient tradition of paying homage to the genitals is kept alive today in some of the most beautiful and playful hula dances.

Your good health, and even your life, may depend upon your knowledge of postpartum pelvic care. Your child's relationship with his or her body will reflect how you feel about the genital region. This chapter is written to help you understand what is happening in your pelvic area during postpartum. I believe talking openly about changes that occur and problems that might come up after giving birth helps women cope with emotional issues as well as the physical aspects of postpartum pelvic health—after all, the physical and spiritual cannot be separated.

Immediately after the Birth

BLEEDING

After giving birth, you will have a vaginal discharge called lochia, which begins as a heavy flow similar to menstrual blood. At first, it may contain small clots. Over the course of several days to two weeks, it turns brown, then yellowish-white or clear. Within six weeks, it should stop altogether.

To prevent excessive bleeding, stay off your feet as much as possible for the first five days postpartum. Nursing your baby also helps prevent excessive bleeding by stimulating your oxytocin, which keeps your uterus tightly contracted. If you soak two large pads in less than thirty minutes after the first twenty-four hours following the birth, or if you pass a clot larger than a golf ball or persistently pass clots twenty millimeters in diameter (about the size of a gum ball), call your health-care giver. Also call him or her if your flow turns back to red after it has been brown. The change in color may indicate you have injured your uterus where the placenta was attached, which usually happens when a mother over-exerts herself. *You are doing too much, slow down!* Your doctor or midwife will want to investigate the cause of this change in your lochia because bleeding is sometimes a sign of uterine infection, and when infection occurs, special care must be taken immediately to protect a new mother's health.

Absolutely do not use tampons in the first few weeks following childbirth. They disturb the vagina's healing tissues and may harbor bacteria, thereby inviting infection. Sanitary napkins should be changed often. Try to choose organic, unbleached all-cotton sanitary napkins. (These are available at health-food stores.) They are kinder to your "scary area" and to our environment. If you tend to get chafed between the legs from commercial sanitary napkins, try making some out of soft cotton fabric. These washable reusable sanitary napkins are less convenient; however, they are more comfortable for many women and more ecological. In recent years cotton, washable, reuseable moon pads have also become widely available.

After giving birth, even if you did not tear or have an episiotomy, it can be painful to pee. Tiny abrasions, bruising, and skid marks are the culprits. Don't be afraid to urinate, no holding back. Simply use a squirt bottle filled with warm water (or warm comfrey or slippery elm tea) to irrigate the area while you pee. If you are having trouble urinating in the first day or two postpartum, your urethra may have been compressed at the time of birth. Again, the warm water squirt bottle is so helpful. Take heart, the perineum, that strong connective tissue separating the vagina from the anus, heals quickly. Gently spread your labia

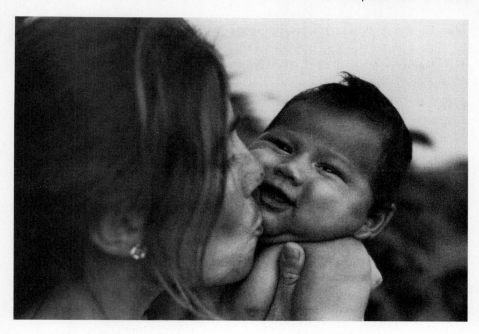

and irrigate the outer vaginal area only. (Do not douche or squirt water into the vagina.) Do this often. Pat very gently from front to back.

AFTERBIRTH CONTRACTIONS

For one to four days after the delivery of your baby, you may experience afterbirth contractions, or afterpains. The intensity of the contractions varies from woman to woman. They will be stronger if this is not your first baby because your uterus has more work to do to regain its pre-pregnancy shape and size. They are also more intense while you nurse. Oxytocin, the hormone responsible for the letdown of your milk (see page 71), also causes your uterus to contract.

The process of the uterus returning to its original condition is called "involution." By about the sixth week postpartum, this process will be nearly complete. Afterpains can come back at any time during involution but usually with less intensity than the days immediately following the birth. The uterus that once housed the baby, placenta, and amniotic waters returns to about the size of your fist.

If your afterbirth contractions are bothersome or painful, gently massage your lower abdomen. You will be able to feel your uterus. During this period, it is easy to distinguish: It is hard and about the size of a grapefruit. Try lying on your stomach with a firm pillow beneath you to keep your uterus pressed against your other organs. Another trick that I've seen women do automatically in response to afterpains, and which you may have already done, is to rest the side of one hand against your pubic bone and, while leaning forward and crossing your legs, press against the uterus with your palm. (Jiggling your belly while in this position helps even more.) Placing a hot-water bottle on your tummy can be a relief. You may also use relaxation and breathing techniques like those used during birthing. Herbal teas that relieve afterpains are motherwort, shepherd's purse, and false unicorn. They are available at many health-food stores. (See chapter 11, Herbs for the Postpartum Woman.) If the contractions become too intense, call your health-care giver.

Now that you have your baby, you may feel it's not fair to be feeling more discomfort. Don't get discouraged. Remember that the afterpains play an important role in your recovery.

UTERINE INFECTION

If you run a temperature over 101° F and your uterus is tender, call your health-care giver right away. This could be a sign of uterine infection. Other indications of infection are foul-smelling lochia, lower back pain, cold sweats, and an elevated pulse. If infection becomes systemic, it can lead to death. Every new mother should take her temperature if she has any indication that infection may be present. To decrease the chance of infection, do not use tampons or insert anything into the vagina while the lochia is still flowing, which may be up to six weeks. Vaginal bleeding means the cervix is still somewhat open, making the uterus vulnerable to bacterial infection.

EPISIOTOMY AND TEARS

If you had an episiotomy, a labial skin split, or a perineal tear, your stitches may be itchy and sore for a few days or weeks following the birth. The discomfort may make you want to avoid moving, but keep in mind that gentle movement stimulates circulation, which facilitates healing. Don't open your legs too wide, as you can disturb your stitches. You may have opted for no sutures. In that case, you will want to be even more enthusiastic about doing sitz baths (see page 39). Also, keep your legs closer together while you heal. Kegel, or yoni, exercises (see pages 112 and 132) also speed up the healing process by stimulating circulation, though they may hurt at first, and you may feel like nothing is happening when you do them.

Exposing your genital area to direct sunlight warms the tender tissues and promotes faster healing. If possible, lie naked in the light of a sunny window or in a secluded corner of your backyard. (Never expose your pelvic area to sunlight if you are suffering from herpes outbreak. The herpes virus thrives on ultraviolet light.) Take your baby along. A little sun is good for newborns, especially if they are jaundiced (see pages 32–33). Remember, babies' skin is very delicate and can tolerate only three or four minutes of direct sunlight at a time.

Try sitting on a pillow or a blow-up doughnut or ring (like a pool toy) to make you more comfortable. Warm water squirted on your perineum while urinating will relieve some of the burning sensation. If you have a great deal of pain, call your health-care giver. Talk to the women who have had episiotomies. Their advice can put your mind as well as your seat at ease.

By week six postpartum and usually sooner, perineal tears, labial skin splits, or espisiotomy stitches should be well healed. Though they may still be tender, many women have resumed sexual activity by this time. If you do so, you must make sure your partner is aware that lovemaking must be very gentle at this early stage of postpartum.

Even if you had an episiotomy this time, take heart, you need not have one the next time. Episiotomy is the most common surgical procedure performed in the United States.[1] According to Sheila Kitzinger, "It is the only surgery likely to be performed without her consent on the body of a healthy woman in Western society."[2]

There are ways to prevent future perineal tears, good nutrition being the number one way to keep perineal tissue strong and supple. Doing kegel exercises regularly is another important way to keep your perineum intact. To prevent future episiotomies, choose a midwife over a doctor as your birth attendant. Though midwives can and do perform episiotomies, they are far more likely to help you give birth gently over an intact perineum.

The Pelvic Floor
(The Bottom of the Scary Area)

The pelvic floor, slung like a hammock from the pubic bone to the coccyx, is a set of interfaced muscles that support the pelvic organs: the bladder, the uterus, and the anal canal. These muscles, also called the pelvic diaphragm, form an interacting figure eight.

Like all other active muscles, they need to be exercised daily to maintain tone and elasticity. Because the pelvic floor is usually covered by clothing and serves no locomotive purpose, we tend to ignore it. Many people forget this set of muscles even exists, except during sexual activity.

A healthy, responsive pelvic floor prevents the bladder, uterus, and bowel from sagging. If the floor gives way, these organs will give way as well. The uterus is then in danger of prolapsing (see below) and urine or excrement may leak. Many people suffer from hemorrhoids, incontinence, and general ill health due to a weak pelvic floor.

Pregnancy and childbirth put great strain on these muscles. Pressure caused by coughing, lifting, running, or straining for a bowel movement further weakens neglected pelvic floor muscles.

At one time the "husband's knot" was a common medical procedure performed following childbirth. An extra stitch was sewn in the perineum while the doctor closed up the episiotomy. The purpose of this stitch was to restore the size of the vaginal opening to a virginal state. By tightening the woman's vagina, it was thought by male doctors, her husband would experience increased sexual pleasure.

Many women have gone through this sexist procedure because they were either unaware that it was being done to them, or they were too tired after childbirth to refuse it. This free service, the husband's knot, can make sex uncomfortable for women, even painful, long after childbirth. Some women have reported discomfort, resulting from the procedure, whenever they sit. Furthermore, it never did solve the problem of a weak pelvic floor. Even so, some doctors continue to perform it.

Fortunately today many health professionals are finding that taking a few minutes to teach new mothers vaginal exercises called kegels, elevators, or yoni exercises (see pages 112 and 132) is far better medicine than the husband's knot. In fact, evidence indicates that avoiding episiotomy and preventing tears by supporting the perineum during delivery is the best form of prophylaxis.

A postpartum woman must take the danger of uterine prolapse, the uterus falling out of position (see below), seriously, especially in the first six weeks following childbirth. Her focus for recovery during those weeks must be strengthening the pelvic floor, not on weight loss, trim thighs, or a flat tummy.

The solution to a weak pelvic floor is simple: Do not jump right back into activity immediately after childbirth. However, you may do yoni exercises. Begin them as you read this chapter. Do them regularly for the rest of your life.

UTERINE PROLAPSE

After birthing, the uterus may be displaced so it lies directly above the vaginal opening rather than tipped forward as it is normally positioned. Improper placement and a weak pelvic floor put the uterus in danger of falling out of the body through the vagina. This experience, called uterine prolapse, can be very frightening.

Prevention is the key. *Do not* strain, overdo it, make pancakes for your family, or resume your household responsibilities too quickly after having a baby. When a woman calls me to say she feels her uterus is prolapsing, the first thing I ask is, "Are you doing too much?" Sure enough, these women have jumped back into activity too quickly.

Rest more. Do kegels frequently. Chapter 8, Toning What's Inside, describes in detail how to do vaginal exercises and other gentle exercises that are safe to do immediately after birthing. Sit-ups, leg lifts, and other strenuous exercises are unsafe in the first six weeks postpartum (and longer for some women) when the danger of uterine prolapse is greatest. If you strain to get back into full activity too quickly, you run the risk of losing your uterus.

The warning signal that you have partially prolapsed is feeling your cervix too low or close to your vaginal opening. If you feel or see your cervix protruding from your vagina, lie down immediately. Don't panic. Lie on your back and put pillows under your buttocks. Call your midwife or doctor; she may want to put your uterus back into its natural position manually. Uterine prolapse does not mean you need a hysterectomy. A skillful health-care giver can help you heal yourself without removing your uterus. You must remain in bed, lying on your back with hips elevated by pillows, for a few days. Do three hundred or more kegels daily (believe me, after having a baby that will wear you out). Contact a health-care provider who is familiar with homeopathy. I had amazing results using a homeopathic remedy, bed rest, and kegel exercises. Soon your pelvic floor and the muscles that hold your uterus in place will regain their integrity. Uterine prolapse increases the risk of uterine infection, so you will need help with your daily health maintenance. You will also need extra help taking care of your baby.

If you have uterine prolapse with this birth, be aware that you run a higher risk of this condition occurring again after subsequent pregnancies than women who haven't had prolapse. Plan ahead: Ask friends and family to help out after your next birth so you can stay in bed a few extra days. While you rest and recuperate, elevate your hips on a pillow and do your kegels!

If your doctor recommends a hysterectomy, get a second and even a third opinion. Even in severe cases of uterine prolapse, it is often possible to save the uterus. Many health-care givers are convinced that a good number of hysterectomies are unnecessary. Your uterus, which has many functions, is essential for your entire life span. Do not allow your uterus to be removed unless there is no alternative and your condition is life threatening.

HEMORRHOIDS

You knew motherhood had its downside, like washing dirty diapers and babies spitting up, but nobody ever warned you about hemorrhoids. Who would venture to bring offspring into this world if they knew ahead of time that hemorrhoids were part of the deal?

Simply put, hemorrhoids are swollen veins that protrude from the anus. They can be extremely painful. Pregnancy and childbirth put immense pressure on the pelvic floor. That, coupled with the increased volume of blood during pregnancy, causes dilation of veins in the rectum, which can result in hemorrhoids. There seems to be a hereditary factor concerning hemorrhoids; I've had five babies and no hemorrhoids. My husband has never been pregnant (though I've tried to get him PG), and he has bad hemorrhoids. His entire family suffers from them. Eating whole foods is one way to prevent hemorrhoids. There are, however, no guarantees; I know women with fantastic eating habits who have gotten hemorrhoids. They, however, recover much more quickly than women with poor diets.

Hemorrhoid pain is greatly relieved by gently pushing the veins back inside. Make sure your anus is thoroughly clean after each bowel movement; this prevents the hemorrhoids from becoming irritated and getting worse. Be careful not to harm the delicate tissues with toilet paper. Rather than abrasive wiping, gentle rinsing with good old warm water is best. Tucks, a nonprescription product, can make you feel more comfortable. Take warm shallow sitz baths for relief (see page 39). Pregnancy-related hemorrhoids eventually diminish and disappear once the excess pressure from pregnancy is gone. Do not let yourself get constipated (see page 114) or strain on the toilet because you will increase the pressure of swollen veins.

YONI EXERCISES

To me, the word vagina is sometimes awkward. It sounds too clinical. I prefer the Sanskrit word for vagina, *yoni*. The vagina as a sacred temple is inherent in the word yoni.

Within a day or two after giving birth, you must start to strengthen your vaginal and pelvic floor muscles. Restoring the integrity of these muscles is the key to a healthy future. Some women feel separated from their yonis after birthing, not wanting to think or talk about the vagina. Others feel very connected to this amazing part of their bodies that allowed their babies entrance into the world.

Yoni exercises, often called kegels or elevators, will make your vagina and pelvic floor feel better and heal faster. You can do yoni exercises at any time or in any place because they can be done while standing, squatting, sitting, or lying down (see page 132). When done correctly, yoni exercises will feel as if you are lifting or elevating your vaginal canal toward your torso. Tighten your pelvic floor muscles as hard as you can; do not push down as you tighten, lift your pelvic floor up. To learn how these exercises feel, you must first isolate the muscles of the pelvic floor. Do this by eliminating other muscles such as the buttocks or the abdomen that you might have a tendency to use instead of the pelvic floor muscles. Use only the muscles of the pelvic floor. Feel the difference? Rest a bit and try again.

You may find that doing yoni exercises makes you tired, and at first you may not be able to hold the muscles tightly for very long. If you *just* had your baby, it will feel impossible. Trust me, yoni exercises work, even if it feels like you are accomplishing nothing. Don't worry; these muscles are highly elastic (look at the size of the baby that so recently came through your yoni!) and respond quickly to exercise. Practice will pay off and soon kegels will be simple and enjoyable. Later, when you're ready, practice this exercise while making love, your partner will be able to tell you how much you've strengthened your muscles.

Men should do kegel or elevator exercises too. Fewer prostate problems are reported in men who do them. By the onset of puberty, all young people should be taught kegel exercises. They should be done daily throughout life, not just by women after giving birth. These exercises can prevent incontinence in later years.

If learned when young and practiced regularly, kegels increase health and awareness of the pelvic region, making it less of a "scary area." The importance of

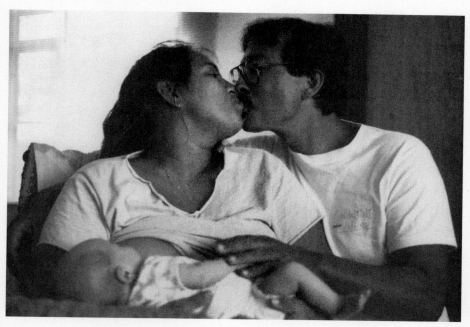

yoni exercises cannot be stressed enough. Lack of time is no excuse for not doing elevators daily. You can do a few while you wait at stoplights, shop for groceries, or while you do the other toners in this book. Do some right now!

Yoni (Kegel) Exercise Guidelines

- Breathe—your breath inspires your muscle tone.
- If you can't distinguish between your buttocks, tummy, and yoni muscles, try this on the toilet: Pee, stop it. Again, pee, stop it. Let some out. Stop it, etc. Do this only to learn the location of your kegel muscles. Don't do your yoni exercises on the toilet.
- Now that you've "got" it, put a pillow between your legs while side-lying, and do some yoni exercises, while squeezing the pillow with your knees. Hold each a few seconds, then release.
- It should feel like you are elevating your yoni, not pushing it down or out. Rather draw it up, deeply into your body. Hold. Release slowly.
- Try doing your yoni exercises quickly and then try doing them slowly, releasing slowly as well.
- Try your yoni exercises in a "plié" type position, knees shoulder width apart and slightly bent, feet slightly turned out.

(See Reading and Resources for information about Beyond Kegels, an interactive treatment program for women with pelvic health problems and/or incontinence.)

Staying Healthy in Your Scary Area

CONSTIPATION

Your pelvic floor has been through a lot. No wonder you may be holding back bowel movements. You may be afraid to have a bowel movement or even to urinate if you had an episiotomy. Try to relax on the toilet. Avoid pushing hard. If you have hemorrhoids, follow the advice given earlier in this chapter.

It is important that you not hold a bowel movement until it becomes hard and even more difficult to pass. Sometimes it helps to apply gentle pressure, using a gauze pad, to your perineum while you have a movement. A squirt bottle full of warm water really helps too. Simply squirt over your sore vaginal opening, anus, and perineum. To prevent constipation, be sure your diet includes lots of fluids and roughage such as leafy greens, hearty mashed potatoes with their skins, bran, and oatmeal or a multigrain cereal. Taking short walks may also help you stay regular. If constipation persists, visit with a reliable homeopathic practitioner; she or he can help you with a constitutional remedy.

Aloe vera juice is often recommended as a remedy for constipation (see pages 152 for quantity and directions on how to take it). Another natural remedy is to put one teaspoon of whole flaxseed in one or two ounces of warm water (add it to your herbal teas when you have just a few sips left). In severe cases of constipation, take flaxseed several times a day. Use commercial laxatives as a last resort and only when prescribed by your health-care giver.

URINARY TRACT INFECTIONS AND INCONTINENCE

Pregnancy increased your blood volume, thereby increasing the stress on your kidneys, which filters waste from your blood. This may have left your urinary system vulnerable to infection. Lack of rest, the strain of birthing on your pelvic floor, and general postpartum stress further increases the risk of urinary tract infection.

To prevent infection:
- Increase your intake of water and unsweetened postpartum herbal teas.
- Wear no underwear or only cotton underwear.
- Pads should be of the highest quality, either unbleached cotton or homemade moon pads.
- Urinate before and after intercourse.
- Wipe from front to back after using the toilet.

If detected early and treated with home remedies, an irritated bladder need not develop into a full-blown infection.

The warning signs of infection are:
- Frequent need to urinate but with little result.
- Burning sensation during urination.
- Dark-colored or red urine.
- Aching in the abdominal area.

Avert an infection in the beginning stages by eating two to three oranges per hour, or drinking the juice and pulp; this natural vitamin C source is very effective. Also drink *unsweetened* cranberry juice, which you can buy in health-food stores, or cranberry juice sweetened only with other fruit juices. (Avoiding juice sweetened with sugar or corn syrup is important as this type of bacterial infection thrives on them.) Drink a minimum of eight ounces of pure water every hour.

Bladder infections can be painful and in severe cases quite dangerous. If you are in pain or have questions, see your health-care giver.

The stress of pregnancy and birthing on your pelvic floor may have compromised your ability to hold urine. This problem becomes more common with women who have had many children. Leaking urine is a signal from your body that you need to pay more attention to strengthening you pelvic floor and vagina. Vaginal exercises (see page 112) must be done frequently to heal this condition. Doing them will improve your overall pelvic health.

VAGINAL INFECTIONS

Yeast is the most common and least serious cause of infection in female reproductive organs. The fungus *Candida albicans* (monilia) is the culprit. If you experience itching, burning, and a mild-smelling (the smell is not bad), white curdlike discharge, you are probably suffering from a yeast infection. Pregnant women have a tendency to get yeast infections because the glucose level in the vagina is increased during pregnancy. Postpartum may also be a time when you are most susceptible to infection because of lack of rest.

Because the fungus responsible for your discomfort does not like an acidic environment, you can try these home remedies. Douche twice daily for about a week with a solution of two tablespoons apple cider vinegar to one quart of warm water. A good alternative to a vinegar douche, especially for women who find vinegar irritating, is a solution of two tablespoons buttermilk or plain, unsweetened yogurt to one quart of water. The latter solution, which should be used twice daily, keeps the yeast population in check. Both yogurt and buttermilk contain *Lactobacillus acidophilus,* a bacteria that promotes the growth of the lactobacilli that normally reside in a healthy woman's vagina. Continue the buttermilk or yogurt douche for a few days after you notice the infection subside. Yeast infections are often caused by the loss of your own lactobacilli, which can be the result of taking antibiotics (especially if you had a cesarean birth) or from routine douching. Routine douching or using feminine hygiene deodorant sprays should always be avoided. They interrupt the balance of your vaginal environment and can lead to an infection.

If the lips of your vagina are tender, apply a soothing ointment like aloe vera gel or comfrey ointment. Avoid lovemaking while you have a yeast infection because the yeast colonies can break up and spread. Your partner can become infected and not know it because men often do not show symptoms. If he is not

Suggestions for Preventing Vaginal Infections

- Never use commercially made douche preparations. Douching is nearly always unwise.
- Do not use tampons while postpartum (they are not a good idea anytime).
- Use white, unscented, unbleached toilet paper.
- Always wipe from front to back. Wiping from the anus forward introduces unwanted bacteria into the vagina.
- Do not wear nylon panties. Cotton underwear is the best because it breathes.
- Avoid wearing tight pants. Pants that bind restrict the circulation of air and blood, creating a perfect environment for infection.
- Avoid commercial bubble-bath solutions. Natural oatmeal and herbal bath preparations are wonderful, and they do not promote vaginal infections.
- Reduce the amount of sugar in your diet. Women who eat a lot of sugar tend to have more frequent and more severe infections.

aware he has an infection and is not treated, he can reinfect you.

If home remedies don't clear up the infection before your discomfort makes you want to say, "I've had it," your health-care giver can prescribe medication.

A foul-smelling, greenish-yellow, foamy discharge and itching indicate you may be suffering from a parasitic infection called trichomoniasis. See your doctor to obtain a prescription medication. If you have foul-smelling discharge but don't itch, you may have a bacterial infection. Bacterial infections, which produce pus, may be located in your uterus, cervix, vagina, or in all three. It is important that you see a doctor to obtain an effective medicine to clear up this type of infection.

HERPES

If you have herpes, talk to your health-care giver. Because herpes is potentially dangerous to your newborn, follow his or her advice carefully.

Do not bathe with your infant while you are having a herpes outbreak. It is also recommended that a herpes-infected mother place a towel over her lap while nursing. This added barrier provides extra protection. After the first few months of life, the risk of the virus invading your baby's nervous system is reduced greatly as his immune system has grown stronger. However, the baby still runs the risk of getting herpes skin lesions. There are still so many unanswered questions concerning this virus, and no cure has been found. Better to take precautions and be safe where your baby's health is at stake.

The added physical and emotional stress in a postpartum woman's life may increase the incidence of herpes outbreaks. Get plenty of rest and eat well to help suppress outbreaks. Avoiding sugar and foods rich in the amino acid arginine is good prevention. Foods rich in arginine include chocolate, tomatoes (the seeds) brown rice, nuts, and fish.

MENSTRUATION

During pregnancy, your periods, or moon-times, were absent. You may resume menstruation as early as a few weeks after the birth. Caution: Your cycles may return to normal quickly, making you fertile again. On the other hand, after childbirth it is not uncommon for your period to remain absent for many weeks, even months, potentially longer if you are exclusively breastfeeding. Mothers who fully breastfeed often do not commence menstruating until the baby begins to eat solid foods. Do not be alarmed if you don't have a moon for a year or more.

Breastfeeding, even if it suppresses your moon, is not a reliable form of birth control. Don't assume you are infertile because you have not resumed your menstrual cycle. It is possible to get pregnant the first time you ovulate (and before having a moon) after giving birth. Do not risk getting pregnant unless that's what you want. (See chapter 18, Family Planning.)

If you do not wish to become pregnant, use a reliable method of family planning vigilantly. Many couples let this slip because they are out of practice from not needing to use contraceptives during the months of pregnancy. If you haven't used contraceptives or family-planning methods regularly since you gave birth and you've not yet had a period but feel the symptoms of pregnancy, you may well be expecting.

PAP SMEARS

It is wise to get a Pap smear, which tests for cervical cancer, yearly. If caught early, cervical cancer need not be fatal. With all the excitement and changes in your life due to pregnancy and the arrival of your baby, you may have let the date for your annual Pap smear pass you by. Postpartum is a great time to reestablish good pelvic health practices.

LOVEMAKING

You may resume lovemaking when you are ready. This means ready emotionally, spiritually, and mentally as well as physically. The physical part is easiest to judge. Most postpartum women do not wait the prescribed six weeks following childbirth. Three or four weeks seems to be the norm. Remember, however, the os of your cervix is still open after childbirth. You are vulnerable to an infection until you have stopped bleeding completely. It is wisest to wait until all lochia has ceased to flow. The tradition of waiting forty-two days before resuming marital relations is followed by many cultures, because it protects postpartum women from infection. If you do make love in the early days postpartum, make sure your partner is freshly washed and very gentle. Your yoni may be sore from tiny tears or stretched places. Stop if you feel discomfort.

If you are breastfeeding, your yoni may be quite dry. This is due to a decrease in estrogen. Dryness does not make you less desirable; according to some men, the hormone prolactin seems to be a potent attractant. Furthermore a breastfeeding mother is oozing with oxytocin, the powerful hormone of love. Your somewhat dry vagina will cause your lovemaking movements to be slower, more gentle. This, in turn, allows for more complete healing. Lovemaking itself wakes the oxytocin in your body, so by making love you set up conditions that cause your yoni to be more lubricated. For more information on the emotional aspects of lovemaking during postpartum, see chapter 16, Issues of the Heart.

Is Your Area Scary?

As a child were you admonished to sit with your legs closed? Were you punished or shamed for touching yourself? Did you ever attempt to see what it looked like "down there"?

What was your first gynecological examination like? Were you frightened? Did your mother go with you or did you go alone? Were you seeking some kind of birth control? Or were you there because you had gynecological concerns or problems? Were you pregnant? Was there someone there to hold your hand? Was the doctor or nurse or midwife kind, understanding, and gentle, or rough and too busy to listen?

Do you recall the first time you made love? Was it pleasurable? Painful? Were you afraid?

Unhealed psychological and spiritual pain from the past has been associated with many vaginal, rectal, and urinary problems. Emotional upset has been the cause of much sexual dysfunction. Fear, pain, and stress do indeed make the pelvic area seem scary. For many women, counseling, either group or one-to-one, has helped immensely. Because the hurts of the past are so painful for some of us, we may not even remember them specifically. The connection between the present disease, unrest, or dysfunction and the past may not be clear until the process of healing is under way.

> "I remember being ten years old and going into my father's bathroom to investigate anatomy with my best girlfriend. We giggled and got naked and sat on the cold tile floor. We faced each other and opened our legs in the same position we'd played jacks in. I'd always wanted to see myself, down there, but never could. Now we each saw 'everything,' and for some reason it was scary. After that day, we never looked each other in the eyes in the same way. It isn't that we thought we'd done anything wrong. But the very act of looking made us feel afraid of each other, or ourselves. Even as I write this my heart is pounding."
>
> *Margo*

Now you are diapering your own child. If you have a boy, he will soon play with his penis. Baby girls will play with their yonis. He might take off his pants and pee on the neighbor's carpet. She may eat her bowel movement or decorate your walls with it. You can be sure that your attitudes about body smells, body wastes, privacy, nudity, intimacy, and sex are already being learned by your baby.

Your feelings about issues concerning all these aspects of your body have been shaped by your experiences. As you begin to shape the experiences of your child, you have an opportunity to examine your attitudes and any inhibitions or sense of shame you may carry. While giving birth, you may have dropped those inhibitions as your body did its sacred job. Postpartum is the perfect time for you to seek nurturing therapy if you have fears, doubts, or concerns surrounding your sexuality and your pelvic region.

As you're looking over this chapter, it may seem like so much can go wrong in the pelvic area during postpartum. Remember, serious physical problems are the exception, not the rule, and many can be prevented when women have adequate knowledge about their bodies. What I have been calling the scary area need not be scary at all.

> "After a long and difficult labor, I was finally in the delivery room. My legs were forced apart, and put into stirrups. The doctor, a man I hardly knew, examined me. He asked if I wanted a boy or a girl. I remember saying, 'I don't care if it's a set of dishes, just get it out of me.'"
>
> *Millie, 1957*

PART II

Postpartum

Toners

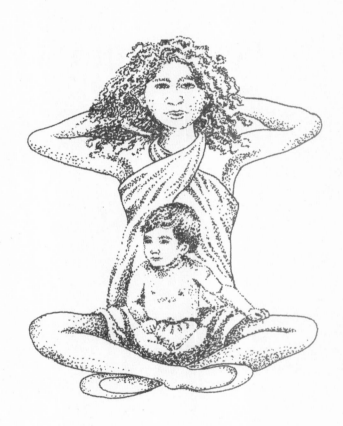

CHAPTER 7

The Importance of Posture

Mothering places new demands on you. All your attention is pulled toward your baby, and if you had a long labor, difficult birth, complications, or surgery, the demands of mothering may be even more challenging. You'll be asked to give more—spiritually, emotionally, physically, intellectually, and possibly financially as well. That *more* will show in the way you carry yourself, and in turn, the way you carry yourself affects your emotional and physical sense of well-being.

The body's dynamic balance deserves our highest respect. As a mother, you experience such joy when your baby first grasps, crawls, or takes a step. You feel the subtle power of unification of mind, body, and spirit with each move your baby makes. This wonder at movement and balance needn't be directed only toward your baby but is ever available for you to celebrate your own body. You need only muster the courage to crawl, walk, run, dance, and fly.

Babies are heavy in more ways than one. Carrying and attending to the daily care of a newborn can, figuratively speaking, be the straw that breaks a badly postured spine. If this is your first child, your body is probably experiencing a type of strain it has never felt before. This subtle tension finds a home in your back. Unless you release it, you may carry this tension for months or even years. Paying attention to your posture now by establishing good habits for lifting and carrying your child will prevent you from forming lifelong patterns of poor posture.

Pregnancy or other life transitions may have taken their toll on your posture. Now, as your body makes its natural readjustments in the postnatal process, you have an opportunity to remind your body that good posture feels good, looks great, and is essential to spiritual well-being.

Evaluate Your Posture

Stand naked in front of a mirror. Alternate between looking at yourself from front and side views. Take an inventory of how your body looks and feels. Note the tilt of your pelvis as well as the "feel" of your hips. Notice how you hold your head and shoulders, your knees and feet. Feel your body. Make slight adjustments until your posture feels right to you. Now ask yourself these questions:

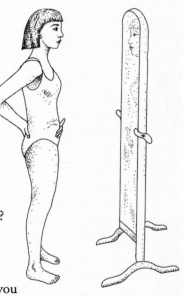

- Do your shoulders lie evenly?
- Is one higher than the other?
- Are they slumped forward or pulled back?
- Is your chest sunken and collapsed or lifted?
- Is your abdomen tense and rigid or soft and full?
- Is your lower back turned up like a duck's?
- Are your hips tense and pulled forward?
- Are your knees leaning toward each other or locked?
- Are your hips directly over your feet?
- Are your feet turned out?
- Do your hands, fingers, and toes look relaxed?
- Does your jaw look tight or relaxed?
- Do you look tense or at ease?
- Do you feel supple or rigid?
- Do you feel lifted or is your weight dragging you down?

Let's examine the elements of good posture to see what you can do to improve your stance. Continue to stand in front of the mirror, again switching between front and side views.

The key to good posture is the position of your pelvis and feet. Bounce lightly on your feet. Position them, facing directly forward, just under your hips, shoulder width apart. Curl your toes up and down. Roll onto the balls of your feet and then onto your heels. Feel the lift in your arches. Imagine you are standing on a cushion of air. Raise your toes and spread them like a fan. Now plant them firmly on the floor. Imagine hot light or energy bursting up from the earth through your arches.

Draw this heat or energy up the inside of your legs, letting it soften your knees so they are slightly bent.

You want your pelvis to be centered, not tipped forward or backward. Try all three positions to feel the difference.

Arch your lower back. Let your buttocks stick out like a duck's tail. Feel how standing this way shortens your back muscles, dropping your center of gravity and locking your knees. It cuts off the energy pathway that flows down your legs and up your back. The duck posture weakens deep-lying muscles, curtails your breath, and by accentuating the curves of your spine throws your ribs and head out of alignment. You make every muscle in your body overwork when you stand like this.

Now tuck in your buttocks very tightly. Feel how your mood shifts. Your mouth seems to grow tight, as tight as your pelvis. You may make your buttocks appear a bit smaller and your thighs a bit slimmer, but this position pulls your shoulders forward, collapsing the space where your vital organs are located, between your pelvis and chest. It also shortens your breath.

In the balanced position, your pelvis is soft; your back is neither arched nor are your hips tightly tucked. Experiment by shifting your pelvis from front to back and side to side in tiny increments until you feel your center. Let heat circulate in your pelvic bowl. Your pelvis, the cradle of your children, is round and full.

Place your hand on your lower back. At the spot on your back that aligns with the top of your hip bone, the spine is about four inches thick. Feel it. Now place the other hand on your belly, right below the belly button. You now have one hand in front and one in back.

As you breathe, let the area between your hands expand from front to back, like a balloon filling. As you exhale, stroke down firmly with the hand on your back. As you inhale, stroke up firmly with the hand on your belly. The hand in front lifts your energy. The hand in back releases tension. Do this several times.

When you do this toner, your strength rises up the front of your spine, in the center of your body. Your back is open and relaxed.

Continue bringing your strength up your spine into your heart area. Be aware of your breath as it enters your body. Relax your rib cage. Think of letting your rib cage hang from a pivotal point at the center of the spine. Do not try to hold your chest up. See your body in your mind's eye as a graceful Christmas tree, with a star at your throat.

Let your shoulder girdle "rest" on the top of your rib cage. Do not thrust your shoulders back or curl them forward. Find the soft place in the center where your shoulders lie evenly and relaxed.

Your spine continues into your skull. Imagine the top of your spine as an oiled pearl. Your skull rotates around this pearl like a ball bearing.

A silver thread reaches out of the crown of your head. Imagine that you are suspended from this heavenly cord. Now let your feet return to Earth. Visualize water trickling down the back of your head. Let it soften and lengthen the nape of your neck. Let go of the grip of your shoulder blades. Feel your spine lengthen. Let the water soften the back of your knees. Let the water trickle through your heels and back into the Earth.

Your Posture and Your Baby

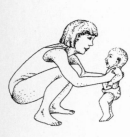

Throughout every age, women have borne children and carried them in their arms. Hold your child with integrity; you are continuing a tradition that precedes history. Always stand tall and easy, and retain your center while holding your baby. Feel in your posture the pride of your job as mother.

Pick up your baby. What happened to your posture as you did this? Did you bend just at the waist and lift? As with all lifting, you must remember to bend your knees. Put your baby back down. Now pick her up again, noticing how you lift her.

Never hyperextend, as the woman in the following illustration is doing, when you pick up your baby. Always bend your knees and use the strength of your legs to lift.

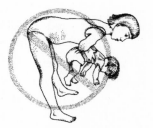
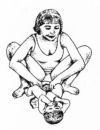

Squatting is the most natural way to do just about anything close to the ground. If you can't squat, sit with legs crossed. If you can't sit cross-legged, stretch out one or both legs. Do this to change diapers, to play, or to pick up your baby.

Try holding your baby on your hip. Look in the mirror, both front and side views. Notice how this position throws your entire body out of balance. In a short period of time, you can damage muscles and nerves by using your hip as a baby chair. If you stand like this over a number of years, especially if you have several children, you can alter your alignment permanently.

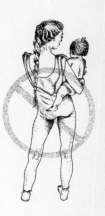

Make it a habit to carry your baby in the center of your body. Baby carriers work great for this. Choose one that does not strain your back and shoulders. Practice lengthening your neck and relaxing your shoulders while carrying your baby. There is absolutely no reason you shouldn't look graceful while holding a child.

Don't slouch, hunch your shoulders, or lean back while breastfeeding. Sitting incorrectly causes the baby to be poorly positioned for nursing, resulting in feeding problems for your baby and aches and pains for you. (See page 79, for more on correct positioning.) You'll be breastfeeding a lot, so set up a few places in your home where you can do it comfortably.

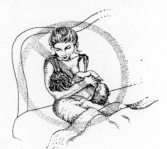
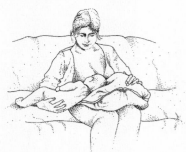
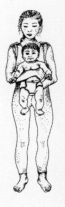

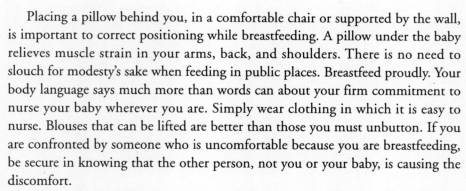

Placing a pillow behind you, in a comfortable chair or supported by the wall, is important to correct positioning while breastfeeding. A pillow under the baby relieves muscle strain in your arms, back, and shoulders. There is no need to slouch for modesty's sake when feeding in public places. Breastfeed proudly. Your body language says much more than words can about your firm commitment to nurse your baby wherever you are. Simply wear clothing in which it is easy to nurse. Blouses that can be lifted are better than those you must unbutton. If you are confronted by someone who is uncomfortable because you are breastfeeding, be secure in knowing that the other person, not you or your baby, is causing the discomfort.

After each nursing session, take the time to counter the tension of breastfeeding. Raise your arms, rotate them easily in their sockets. Reach around and rub your upper back. Look up. Stretch your spine. Take a deep breath and relax. To recharge your battery after breastfeeding, you may also wish to get into the Constructive Rest Position (see page 130).

Whenever possible throughout the day, stretch your back over a pillow or two. Let your head hang over the edge. Allow your chest to relax and your heart area to open.

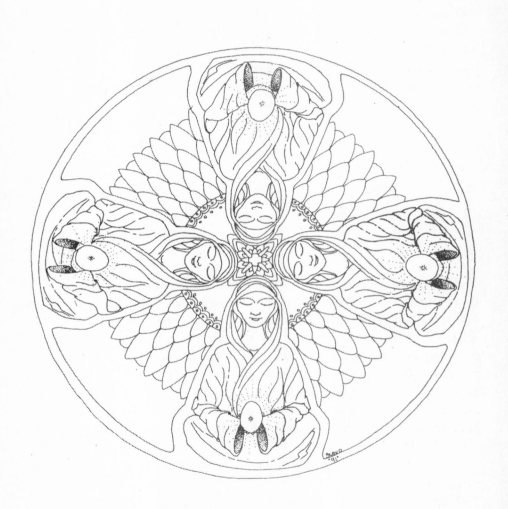

CHAPTER 8

Toning What's Inside

Just for fun, let's go on a journey into the interior of your baby's body as well as your own.

Close your eyes. Breathe deeply. You can see clearly inside your body and inside your baby's. You look through skin and see muscles, tissue, and organs. Even breath is visible to you. Slowly open your eyes…look at your baby. See the tiny skeleton that protects his miniature organs and gives his muscles structure to make movement possible. The bones are not hard and stiff, but flexible, strong, and composed of living substance. Visualize your baby's small, small heart…pumping his blood, maintaining life in every cell. Look at the bones in the newborn's foot—bones he will someday dance upon.

Now turn your vision upon yourself. Look at your body, each bone and muscle and organ working in harmony. Not so long ago, two lives existed within your body. Remember the work you did birthing, the strong contractions. You are truly amazing, and this body of yours has served you well. Are you ready to tone it up?

This chapter and the two that follow it offer you gentle step-by-step guidelines for rebuilding your body. Your body is a beautifully balanced system. During your pregnancy you experienced firsthand just how well it functions. To sustain pregnancy, you had to be strong. Yet, in order not to reject the baby growing inside, your body had to be flexible and yielding. In the postpartum period, you are virtually starting from scratch; your body, after being pushed to its limit, is ready to begin a new wellness program.

Immediately after delivery, you are very vulnerable. You are literally "open" to infection and chronic fatigue. That wobbly feeling you may have felt after the birth is due partly to the limp condition of your muscles. Hormonal changes and extreme stretching have taken place. Your return to full strength will be gradual. Do not push yourself to regain your pre-pregnancy body too quickly. If you do, you risk injury. Before beginning this or any other physical fitness program, you should consult your health-care giver.

I cannot stress too much how important it is not to strain while toning your body. Overactivity and stress cause your adrenal glands to overproduce adrenaline, which inhibits the action of oxytocin, the hormone responsible for uterine contraction during and after birth and for milk letdown.

Toning Your Body in the First Six Weeks Postpartum

These body-toning exercises can be done during the first six weeks of recovery. They can be done while you are in bed or lying on the floor. Begin slowly. Add exercises gradually, in the order they are presented. Be conscious of your breath while you do them. Your breath should be full, deep, and vital at all times.

Never exclude your baby. If your baby cries or needs your attention, do not hesitate to give it to her. The keys to your recovery program are your spirits and emotions. If you allow your baby to cry so you can get through your entire routine, you will feel down, which diminishes the benefits of exercising.

This is a simple framework for you to build your individualized postpartum exercise program upon. *In the first six weeks, do only the toners in this chapter!* As your strength grows, you can add more challenging and creative movement exercises. For now, the glow of heightened awareness surrounds you; don't break this magical bubble by straining or jumping back into full activity too quickly.

Constructive Rest Position

Constructive Rest Position (CRP) is designed to take pressure off your spine. In CRP, you simply do not have to hold anything up. This position, which can be used either in bed or on the floor, minimizes tension in the body and facilitates deep, relaxed breathing.

During pregnancy, it should be maintained for short periods only (three to five minutes at a time), as the increased weight of the uterus can compress your inferior vena cava, the great vein that receives blood from all veins below the diaphragm, constricting the return of blood to the heart. In the postpartum period you can maintain this position as long as it is comfortable. You will find CRP helpful for replenishing the vitality that's lost when caring for your newborn in the night.

GETTING INTO CONSTRUCTIVE REST POSITION

- Lie on your back. Adjust your position so your spine is as long and straight as you can make it. (Keep in mind that your spine begins at your tailbone and reaches deep into your skull.)
- Straighten your head if it is turned to one side.
- Allow your neck to be long.
- Your chin is neither tucked nor your neck arched.

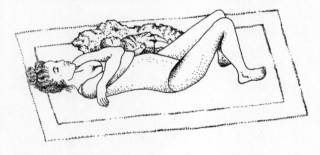

- Bend your knees. Feet can be placed on the floor or you may try putting cushions or a chair under your legs.
- If feet are on the floor, they are shoulder width apart. The position of your feet is important for obtaining maximum relaxation. The heels are not pulled in close to your buttocks, nor are they extended so far from the buttocks that you feel your lower back begin to lift from the floor. To find the correct position, bend one leg at a time. Place the foot of the bent leg in line with the knee of your straight leg. Then bend the other leg to match.
- Allow your knees to flop together. If they do not meet, relax your legs even more and give it time.
- Rest one arm across your upper chest and the other on top of it. If this is uncomfortable due to fullness in your breasts, simply allow your arms to rest easily across your tummy.
- Let your hands fall free. Do not grip; let your fingers go.
- Allow your breath to flow easily.
- Let your mind float on uplifting thoughts. While in CRP, you may wish to meditate or pray, for this is sweet, quiet time.

HOW TO GET UP FROM CONSTRUCTIVE REST POSITION

*Because CRP is meant to be relaxing, it is not wise to jump from it directly into activity. Ease yourself up and back into activity. Even if the phone rings or you need to get up to attend to your baby, please remember to **roll up** rather than jump up.*

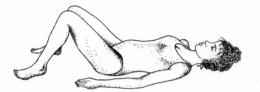

- Press down through your left foot. This will roll your body onto your right side. (Rolling in either direction is fine. Press through your right foot to roll onto your left side.)
- Draw your knees up to your chest.
- Roll over onto your knees, keeping your back curled and head down.
- Uncurl your spine with you head coming up last. Now you are sitting on your knees.

Yoni Exercises

Toning your pelvic floor is essential for recovery from childbirth. Yoni, or vaginal, exercises are the best way to do this. Many people call these exercises kegels or elevators. Make sure you isolate your vaginal muscles. Distinguish them from the buttocks, inner thighs, and the abdominal muscles. You may wish to do kegels while lying flat or in CRP. You can and should do them any time and any place. Do them while squatting, driving, doing the dishes....

Begin with as many repetitions as you can do, and stretch your endurance a bit each time. Do yoni exercises many times a day, every day, until it becomes second nature to do yoni sessions throughout the day.

- Contract and lift the muscles of your pelvic floor. (Visualize your vaginal muscles as an elevator moving up through your torso.)
- Feel the gradual ascent of your muscles as the contraction reaches deep into your yoni.

- Hold, varying the length of time you hold, from a few seconds to one or two minutes.
- Release *slowly,* controlling the release.
- Then try squeezing and relaxing quickly.
- Breathe deeply.
- You may wish to check your pelvic strength by inserting two fingers into your vagina and then squeezing. Feel your ability to tighten and relax. You may also wish to ask your lover to check your yoni strength using this method.

NOTE: In the first few weeks postpartum, you may feel no strength at all in your yoni. When you do yoni exercises, you may feel exhausted. Don't get discouraged, in time your yoni's tone will return and be better than ever.

Belly Squeeze

This toner can be done while lying in bed. Try alternating it with kegels.

- Slowly tighten your stomach while breathing in deeply.
- Release your stomach a bit at a time. Gradually release your breath.
- Try squeezing and releasing your stomach quickly and rhythmically, using your breath to feel the rhythm.
- Lay your hands on your abdomen and feel your healing energy as it reaches deep into your tissues when you contract and relax your muscles.

Recti Persuasion

Sometimes during pregnancy, the vertical seam in the abdomen's midline where the recti (two long bands of abdominal muscles) come together becomes separated. To check for split recti, lie in CRP, tuck your chin toward your chest, and slowly lift your head and shoulders until you can see your navel. Hold this position while you examine the area around your navel. If you feel a soft gap more than two fingers wide, you have split recti. If this is the case, the recti persuasion is a very important toner for you. While you do this toner and any other abdominal exercises, always support your abdominal muscles by pressing your recti toward your midline with your hands. The gap should begin to close up almost immediately once you are postpartum. If the gap widens or persists past month two postpartum something is wrong, and you should consult your health-care giver.

- Start out in CRP.
- Cross your arms over your abdomen.

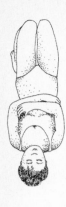

- Breathe in deeply. As you exhale, pull your hands across your abdominals toward your midline and gently squeeze the recti back together.
- Begin with only three to five, and increase at a comfortable pace. Repeat as often as you like. Never strain yourself.

Gravity Helper

This simple exercise employs gravity in the bringing together and healing of the recti muscles.

- While on your hands and knees inhale normally/exhale normally.
- Exhale forcefully the remaining air in the lungs and tighten your abdominal muscles.
- This exercise doesn't feel particularly nice, but it is very effective.

Hip Curl

Hip curls, or pelvic tilts, help to release tension buildup in your lower back. The weight of pregnancy may have left this area quite sore. Avoid lifting rigid sections of your spine; roll your spine up one vertebra at a time.

- Begin in CRP. Arms are by your side, palms facing down. Your knees are bent, feet flat on the floor or bed and shoulder width apart.
- Keeping your lower back planted firmly on the floor or bed, exhale and curl your pelvis up. *Lift only three inches.* Hold this position as long as you can, but do not strain.
- Inhale as you release your pelvis back onto the floor or bed.
- Repeat five to ten times a day in the first week. As you regain strength, you may do as many as you like.

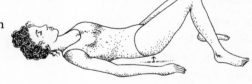

- Do not strain. Though very small and easy, this movement is effective.

Knee Hug

The knee hug warms and relaxes the lower spine. The rolling motion is borrowed from hatha yoga. In that tradition, rolling is considered an essential part of the daily health routine. Be sure to do this on a cushioned surface.

- Begin in CRP, with your arms by your sides.

- Exhaling with a strong hiss and bending your legs, bring both your knees into your chest. Avoid arching your back as you lift your legs. (Hissing as you exhale and lift should keep your lower back pressed into the floor.)

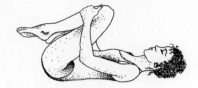 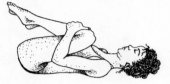

- With your arms, hug your knees to your chest.
- Rock on the bottom three inches of your spine several times so you feel this portion of your back and bring warmth to it. Feel kinks and tension unwind.
- Gently, roll easily onto your right side.
- Roll back to the center.
- Roll onto your left side.
- Repeat often without straining.

Side-to-Side

Your abdominal muscles can be thought of as a team, crisscrossing your entire torso. They are like hands reaching across and around your body. The side-to-side enlivens and strengthens this team of muscles.

- Begin in CRP, arms at your sides.
- On the exhale, lift your head and arms simultaneously, reaching toward the right side of your knees. Keep your chin tucked into your chest.
- On the inhale, release back down to the floor.
- On the exhale, lift your head and arms again, reaching to the left side of your knees this time.
- On the inhale, release back down to the floor.
- Repeat. Stop at the first feeling of strain.

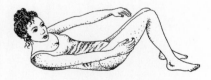 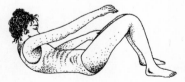

After this or any other body-toning program, take a few minutes when you are finished to stretch gently. Get up slowly.

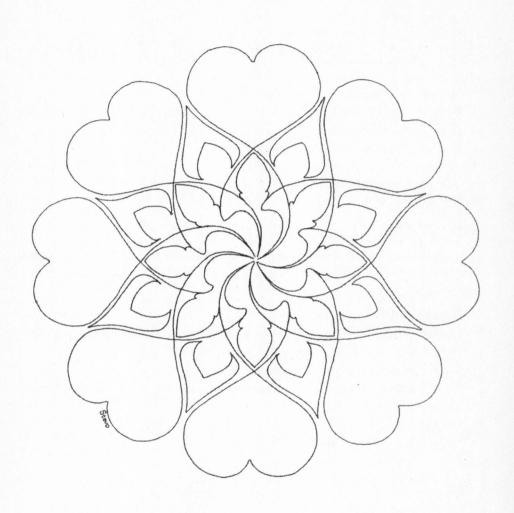

CHAPTER 9

More Movement for Mothers

These body toners will help you remember the parts of your body you may have "forgotten" during pregnancy. Get up and put on some music, or go outside and move.

The Face

When making faces, you use a wider range of motion, increasing circulation in the face. This brings the glow of health and beauty. One's face should not be blank, but should map subtle shifts of feeling. Playing at making faces inspires just this. Yogis and yoginis make wonderful faces as part of their daily regimen.

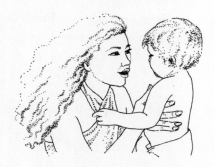

Make faces. It's fun.
Your baby will love it.

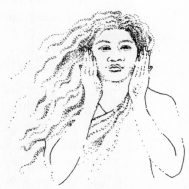

Gently pat your face.

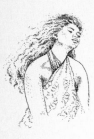

The Neck

Gently roll your neck in a complete circle, first one direction and then the other. Feel it lengthen, getting stronger. Feel any tension you may be holding float away.

Releasing the Neck and Upper Back

Supported by your elbows, which are aligned directly under the shoulders, stretch out facing skyward. Place your hands on either side of your bottom and let your head fall back gently. Feel the stretch in the front of your body and try to feel the shape of your upper back.

Lying flat, clasp your fingers together and cup your hands behind your head. Gently draw your elbows together; raise your shoulders slightly off the floor and roll your head forward, keeping your lower back pressed to the ground.

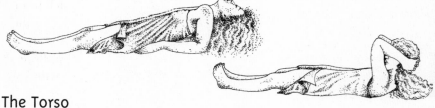

The Torso

Sit comfortably on the floor with your knees bent and the soles of your feet together. Draw your heels up close to you.

Let your chin curl and your shoulders round as you allow the top of your head to drop forward.

Stretch your right arm over your head and reach to the left. Stretch your left arm over your head and reach to the right.

You can feel the stretch in your torso with your opposite hand. Be sure to keep both your buttocks planted firmly on the ground, so you attain an optimum stretch.

The Fingers, Hands, and Wrists

Put your palms together. Spread your fingers apart. Move your palms apart and push your fingers together. Feel the life in your hands.

Make loose fists. Beginning with your thumb, unfold your fingers, one at a time. Again, fold your fingers together, starting with the thumb. Do this slowly and gracefully while rolling your wrists in the direction your fingers are moving.

The Arms

Stand with your feet shoulder width apart. Hold your arms out to the sides at shoulder level. Your palms are turned up as if you are receiving the sky. Let your neck be long. Your shoulders are down (not up around your ears) and arms are soft, rather than held stiffly. Inscribe tiny circles with the tips of your fingers. Slowly, increase the size of the circles until they are gigantic. Reverse the direction of the circles and gradually make them tiny again.

The Arms, Torso, and Back

Stand with your feet shoulder width apart; your knees are soft. Stretch your right arm over your left side, supporting yourself by placing your left hand at or slightly above knee level on the outside of your left leg. Feel the stretch from the arch of your right foot, through the leg, waist, arm, and all the way to the fingertips. Hold the stretch as long as you like, the longer the better.

Now bend your knees and allow your right arm to drop and cross in front of you in a giant half circle. Exhale vigorously, making a swishing sound with your breath. Repeat on your left side.

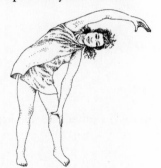
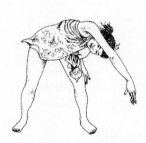

Tai Chi Warm-Up

While standing with your feet shoulder width apart, raise both arms in front of you to shoulder level. Let them be soft. Bend your knees slightly, keeping them soft. Twist your entire upper body as if you are attempting to look behind you. Do not hold this position; allow yourself to unwind in the opposite direction. Your arms will follow behind; you want them so loose they feel as if they're boneless. Twist in one direction and then immediately go the other direction, as if it were one continuous movement. Breathe deeply.

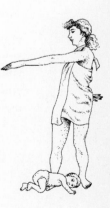

The Buttocks

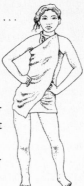

Stand with your knees soft and your feet shoulder width apart. Imagine you are standing inside an almost empty jar of peanut butter. You are going to scrape the insides of that jar with your *okole* (Hawaiian word for buttocks) so you can get the last of that delicious peanut butter. Circle your bottom and hips in one direction, then the other. You can put your hands on your hips.

Try doing kegel exercises while you do this toner. Now try inscribing a figure eight inside the jar with your hips.

Now for the Legs

Stretch out on your side, propped up on your elbow. Cross your upper leg over the leg that is closest to the floor. Grip the ankle of the crossed leg. Flex the foot of your outstretched leg. Make sure your inner thigh is facing the ceiling. Now lift, lift, lift, lift the foot of your outstretched leg. The lift need not be large to feel the work in your inner thigh. Try not to let the foot touch the floor between lifts.

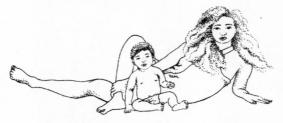

Roll over and do the same number of repetitions on the other side. Do kegel exercises while you are lifting, lifting, lifting.

The Toes and Feet

While in a squatting position with your palms on the floor in front of you, roll onto the balls of your feet. Dig your toes into the rug. Settle your weight back onto your heels and move your hands behind you, letting them take your weight. Curl your toes, stretching the tops of your feet. Wiggle your toes.

From Head to Toe

Stand with feet shoulder width apart. Relax everything. Now shake every part of your body. Allow a "haaaaaa" sound to come from deep within.

Swimming

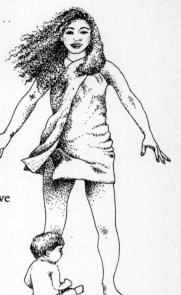

Water is nature's revitalizer. Take every opportunity you can to swim. Feel the water wash away worry and fatigue. Feel the stretch and strength of each stroke. Feel the buoyancy of your body as it is cradled by the water.

Introduce your baby to the water when he's in the mood. He'll love it if you do not force him and he feels safe.

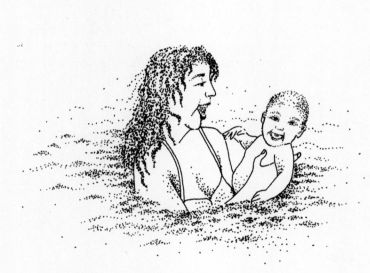

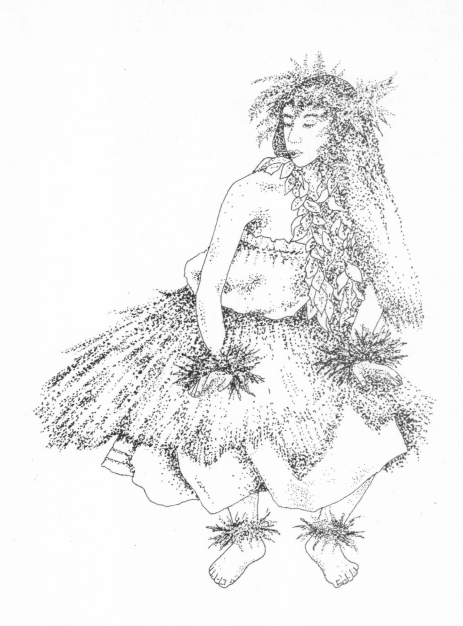

CHAPTER 10

Toning Your Body
As You Play with Your Baby

Part of the fun of getting in shape is doing it with someone. That "someone" can be an entire dance class, one good friend, or, believe it or not, your baby. Now that the first six weeks postpartum have passed, you may wish to add some new toners to your daily routine. One mother called this period of her recovery "the space between heaven and Earth." She spoke of how quickly her baby was developing. She felt her emotions surge from the doldrums to elation. She felt her body wanting to move in new ways.

In this space between heaven and Earth, you can become more active with your baby. This can mean simply holding and cuddling with the intention of making your body, as well as the baby's, feel good, or it can mean adding the toners in this chapter. However, don't jump into full activity too fast. By now, you'll be going out of the house with your baby more and resuming many of your prepregnancy activities. These can wear out you and your baby, so do these toners when neither of you are tired or hurried and when you can enjoy each other.

Inventory the parts of your body that you don't use every day. Think of the muscles you haven't stretched or really moved in a while, put on some music, grab your baby, and move those parts. Make sure you always warm up your muscles before doing strenuous exercise. Hug Rolls and the Halloween Cat, the first two exercises in this chapter, are perfect to begin any exercise routine.

Follow These Important Rules Before Beginning Body Toners with Your Baby

- Hugging and cuddling are in themselves good exercises for you and your baby. When you tone with your baby, use the same caution you observe whenever you hold her.
- Use a quilt, mat, rug, or blanket to cushion the floor. To prevent falls, never put your baby on a table or a chair when you exercise.
- Take into consideration your baby's development and never push beyond what he can do naturally on his own. Never bend his limbs or torso in unnatural ways or beyond his natural extension. Check with your pediatrician before exercising with your baby.
- Never jiggle your infant or jar her roughly as this can be stressful or harmful to her neck and spine.
- A hungry, tired, or wet baby won't be in the mood to be active. Make sure your baby is completely comfortable before you begin. Most of these toners do not require the presence of your baby except, of course, for inspiration. Include your baby in this or any activity, only if she is physically and emotionally ready to enjoy it.
- If your baby cries, he is letting you know that it's time to do something else. Try a different exercise, or find out if he is hungry, wet, or just bored. Lots of hugs and kisses will make any activity more fun for both of you.
- Be inspired to make up your own program of movement and play that is tailored by you and your baby. Your program will change as the baby grows and as your energy and strength return.

Hug Rolls

The spine stores much of a mother's tension. By simply hugging your baby, you can release this tension. As is often the case, nature makes the most essential things the simplest.

- Lie on your back on a cushioned surface, with knees raised and baby in arms.
- Gently and slowly, roll with your baby. Roll first to one side, then to the other. Feel your vertebrae let go of tension.
- Repeat as often as desired.

Halloween Cat

This is another good exercise for relieving "mother's backache"; you also strengthen your back while you relax these muscles.

- Get onto hands and knees. Baby does whatever he or she wants to do.
- Exhale as you arch your spine toward the sky by tucking under head and bottom.
- Hold.
- Inhale as you release the position, letting your back relax. Don't allow back to sag like an old horse and do not force or press it toward the floor.
- Repeat as often as you like when your lower back needs a good stretch. Let your movement be fluid.
- During pregnancy, be extra conscious of concentrating on the upward movement. The extra weight of pregnancy already curves the back, which shortens the muscles in the area of the lower spine, so release from the arch gently. Even when not pregnant, the emphasis is on the upward stretch.

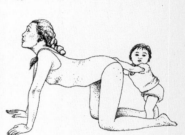

Upside-Down Baby

This gives baby's spine a gentle stretch, which also strengthens the front of her body and will help her learn to roll over and lift her head and shoulders (precursors to crawling). Upside-Down Baby strengthens mother's pectoral and arm muscles and gives her a good giggle.

Check with your health practitioner or a chiropractor before you attempt to do this toner. Very small babies should not be hung upside down, certainly not soon after birth. Wait until your baby is about two months old before trying this. Go very slowly and gently, remembering humans have only two innate fears: the fear of falling and the fear of loud sounds. The first few times you hang your baby upside down, ask your partner to help when you pick up and lower the baby.

- To begin, sit comfortably on the floor (not on a chair) with your legs extended.
- Baby is lying on your legs on her tummy.
- Firmly grasp your baby's legs just above the ankles.
- Lift her up slowly.
- Hold her up for a few seconds.
- Gently lower your baby.

- If your baby arches her head back and reaches for the floor, lower her face-down. This will soon be her preferred method of being put down.
- If at first baby tucks her chin, lower her carefully facing up. If you ask your partner to place baby's hands on the floor while she is in the raised position, soon she will be reaching for the ground herself and arching her head to be lowered facedown.

Pony Ride

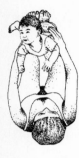

This ride is great fun for baby and will tighten and strengthen your buttocks and thighs. Wait until your baby is two months old to do this one; before that age, many children may not enjoy this movement.

- To begin, lie on your back with your upper legs at a right angle to your torso. Your baby, lying tummy down, is balanced on your shins.
- When baby is comfortable, gently give him a ride up and down by raising and lowering your feet about six inches each way. Be sure to hold him carefully. (Singing a silly song while doing the Pony Ride is very important.)
- Be very careful not to put strain on your knees.

Seat Walks

This movement will slim your thighs and tone your buttocks.

- Sit on the floor with your legs extended in front of you.
- Rock back and forth on your buttocks, reaching with your right hand while "walking" your right foot forward. Then, reach with your left hand while "walking" your left foot forward. In this way, seat-walk across the room.
- Moving backward, seat-walk yourself back to starting place.
- Accentuating the movement of your arms back and forth will make this exercise more beneficial, engaging and strengthening your torso and tummy while tightening your upper arms.

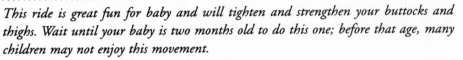

- Repeat as desired.

Out and Cross

While you are on the floor stretching your legs, roll onto your back. Gently rub your calves and thighs to warm your muscles. You will tone your inner thighs and buttocks with this exercise.

- While lying on the floor, let gravity gently pull your legs apart.
- Close and open your legs like a pair of scissors. (Do this with your feet flexed, then do it with your toes pointed.)

- Repeat daily and increase the number of
repetitions as your strength improves.

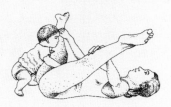 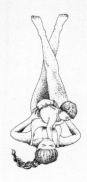

Baby Boogie

If you are in a playful mood, put on your favorite upbeat music. If you are feeling
quiet, put on something classical. Be sensitive to your baby's mood also when you
choose the music. There is no starting position, nor do I suggest any specific
action, just go for it. Judge how vigorously you move with your baby by her
responses: smiling and laughing mean "yes, more"; fussing or crying means
"slow down" or "stop." Be creative with your movement. Dance with your
baby in your arms, or put the baby down and keep dancing. Ham it up.
Your baby is a terrific partner and audience.

Dancing, playing, and singing are essential parts of growing up. Your baby
first learns these activities and how to appreciate them from you. Traditionally
dance and music originated in the home. Our culture puts them on stage, which
is nice, but they belong at home too.

Playing is good exercise. Pretend you are harvesting or hunting. Growl like a
lion. Sing out at the top of your lungs or very softly. Two sticks become rhythm
instruments. An oatmeal box is your baby's drum. Go ahead, get crazy. Get
sweaty. Be a child with your child.

Stretches

*Flexibility allows you a greater range of movement, and you will be more comfortable
in a body that is supple. Stretching does not mean straining. You will progress faster if
you do not hurt yourself while stretching. Described here are just a few ways in which
you can stretch with your baby close to you, providing inspiration.*

- Sit on the floor with your legs spread apart comfortably. Do not lock your
knees. Body is lifted, spine long and open. Breathe in deeply.
- Without bouncing or forcing, lower your torso toward the floor, feeling the
stretch in your legs and back. Exhale as you come down.

- Alternately flex and point your toes.
- Stretch over one leg and then over the other.
- Stop in the middle to cuddle your baby if he or she is there.
- Stretch with a flat back and then try it with a rounded back.
- Walk your legs together and stretch your torso down over your extended legs, remembering to keep knees unlocked.
- Repeat daily.
- Hold stretches for twenty to thirty seconds or longer.

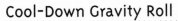

Cool-Down Gravity Roll

Just as you must always warm up before vigorous activity, you must cool down before you stop. Do this gravity roll. Then rub your muscles, stretch, walk around a bit, and end your workout with a few minutes of CRP (see page 130).

- Stand tall and easy.
- Drop the weight of your head forward. Take a breath and relax. Feel the pull.
- Let the weight of your head and gravity draw you downward slowly. Breathe. Go as far as you can without straining.
- Hang there. You can make a loud "bbllahh" sound if you like.
- Roll up, one vertebra at a time, beginning at your tailbone.
- You will feel like you are uncurling.
- Let your head come up last.

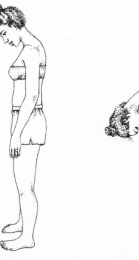
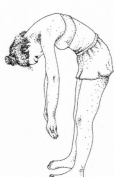

PART III

Good Health Now
and for
the Rest of Your Life

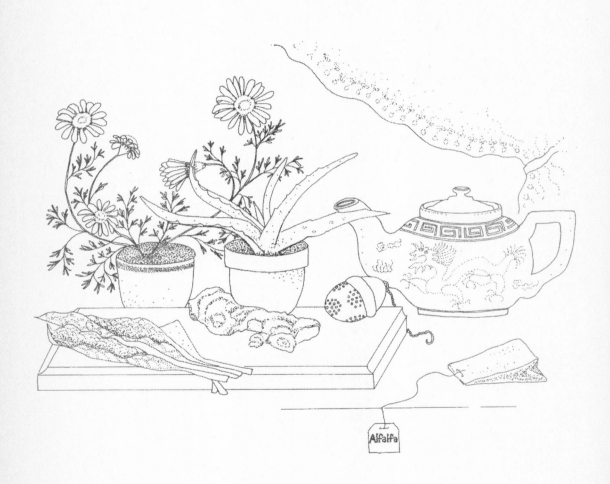

CHAPTER 11

Herbs for the
Postpartum Woman

Before there were drugstores, people looked to their gardens for remedies. In many parts of the world, both in traditional and modern cultures, growing herbs for home remedies is part of life. In Switzerland, family herb plots are not at all an uncommon sight. Herbs have been our partners in daily health care for thousands of years. Described here are just a few of the many members of the plant community that are known for their ability to improve the vitality and hasten the recovery of women after childbirth.

You can obtain herbs by growing them yourself, by checking with neighbors and friends who have gardens, or by looking in grocery or health-food stores. They can be purchased fresh, dried, or as prepared teas. Many medicinal herbs are available as tinctures and packaged in eye-dropper bottles; in this form they are very potent and convenient to use.

Herbs may be steeped into teas and taken as a drink, made into compresses and applied externally to sore or wounded areas of the body, used to flavor foods, or nibbled fresh from the plant. The aroma of some herbs is healing and curative; in Eastern cultures, their cultivation is said to increase well-being. Scientists have found that herb plants increase negative ions, which are known to purify the environment and also to lift our moods.

Today many health practitioners prescribe or recommend herbs. If you have specific questions, you can talk to a midwife, a doctor of Chinese medicine, a homeopathic physician, a nurse, or a physician associate, or a doctor who prefers natural remedies.

The herbs in this chapter are a few of my favorites for new mothers, because they are effective companions during postpartum. I have only included those that are known to have no negative side effects. However, treat your herbs as a medicine. Try them in small amounts to determine which ones work well for you and your family. Gradually collect a basic herbal pharmacy so you will have these natural remedies on hand when you need them.

ALFALFA *(Medicago sativa)*

Alfalfa is high in vitamins A, D, E, and K, all of which are beneficial to the baby as well as to mother. (If you are breastfeeding, your baby will derive the benefits of the herbs you take through your breast milk, so do not give your newborn herbal teas directly except under the supervision of your health-care giver.) Alfalfa also contains folic acid as well as eight important digestive enzymes. It stimulates the cell growth of supportive connective tissue. Alfalfa and kegel exercises are a winning combination when you're working to get your pelvic floor strong again. Drink the tea or eat the sprouts. *Alfalfa greatly increases a mother's milk quantity,* so you may want to take it if you are afraid you are not producing enough. Do not use this herb until initial engorgement of the breasts has subsided.

ALOE VERA *(Aloe; Liliaceae)*

What a friend this succulent plant is! Every family should have aloe vera growing in the yard or potted in the kitchen. It is excellent for soothing and healing minor burns, insect bites (yes, it relieves itching), sunburn, and it heals and soothes diaper rash. Put aloe vera gel on your face instead of buying expensive creams. (Before applying it to your face, test it on another area. Don't be alarmed if the treated skin turns burgundy. Some individuals' skin reacts this way to aloe vera. Skin stains usually fade within a few hours.) Simply break off an arm of the plant, peel back the outer layers, and apply the gel directly to your skin. Aloe vera can stain clothing as well as skin, so take the necessary precautions.

For treatment of a torn perineum, scrape the gel out of the plant, place it on a sanitary pad, and apply directly. This helps relieve the pain. When pain returns, apply a fresh aloe vera gel poultice. Aloe vera can also be used to combat vaginal yeast infections. For this, peel off the plant's skin, being very careful to remove all the spines, and insert as a vaginal suppository.

Drinking the juice in small amounts (approximately two tablespoons a day) works as a laxative and, in the experience of some midwives and doctors, is an excellent guard against postpartum infection. However, you should drink ginger tea with the aloe vera juice to prevent stomach cramping. Aloe vera applied

Making Herbal Teas

To prepare teas, put approximately one ounce of dried or an equal portion of fresh herbs in a pot containing one quart of cool water. Slowly bring to a boil. Cover the infusion and let it steep for a few minutes. For full-strength herbal infusions, steep for four hours. If you are using loose herbs, you may need to strain your tea before drinking it. Herbal tincture teas are prepared by pouring warm water into your cup and adding the number of drops recommended on the tincture package or by your health-care giver.

You may add honey to your tea, but don't boil tea once honey has been added, as boiled honey may be toxic. Never give honey or tea with honey to babies less than a year old because bacteria in honey poses a known health risk to infants. Herbs may also be prepared in warm milk, instead of water, with ghee and honey (see chapter 15, The Ayurvedic Lifestyle, page 203). Keep a pot and cup by your bedside and sip often. During the first days postpartum, it is best to take the teas warm to promote healing, but room temperature is also fine.

externally is a curative for hemorrhoids; however, avoid taking aloe vera internally if you are suffering from hemorrhoids as it may aggravate the problem. Apply to cracked nipples for fast healing.

BORAGE *(Borago officinalis)*
Borage leaf tea will increase your milk. If you already have a copious flow, you may wish to steer clear of this herb. Borage also contains much potassium, which helps you think clearly. It is mildly laxative and soothing to jangled nerves. The blue flowers may be added to salads.

CHAMOMILE *(Matricaria chamomilla)*
Drinking tea brewed from this herb's flower will help you fall asleep, brighten your eyes, and relieve the crankies. Try giving the tea to "super active" or teething children.

If you are feeling mentally restless, worried, or sleepless, briefly steep chamomile flowers and drink several cups of this aromatic tea. Not only is it a calming herb, chamomile works great as a hair rinse.

COMFREY *(Symphytum officinale)*

Comfrey is also called "bone knit" because it contains allantoin, which speeds the healing process. It literally grows like a weed. Just like a woman who has found her home, she flourishes, but comfrey simply won't grow in a spot where she's unhappy. The leaves, fresh or dried, as well as the ground root, can be made into a tea. The tea works great as a douche to combat yeast infections. A comfrey compress relieves itchy stitches and keeps perineum tissue soft and pliable while it heals. To make a soothing compress, soak a couple of handfuls of fresh comfrey leaves in four ounces of hot water for ten minutes or longer, or make a paste with the powdered root. Apply the compress directly to your pelvic floor for up to five minutes. You may also take a comfrey tea sitz bath or make comfrey tea, soak a cotton cloth in it, and apply this to the area. If you're suffering from sore breasts due to engorgement, a hot comfrey compress will soften your breasts and reduce the pain.

DANDELION *(Taraxacum officinale)*

Leaves, roots, and flowers are healing and improve the function of the liver and kidneys. You may use the dried leaves or root or find it in tincture form. However, the best way to benefit from dandelion is to pick it from your lawn, cook it like you would any vegetable and enjoy. I feel that people are dying of cancer because they neglect to eat the weeds in their own backyards.

Because dandelion contains vitamins A, C, B_1, and B_2 plus calcium, iron, potassium, choline, and trace minerals, it helps prevent and treat preeclampsia in pregnancy.

I prepare dandelions in this way: I pick the leaves and sometimes dig up the roots as well. The flowers are also good. These I wash and throw in a hot iron skillet with a dash of sesame oil, a splash of tamari and vinegar. I serve it over a bowl of steaming rice, sprinkled with sesame seeds. *Masarap!*

ECHINACEA *(Echinacea agustifolia)*

Echinacea is one of nature's antibiotics. It cleans the blood and lymph systems. The herb is good for treating colds and flu and is also known to clear up vaginal infections when an infusion is used as a sitz bath. Echinacea is best purchased as a tincture because the dried herb loses its potency quickly.

After birthing, some women are susceptible to infection. There was a time when childbed fever claimed the lives of many new mothers who gave birth in hospitals. If your midwife feels you are at risk for infection, as a preventive measure in the first few days postpartum, you can take ten to fifteen drops of echinacea tincture twice a day in warm water or with your postpartum brew (see page 158). Some people feel dizzy when taking echinacea. This side effect can be alleviated by preparing it with licorice.

Mastitis, or inflamed breasts, can be treated effectively with echinacea. However, large doses (one drop of tincture per two pounds of body weight) must be taken three to four times daily until the fever is gone. Then continue with smaller doses (one drop of tincture per five pounds body weight) for five to seven more days. In the case of serious infection, echinacea should be taken under the guidance of a trusted health-care giver. Until more research on echinacea has been done, it is advisable not to use it for extended periods (no more than three weeks unless your health-care giver advises longer). This will prevent any possible side effects such as changes in one's intestinal flora or liver irritation. People with immune deficiencies or lupus should consult a health-care provider before taking echinacea.

FALSE UNICORN *(Chamaelirium luteum)*
The root of false unicorn is a powerful uterine tonic and therefore is a main ingredient for postpartum brew. It is used to treat afterbirth contractions as well as menstrual cramping. False unicorn increases fertility in women, prevents miscarriage, and reduces nausea during pregnancy.

FENNEL *(Foeniculum vulgaris)*
The seed of the fennel plant, which has a lovely scent, is known for increasing the amount and wholesomeness of breast milk. If your baby has colic and you are breastfeeding, drink fennel tea and see the soothing effect it has on her. This is due to fennel's talent for aiding digestion. The sweet herb calms nerves and promotes menstruation. It also causes one to urinate more, therefore is cleansing and helpful in reducing water weight.

To relieve painful after-contractions, boil one half cup barley and one teaspoon fennel seeds in three cups of pure water for one half hour. Strain and sip, warming, soothing, and strengthening.

GINGER *(Zingiber officinale)*
This lovely root is terrific in teas and will add super flavor to your cooking while aiding your digestion. It is commonly used in the Orient to relieve menstrual cramping and to increase energy.

A ginger compress soothes stitches from a cesarean section. It is an excellent treatment for pain from an episiotomy or torn perineum. Ginger compresses are also good for soothing engorged breasts. To make a ginger compress, soak a clean cotton cloth in approximately one half quart of boiled water with one to two inches of grated ginger. When cool enough to handle, apply directly to the sore area.

LEMONGRASS *(Cymbopogon citratus)*

Lemongrass promotes good kidney function and literally washes one clean. Drink lemongrass tea while in labor as well as after birthing. The nice lemon flavor will convince you to combine it with other teas for a real treat. Don't toss out the leftover tea; use it as a hair rinse, or splash it on your face and body. You'll feel and smell wonderful.

LICORICE ROOT *(Glycyrrhiza glabra)*

Use licorice root instead of sugar to sweeten tea. Sugar should be avoided in the postpartum period as it slows the healing process and feeds infection. Licorice acts as a mild laxative, which is very important after birthing when you want to have regular bowel movements, and when many women find they are constipated due to trauma of the pelvic floor. (If you are having trouble moving your bowels, be sure not to strain.)

Because it contains estrogen, licorice root is a hormone balancer. Although in rare cases, this herb can cause water retention and elevated blood pressure (symptoms many women experience just before the onset of menstruation) because it increases the body's level of estrogen, there is little need for concern during the postpartum period. Licorice root is relaxing, soothing, and cleansing. The ancient Egyptians and Chinese considered licorice root a cure-all. The tea can be taken for coughs and fever. Sip it to combat the "baby blues."

MOTHERWORT *(Leonurus cardiaca)*

This uterine toner is very beneficial for treating painful afterbirth contractions or menstrual cramps. It is also given to women who have a great deal of pain in early labor.

Women who suffer with symptoms of premenstrual syndrome may take this herb to avoid feeling overwhelmed. People with stressful lives can take motherwort to help prevent heart attack because it has an antispasmodic effect on the heart muscle. Motherwort is not a casual herb. If taken in large doses over a long period of time, it can cause mental dependence, so use it only as you would a medicine. This advice should not be too difficult to follow because motherwort is bitter.

Motherwort is invaluable for preventing hemorrhage and treating shock. However, repeated doses have been known to inspire more bleeding. So, once again, remember that this herb is a powerful medicine and a little goes a long way.

Mugwort is not the same herb but has many of the same properties. Both motherwort and mugwort are good for treating suppressed menstruation.

NETTLES *(Urtica dioica)*
Nettles are nourishing, high in chlorophyll, vitamins A, C, D, K, calcium, potassium, phosphorus, iron, and sulphur. The calcium in nettles can decrease muscle cramps, even those awful leg cramps. It is know for its ability to cleanse the kidneys. If taken before childbirth, it decreases a woman's risk of hemorrhage. By strengthening blood vessels, nettles helps heal hemorrhoids and it is mildly astringent. New mothers will find that nettles increase their milk supply.

RED RASPBERRY *(Rubus stigosus* or *Rubus idaeus)*
The perfect pregnancy herb, red raspberry contains vitamins C, A, B complex, E, and many minerals as well. It is high in readily absorbable calcium, making it a wise lifelong uterine and bone tonic tea for women. It can help lessen nausea and prevent miscarriage and hemorrhaging. This herb is known to make birthing easier, so it is good to drink a lot of red raspberry leaf tea in the last months of pregnancy. After birthing, it reduces cramping and regulates vaginal discharge. Red raspberry is wonderful for increasing milk quantity and quality. Stomach problems like indigestion, cramping, diarrhea, and flu symptoms are often treated with raspberry leaf and chamomile tea combination. Let tea water cool a bit before putting in red raspberry leaves because boiling reduces this herb's effectiveness.

SHEPHERD'S PURSE *(Capsella bursa-pastoris)*
Shepherd's purse, which contains vitamins C and K, aids blood clotting. The antihemorrhage effect of shepherd's purse is immediate. It may be used to control bleeding during miscarriage and is a favorite afterbirth herb as it promotes the afterbirth contractions that cause the uterus to return to its pre-pregnancy shape and size. It was used traditionally by Native Americans to stop internal bleeding.

Children who have trouble with bed-wetting may benefit from shepherd's purse tea because it has a soothing effect upon the elimination systems. This herb is an excellent diuretic, clearing up diarrhea, which is a problem for some women during menstruation. Shepherd's purse tastes somewhat like cabbage and may be added to soups.

VALERIAN ROOT *(Valeriana officinalis)*

This herb tastes very strong and bitter; however, it is a powerful painkiller. It also stops trembling and relieves tension. If you suffer from headaches, painful after-birth contractions, or insomnia, the nervine properties of valerian may help you get some peace and quiet. Valerian root is an excellent herb for mothers who had cesarean births because it helps reduce the severe gas pains that frequently accompany recovery from a cesarean section.

YELLOW DOCK *(Rumex crispus)*

Yellow dock root is the midwives' favorite absorbable source of iron. It is also nonconstipating. Some pregnant and breastfeeding women with anemia have found that taking iron tablets does not bring up their hemoglobin, while taking tincture of yellow dock root will do the trick. A quick way to check for anemia is to peek at the inside surface of your lower eyelid, if it is red, you're fine. If it is pale pink, worse even—white, you are anemic. If your midwife or doctor feels concern that you had significant blood loss after childbirth, please take twenty-five to thirty drops of yellow dock root tincture, three times a day. You will definitely feel stronger and have more energy as your hemoglobin returns to normal.

Maui Midwives' Postpartum Brew

Tina, a midwife on Maui, like many midwives there, tells her postpartum women to sip this brew throughout the day and when they wake at night. She asks them to continue drinking the tea for the first four days postpartum, or until the lochia ceases to flow. During this time, she asks them to do nothing except tend to the baby and take care of their basic grooming (brushing teeth and hair, showering, and changing into fresh pajamas every day). She enlists the new mother's friends and family to help with meals, take care of the other children, and do the housekeeping. In general, women who follow her wise instructions stop bleeding within the first week postpartum. They heal quickly, have fewer breastfeeding problems, and feel good overall.

To one gallon pure water, add a generous pinch of each of these dried herbs and bring to a boil:

False unicorn
Licorice root
Shepherd's purse
Red raspberry leaves (add last, when cooled, as boiling reduces effectiveness)

Steep fifteen minutes or longer. Strain, sip often throughout the day.

Health-food and herb stores sell tinctures of these individual herbs, which you can combine to make this brew. This form is convenient when you wish to make the tea one cup at a time. However, postpartum women need lots of this nourishing liquid, and they don't have time to make a cup whenever they're thirsty. Making it by the gallon keeps the supply flowing and costs much less. (When available, choose fresh herbs over dried, using in more generous amounts than those given here.)

This naturally sweet postpartum brew will tone your uterus, control bleeding, promote regular bowel movements, increase milk supply, and relieve afterbirth contractions.

Remember, herbs are powerful; a little goes a long way. Experiment with combinations of your favorites and come up with a few that please you and your family. Children over one year of age may be given herbal teas half strength. Consult an herbologist or health-care giver about giving herbs to children younger than one. The milder herbs like chamomile, lemongrass, licorice root, and red raspberry are easily taken by children. My children will drink room-temperature herbal tea blends as readily as they will drink juice, and they don't get that sugar rush from the tea.

When friends come to visit, get out your teapot. Postpartum is a good time to establish partnership with the healers of the plant kingdom.

Uplifting Tea

This caffeine-free brew will lift your spirits, lessen fatigue, and give you additional iron, which all new mothers need.

1 teaspoon red raspberry leaf

1 teaspoon nettles

1 teaspoon yellow dock

1 teaspoon shepherd's purse

1 teaspoon motherwort

Add herbs to one gallon of pure water at room temperature. Allow to sit for up to four hours in the sunshine, allowing the healing rays to infuse with the herbs. Enjoy!

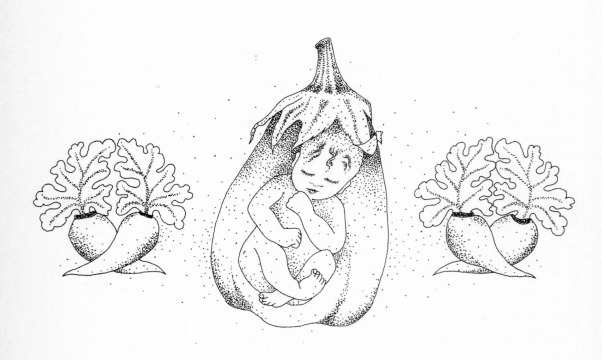

CHAPTER 12

Making Friends with Food

This is the perfect time for you to make friends with food. You have a new baby who will soon begin to eat solid foods. You want your child's relationship with food to be healthy right from the start. Providing a good example for him or her is a great incentive for you to reshape your own relationship with what you eat. Good eating habits are important now, especially if you are breastfeeding, because you want the best for your child and deserve the best for yourself.

If during pregnancy you gained somewhere around thirty-five pounds and then gave birth to a six- to eight-pound baby, shedding ten to fifteen pounds with the waters, placenta, and the sweat you lost during labor, you weigh over ten pounds more than your pre-pregnancy weight. Don't be disappointed. Almost no one returns to her pre-pregnancy weight right away. It may be little comfort, but those extra pounds are part of nature's blueprint. If you're breastfeeding, your baby will need those stored nutrients in his first six months of life.

When your milk comes in a couple of days after giving birth, your breasts are so laden that they weigh an extra one to three pounds. In full-breasted women, the additional weight in the breasts can be even more. It's no wonder women carry some extra weight after having a baby. Water retention also accounts for a few pounds. As your body comes back into its pre-pregnancy hormonal balance, you will shed these pounds.

Dieting is out of the question for breastfeeding mothers! Don't do it. You don't want to undermine both your health and the nutritional needs of your baby. Your baby will thrive on milk produced by a mom who is eating well. Even if you are not breastfeeding, caring for an infant will tax your energy, so you need to eat nutrient-rich foods to prevent feeling run down.

It is estimated that breastfeeding women require between 1,000 and 3,500 additional calories a day. In order to maintain your own good health and provide your baby's nutritional needs, you must get almost as much protein as when you were pregnant and *more* of many nutrients, including calcium, vitamins A, C, E, B1, B2, zinc, niacin, and iodine. Your body requires the same amount of iron,

Tips and Tricks for Maintaining Your Optimal Weight

- **Brush your teeth immediately after dinner.** Do this to avoid snacking during the evening when you don't need extra calories. Make yourself a deal: You won't have to brush your teeth before going to bed, when you're tired, if you don't get food on them again.
- **Eat your evening meal as early as possible.** Parents of small children know that children eat better if served before dark. The entire family will enjoy having more active time between eating and going to bed to digest the food.
- **Take a walk after meals.** The excess body heat induced by exercising on a full stomach actually melts fat. A sunset stroll with the entire family can be so enjoyable it won't even feel like exercising.
- **Don't skip breakfast.** It has been found that people with weight problems have a history of skipping breakfast. Eating a nutritious breakfast prevents uncontrolled eating at night.
- **Skip cocktails.** They're loaded with calories, and alcohol is not recommended for breastfeeding mothers.
- **Desert desserts!** Easier said than done. When your mother-in-law bakes her famous apple pie, which happens to be your favorite, go for it. But skip the scoop of ice cream she offers to dump on top. One cookie won't hurt; it won't help either. One sweet treat a day adds a lot of empty calories to your intake. Don't martyr yourself, but try to get into the habit of eating a piece of fruit instead of a pastry.
- **Treat yourself to a new movement outfit.** A leotard in your favorite color will inspire you to dance around the house.
- **Remember your triumphs.** You are going to cheat, so don't focus on your failures. So what if you didn't lose twenty pounds in a month;

magnesium, phosphorus, and vitamins B$_{12}$ and D as when you were pregnant. For specific quantities of these and other nutrients, see the Women's Essential Daily Nutritional Needs chart on pages 186–187. You can see how important it is to eat wisely during postpartum, so please don't starve yourself. Appetite is greatly increased while you breastfeed. You're hungry because you need to eat more. Listen carefully to what your body tells you. Eat when you are hungry; drink when you are thirsty.

rejoice if you lost three pounds. Forget that ham sandwich you had downtown at the deli. Make up for it by having a nice salad for dinner. Be a reducing saint during the week and a devil on the weekends. Eventually you'll find you won't feel like indulging at the ice cream shop on Saturdays.

- **Set reasonable goals.** It's impossible to lose fifty pounds in a month, even if your high school reunion is coming up. Lose five pounds by eating well and getting some exercise, and with the glow from your confidence you will look better than ever.
- **Be sure to drink plenty of pure water between meals.** Water washes out the toxins that may be left in your body from junk foods, stress, and environmental pollutants.
- **Imagine yourself as you wish to look.** Your thoughts can make anything possible. By holding a beautiful image of yourself in your mind, you instantly begin to look more beautiful. Positive self-image is very powerful.
- **Bless your food.** The gift of food is meant to nourish, strengthen, and beautify you. A moment of silence or a prayer before meals serves as a reminder of food's divine nature.

Your body belongs to you. Sculpt it as you wish, but treat it with kindness and love. You deserve to be physically beautiful by your own standards, not society's. Nurture your body as you nurture your precious children and anything is possible.

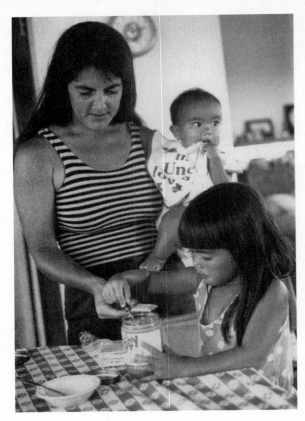

Two groups of pregnant and lactating women must pay even closer attention to ensure they receive enough nutrients: mothers under twenty-three years old and women who are vegetarians. Women under the age of twenty-three have not reached full physical maturity and need higher quantities of the nutrients listed on the chart. Check with your health-care giver who will be able to tell you the levels required to meet your needs while pregnant or nursing. Vegan and strict vegetarian (who eat no animal products) mothers should ask their health-care giver about a good supplement for vitamin B_{12} and other nutrients vegetarians may not obtain through their diet. Vegetarian women may need to eat a greater volume of food to get all the nutrients they need to maintain health and to feel strong and vital. They need not worry about weight gain from increasing the amount of food because the foods they eat are generally lower in fat than meat and other animal products.

Don't worry about the extra weight you may be carrying. Breastfeeding and the demands of mothering seem to be the best reducing plan. As a matter of fact, it is not uncommon for women to get too thin after a few months of breastfeeding. If this is the case with you, see your health-care giver and discuss your weight loss. You do not wish to rob your body of its health and vitality by not eating enough of the right foods. Again, as your body's hormonal activity returns to its pre-pregnancy state, your weight will stabilize.

This natural, gradual return to pre-pregnancy weight sounds wonderful, but some of us will still be dissatisfied with our weight after having a child. Unfortunately, the svelte, even emaciated, modern version of the ideal woman has been ingrained in us through the media. If it were realistic for all women to be skinny, we would not see so much suffering associated with the issue of body weight. Weight, like stature, is largely genetic. You may come from a family that tends to be heavy. Harmful crash dieting, addiction to diet pills, bulimia, and anorexia have become an epidemic among women. Too many of us are striving unrealistically and pointlessly for an unnatural look.

Look in the mirror. You may be seeing many more pounds than actually exist. It is possible to overlook your own beauty. If you believe that perfect means having not one extra ounce of fat, or a pimple, dimple, or sag, you'll probably never be perfect. Don't be so hard on yourself.

Visit a museum; look at the Greek and Renaissance standards of beauty. By modern standards, Greek goddesses are fat. Don't judge yourself by how much you weigh when how you feel is what counts. In ancient Greece, it was easy to be plump and feel terrific. The Hawaiian culture, both ancient and modern, honors the beauty of large women.

Remember, your body is not you, but the vehicle you've been given with which to move through life. St. Francis of Assisi called his body "brother donkey." It's a gift. Would you complain if you were given a Mercedes-Benz instead of a Rolls-Royce? Then why wish for a different model body than the one you've got? During pregnancy and after giving birth, women question the beauty of their bodies. The body has just facilitated the miracle of birth. See the beauty in that and your *personal,* very individual physical beauty will unfold.

How do you become friends with food? Enjoy it. It is a wonderful part of life. Available to you is a vast variety of foods. You have the creativity and resources to make food delicious and beautiful as well as nourishing. Respect the food you eat and you won't abuse the privilege of its abundance by overeating. Remember, too much of a good thing only lessens its value.

A good step toward good eating habits is getting some physical activity. Substantially overweight people who begin exercising do not necessarily end up eating more. Though calories have been expended, appetite is not increased. If you don't increase the amount you eat, you will lose weight. If you are not over-weight, exercising increases your desire for food, keeping your weight stable.

Wise Nutrition and Growing Older Gracefully

Childbearing puts such great demands on your body that you may be feeling your own mortality. Indeed, we all grow older each day, but if you maintain yourself physically and spiritually, you can look forward to growing stronger and wiser with age rather than weaker. Eating well and getting plenty of rest and regular exercise are the keys to growing older gracefully.

In their later years, women are prone to osteoporosis, demineralization of the bones that can lead to fractures, shortening of the spine, and dowager's hump. This condition occurs more frequently in women than in men because women's bones are less dense. In addition, pregnancy and breastfeeding increase the body's need for calcium. And while lactating (and again after menopause), the amount of the hormone estrogen, which helps the body assimilate the minerals necessary for bone regeneration, decreases.

An inadequate diet now can lead to health problems in the future. A postpartum woman may feel that being concerned at this time in her life about the effects of bone deterioration is premature, but to reach your golden years standing tall you must take good care of yourself now. Extra care must be taken to eat mineral-rich foods to obtain enough calcium. A breastfeeding mother requires 500 milligrams more calcium each day than the average woman; this is even more than she required while pregnant. Dairy products, soybean products, nuts, and fresh, cooked leafy green vegetables (and in particular, mustard and turnip greens) are excellent sources of calcium. You may want to use blackstrap molasses as a sweetener because it is high in calcium. To make things more complicated, the body needs the mineral magnesium to absorb calcium. Luckily, sources rich in calcium also provide magnesium: nuts, soybeans, and leafy greens. Watch out for caffeine, found in chocolate and many soft drinks as well as in coffee, because it decreases your mineral absorption. Some prescription and over-the-counter drugs like steroids and antacids contribute to loss of calcium through the urine. Always tell your health-care giver that you are a breastfeeding mother before she or he prescribes medication for you.

To ensure healthy, strong bones and great posture at any age, you must also get regular exercise. The simple exercises found in this book, if practiced routinely throughout your life, will help slow the aging process. Walking, stretching, dancing, and swimming inspire good circulation, flexibility, muscle tone, and fullness of breath, all of which are essential to the regeneration of your cells.

Your outlook on life will also fashion your future. To age gracefully, let go of tensions and laugh. See the world through your child's eyes; get down on the floor with your child and have a great time. Feeling young is as much in the heart as in the body.

Caffeine, Drugs, and Postpartum

If you are breastfeeding, try not to eat, smoke, drink, or take anything that you would not give your baby directly. Remember, what you ingest ends up in your milk. Your breasts are designed to pass nutrients and antibodies to your baby through your milk. The breasts do not have the capability to selectively filter out those elements you would rather your baby not be exposed to; therefore, you must act as the filter by not ingesting them.

Just as you limited your intake of caffeine carefully during your pregnancy, you should limit it during early postpartum. Even if you are not breastfeeding, you should cut back on the amount of caffeine you take into your body. Postpartum women have extremely sensitive nervous systems and will feel the effects of caffeine profoundly. Chocolate and beverages containing caffeine may give you lift for a short time but tend to let you down fast, leaving you feeling that you've crashed and burned. Herbal teas without caffeine can be just as enjoyable as coffee, black teas, and caffeinated soft drinks. Remember, though, that herbal teas are medicinal and some must be ingested with reverence. Read the packages or talk to your health-care giver about which teas to avoid during postpartum. Most herbal teas found in grocery stores have no harmful side effects and may be enjoyed freely.

All nonprescription drugs should be avoided while you are pregnant or lactating. This includes any over-the-counter remedies, recreational drugs, cigarettes, and alcohol. I have talked with many women who sneak an occasional cigarette or smoke a bit of marijuana. Afterward some of them experience extreme guilt over what they are passing through their milk to the baby. I am not sure which is worse for the baby, the chemicals or the guilt. Don't judge yourself; just do your best. If you must smoke, do it outside the house, away from your baby. Never smoke while you are breastfeeding.

If your health-care giver prescribes drugs for you, let him or her know that you are a breastfeeding mother and are concerned about what could be passed through your milk to your baby. If you don't feel your doctor is listening, say it again. If you're still not convinced that the prescribed drug is safe to use while nursing, ask your favorite pediatrician and talk to your pharmacist. Many books, available at your public library, provide detailed descriptions of the effects of prescription and nonprescription drugs.

If you or your partner has a problem with alcohol or drug abuse, look in your phone directory for a local Alcoholics Anonymous or Narcotics Anonymous group. They provide nonjudgmental support for people who wish to be drug free.

New Recipes for New Mothers

With the many theories and philosophies about eating that are popular today, you may be wondering what commonsense eating truly means. You now have a child and may be thinking about eating family style for the first time in your adult life. And this comes at a time when you already may feel overwhelmed by the responsibility of your emerging role as mother.

Think about what your grandmother and mother cooked for their families. Take into consideration what you and the other members of your family like to eat. Add to that what you've learned about nutrition from your own experience, books, and friends, and you will have an eating philosophy that is uniquely your own.

I've chosen these recipes to help you get started because they're easy to prepare, the ingredients are readily available, and they provide a postpartum woman and her family with the nutrients they need.

Healthy Snacks

In the morning while you prepare breakfast, put on a medium-sized pot of brown rice, buckwheat, barley, or quinoa. (Quinoa is a grain from South America that is becoming more available in the United States. Try it. It's delicious and high in nutrients, and it cooks quickly.) This pot of hearty grain can sit on the stove, ready for you and your family to enjoy. Serve it with a dash of tamari soy sauce as a mineral-rich energy booster. Besides being high in fiber, which relieves constipation so common to new mothers and possibly prevents cancer of the colon over the long term, whole grains take away sugar cravings. Unlike sweet snacks, grains will not cause your blood sugar to soar, which generally means your energy and emotions will crash when your body tries to readjust.

Do not forget about popcorn for a fast and fun anytime snack. High in fiber, popcorn contains zinc; and if you sprinkle a couple of tablespoons of nutritional yeast, which you can buy at health-food stores, and tamari soy sauce to taste, you will also be adding other minerals and B vitamins to your diet.

Keep a large bowl, half filled with water, stocked with carrot sticks, cucumber, and green pepper slices, whole green beans, cherry tomatoes, and other ready-to-eat fresh vegetables. When you are hungry between meals, a quick snack will be waiting in your refrigerator.

Why Eat Organic...

While working as a midwife in the Philippines, I found that women who lived far up in the Cordillera mountains, often in villages beyond the roads, had considerably less blood loss after childbirth than women living in or near the cities. These women worked hard and ate less. What was their secret? Because it was necessary to hike to their villages, pesticides, herbicides and chemical fertilizers were not used. They could not afford these "modern" luxuries, nor did they wish to carry them over the trails to their villages. These women and their families grew their food organically.

We live in curious times. Food is being genetically altered. Clearly it is necessary to protect our families from chemicals and genetic tampering with our food. Eating organically and carefully is more expensive. However, we must ask ourselves: "What does cancer cost?" As new parents, it is our responsibility to protect our children's health by eating organic whenever possible.

Almond Banana Smoothie

SERVES 4

Almonds are nearly 20 percent protein. They are high in vitamin E and calcium, as well as vitamin B, copper, iron, zinc, potassium, phosphorus, manganese, magnesium, and selenium. According to Chinese medicine, almonds cure hemorrhoids. Ayurvedic healing (see chapter 15) teaches us that almonds are warming, tonic, and reduce Vata (wind and space in the body). Bananas provide potassium, iron, magnesium, and selenium.

4 to 5 ripe bananas (more if they are a small variety)

5 to 6 tablespoons roasted almond butter

2 teaspoons almond extract (natural variety sold in health-food stores)

Pure water, enough to fill blender two inches below brim,
after other ingredients are already inside

Freeze the bananas the day before; this is a perfect way to use your overripe bananas. In the first six weeks postpartum, avoid overly cold foods: Make the smoothie with three to four unfrozen bananas, and one frozen one. Place in blender with almond butter, almond extract, and water. Blend until smooth and creamy.

Sesame Gomazio

USE AS A CONDIMENT

Sesame seeds are rich in calcium, something every woman needs.

1 cup of white or light sesame seeds

½ teaspoon salt

In an iron skillet, dry-roast sesame seeds, stirring constantly, until golden brown. Add salt. Let cool. Store in an attractive jar, right on your table, so you use it generously to flavor your food.

Beet Salad

SERVES 2

This calcium-rich salad-snack is also a liver cleanser. The omega-3 oil of flaxseed oil is good for brain development, so eat this often the next time you're pregnant.

  1 large beet

  1 tablespoon flaxseed oil

  ½ teaspoon lemon or lime juice

  ½ teaspoon tamari soy sauce

  2 sprigs of mint

Peel and grate the beet. Add flaxseed oil, lemon juice, and tamari, toss, divide in two. Garnish with a sprig of mint and share with your partner.

A Different Kind of Spinach Salad

SERVES 2 AS A MEAL, 4 AS A SIDE DISH

  4 big handfuls spinach leaves, broken into bite-sized pieces

  1 (8-ounce) can mandarin orange slices

  ⅓ pound Monterey Jack or provolone cheese, cut into small cubes

  ½ cup slivered almonds

Toss all ingredients together with the Oriental Salad Dressing that follows. Or try your favorite dressing with this salad.

During pregnancy your calcium needs rose from approximately 1,000 to about 1,300 milligrams a day. Now, if you are breastfeeding, your body requires 1,500 milligrams of calcium daily, plus additional amounts of most other nutrients. This salad contains cheese, almonds, and leafy greens—all good sources of calcium. Vegetarians may wish to substitute tofu for the cheese. Not all spinach salads need to look and taste the same. This one is lovely and will add variety to your table.

Oriental Salad Dressing

MAKES ABOUT ¾ CUP (WITH PAPAYA, 1 CUP)

Serve this sweet-and-sour dressing over A Different Kind of Spinach Salad or with your own salad combination. This dressing poured over sprouted mung beans makes a simple and delicious side dish.

½ cup olive oil

¼ cup sesame oil

Juice of ½ lemon

2 tablespoons apple cider vinegar

1 teaspoon honey

2 tablespoons tamari soy sauce

Pepper

Papaya (optional)

Ginger, ½ inch (optional)

Mix all ingredients in a jar with a tight-fitting lid. Shake well. If you want to be more creative, add the meat and seeds of half a ripe papaya and half an inch of fresh gingerroot. (The papaya and ginger aid digestion.) Put all ingredients in a blender and blend until smooth and creamy.

Greek Salad

SERVES 4

This is one of those salads that is a meal in itself. You can make a lot, serve some immediately, and store the rest in the refrigerator so you can snack on it all day. Whole-grain pasta is a good source of fuel for new mothers because it is a complex carbohydrate and contains many essential nutrients.

- **1 pound rainbow or whole-wheat pasta curls or shells,** cooked and cooled
- **½ pound feta cheese,** cut into bite-sized cubes
- **1 large tomato,** cut into bite-sized pieces
- **1 generous handful fresh basil leaves,** torn into pieces
- **½ cucumber,** peeled and sliced
- **½ zucchini,** sliced
- **¼ cup pitted black olives**
- **¼ cup pitted green olives or pimentos**
- **¼ cup Parmesan cheese**
- **⅓ cup of your favorite Italian dressing**

Toss all ingredients together.

Pumpkin Soup

SERVES 4 TO 6

In Japan shiitake mushrooms and ginger are known for their healing powers. This soup will warm your bones and soothe your spirits.

6 to 8 dried shiitake mushrooms

1 small pumpkin or acorn squash, peeled and cubed

1 inch fresh ginger, peeled and grated

1 (8-ounce) can coconut milk (organic is available in health-food stores)

Salt or tamari to taste

Soak the shiitake mushrooms 1 hour or more in 1 liter of pure water. Save the shiitake water to make the soup. With kitchen shears, cut softened shiitake into strips. Bring mushrooms with water, pumpkin, and ginger to boil in the same water used to soak the mushrooms. Lower heat and simmer until pumpkin is easily mashed. Turn off heat. Add coconut milk then add salt or tamari. Serve steaming hot with Sesame Gomazio garnish (page 170).

Maggie's Sweet Potatoes

SERVES 4

Sweet potatoes are a super energy-boosting food. My grandmother, who was a midwife in the Philippines, was able to keep her ten children from starving during World War II because they were able to find wild sweet potatoes. In addition to providing calcium, the rosemary will increase your milk flow and help relieve intestinal gas.

3 to 4 cups sweet potatoes, cubed (about 3 large sweet potatoes)

1 tablespoon tamari soy sauce

1½ teaspoons rosemary, fresh or dried, crushed

1½ teaspoons lemon juice

3 tablespoons olive oil

1 cup sweet onion, diced

Combine ingredients in a large baking dish. Cover and bake for 1 hour at 350°.

Ibu Ana's Roasted Vegetables

SERVES 6 TO 8

What could be more nourishing or healthy than roasted vegetables?

6 yams, cut into 1-inch cubes

2 large beets, cut into 1-inch cubes

4 potatoes, cut into 1-inch cubes
(omit these in the first six weeks postpartum)

12 to 15 baby carrots

2 large red onions, quartered (optional)

Olive oil

Salt

Herbs, dried and ground (any herbs you love, such as oregano,
basil, rosemary, tarragon, marjoram, or others)

2 garlic bulbs, broken into cloves, unpeeled (optional)

12 or more fresh, whole button mushrooms

Preheat oven to 350°. Prepare the vegetables as suggested above, coat with olive oil, spread out on cookie sheets (except garlic cloves and mushrooms), sprinkle with salt and herbs. Bake, turning vegetables with a spatula every 30 minutes. When potatoes are nearly tender, add the whole mushrooms and garlic cloves, return to oven, and roast until all are tender.

Serve warm. Our children love it with sour cream. This makes a great summertime food to eat out on the picnic table.

Can't Beet It

SERVES 4

Root vegetables grow right in Mother Earth, where she packs them with vitamins and minerals. Just look at them. You can see they are nutritious by their vivid color. This side dish combines hearty beets with cheese and leafy green vegetables for added calcium and minerals.

1 tablespoon olive oil

3 medium or 4 small beets, halved and thinly sliced

1 large bunch kale or your favorite green (approximately 4 cups packed), washed and cut into pieces slightly bigger than bite sized

1 tablespoon tamari soy sauce

½ cup sharp Cheddar cheese, grated

In a wok or large frying pan with a tight-fitting lid, put approximately ½ to 1 inch of water. Add oil and beets. Cover. (If your beets are fresh from the garden and still have their tops, don't discard them. Cut them up and cook them with the kale.) Simmer on medium heat until beets are tender, approximately 10 minutes. Periodically check beets to be sure the water has not cooked off; add water as needed to avoid burning. Add kale or other greens, cover, and let greens steam until just done. To avoid overcooking, remove kale from heat while still bright green. Toss with tamari soy sauce and cheese and serve.

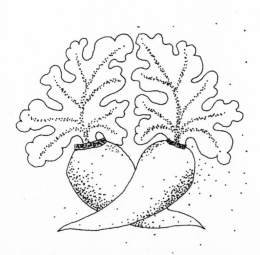

Gado-Gado

SERVES 4 AS A MAIN DISH, MORE AS A SIDE

Peanuts provide protein, tofu is calcium rich, and yams are nourishing for the female reproductive system. This nutritious recipe is a traditional Indonesian medley of flavors.

1 carrot

¼ pound green beans, halved, strings removed

¼ pound Chinese peas, strings removed

1 broccoli stalk and head, peel stalk and reserve for another use (don't waste it)

1 celery stalk, cut in 1 inch lengths

¼ pound mung bean sprouts

1 large yam, cubed

1 large potato, cubed

½ pound firm tofu, cubed

SAUCE

½ cup natural peanut butter

¼ cup pure water

1 tablespoon tamari soy sauce

¼ teaspoon chili powder

½ teaspoon organic brown sugar

½ inch fresh ginger, peeled and grated

Cut vegetables into bite-sized pieces. Steam a few minutes until tender, not soft. Tofu may also be steamed along with the vegetables. Arrange on a platter.

Combine the sauce ingredients using a fork to stir until smooth. Add more water if necessary, so you may pour it over the steamed vegetables. Pour peanut sauce over the entire lovely mess.

Chicken Adobo

SERVES 6

Many cultures the world over believe that chicken soup is a cure-all. This dish is a specialty of the Philippines. Almost every family there whips up a hearty pot of chicken adobo. This version is my grandmother's; she passed it down to my mother.

2 pounds chicken, cut into parts with most of the skin removed

1 to 4 cloves garlic

1 quart water

4 to 6 potatoes, cubed

2 carrots, cut into thin rounds

½ cup apple cider vinegar

⅓ cup tamari soy sauce

Pepper

5 to 7 cups cooked rice

In a big pot, over medium heat, brown chicken parts in their own juices, stirring frequently. Add a little water or oil if needed. While chicken is browning, peel and crush the garlic. (If you're breastfeeding a young baby who is sensitive to the foods you eat, start with a small amount of garlic. When your baby is older, you may increase the amount.) Toss the garlic into the pot with the chicken, and continue to stir. Put on a quart of water to boil. When chicken begins to look browned on the outside, throw in the cubed potatoes and sliced carrots; also add the vinegar and soy sauce now. Simmer chicken, potatoes, and carrots in vinegar and soy sauce for 5 minutes, then add the boiling water. Let cook over medium heat until the chicken is tender and cooked through, and the potatoes are very soft. Add pepper to taste, and serve over rice.

New Mother Pesto

. . . .

SERVES 4 TO 6

Basil is called tulsi *in India. A highly regarded healer from the plant kingdom, basil improves elimination; strengthens the nervous system; reduces fever; hastens healing; relieves spasms; dispels colds, coughs, congestion, and headaches; and tastes wonderful! This herb is said to be life giving—opening the heart and mind as well as increasing love and devotion. (Feed this recipe to your husband!)*

The cheese and nuts provide protein and calcium along with many other nutrients. Garlic is a powerful detoxifier and rejuvenator. Serve over hot pasta with a vegetable side dish. Refrigerate remaining pesto; spread on toast and eat it as a snack. For a quick, high-energy lunch, use pesto as a topping over brown rice or any other whole grain.

1 cup olive oil

1½ to 2 cups firmly packed basil leaves (more if it's in season and inexpensive at the store or abundant in your garden)

½ cup pine nuts, walnuts, cashews, or almonds (almond butter may be substituted)

½ cup grated Parmesan, Romano, or feta cheese

3 cloves garlic

Juice of ½ lemon

Tamari soy sauce

1 pound whole-grain pasta

In your blender or food processor, begin blending the olive oil and basil. Gradually add nuts, cheese, garlic, lemon juice, and tamari soy sauce to taste. Blend until smooth.

Fried Rice

SERVES 4

This no-meat version of a traditional recipe is a favorite with my children. Mothers who wish to increase their vitamin B₆ intake should make this dish with brown rice.

¼ cup olive oil

2 tablespoons sesame oil

2 cloves garlic, minced

½ inch ginger, freshly grated, or ½ teaspoon ground ginger

1 carrot, diced

¼ sweet onion, diced

1 stalk celery, diced

½ cup slivered almonds

½ pound green beans, trimmed and thinly sliced

1 small zucchini, diced

4 cups cooked rice (brown, basmati, or white)

Tamari soy sauce

Pepper

In a large frying pan or wok, heat oils with garlic and ginger. Over medium heat, add carrot, onion, celery, almonds, and green beans. Sauté until onions are transparent and carrots are tender. Add zucchini. When zucchini is tender, add rice, soy sauce, and pepper. Mix well. Serve with mung bean sprouts and Oriental Salad Dressing (page 172).

Stir-Fried Tofu

SERVES 4

Tofu is an excellent source of protein, which is essential for milk production, and is high in fiber. In addition, it contains calcium, as do the sesame seeds used in this recipe. Green pepper provides vitamin C, but don't overcook it because the vitamin is unstable and can be destroyed in the cooking process.

2 tablespoons sesame seeds

¼ cup olive oil

1 tablespoon sesame oil

1 pound firm tofu, cubed

2 cups mixed vegetables of your choice, steamed

1 green pepper, cut into bite-sized pieces

3 tablespoons tamari soy sauce

1 tablespoon cornstarch

1 teaspoon ground ginger

1 cup water

2 to 4 cups cooked couscous

In a wok or large frying pan, heat sesame seeds in oils. Add tofu. Stir-fry until slightly golden, then add mixed vegetables and green pepper. You want the pan hot enough to make the ingredients dance as they sauté. In a bowl, mix tamari soy sauce with cornstarch and ginger, then slowly add water and stir until there are no lumps. Add this mixture to the pan. Simmer until sauce is thick. Serve over couscous. This dish is great with A Different Kind of Spinach Salad (page 171) served on the side.

Hawaiian Tempeh

SERVES 4 TO 6

Tempeh is an Indonesian staple made primarily from cultured soybeans, but some-times other whole grains and seaweeds are added. This cholesterol-free food is high in protein, making it an excellent meat substitute.

An island-style version of tempeh, this dish features ginger, which aids digestion and is helpful in relieving menstrual cramps or afterpains. Burdock is a cure-all widely used in Oriental medicine to restore health, purify the blood, and dispel fever.

1 package (6 to 8) dried black (shiitake) mushrooms, or 8 ounces fresh mushrooms

1 package (8-ounce) natural tempeh

½ cup olive oil

1 inch fresh ginger, grated or sliced thinly

6 inches burdock root *(gobo),* if available, tough skin scraped off and cut into small pieces

¼ cup tamari soy sauce

½ cup water

½ cup red wine

1 (8-ounce) can sliced lotus root and/or 1 can (8-ounce) sliced water chestnuts

1 (8-ounce) can sliced bamboo shoots

2 medium carrots, diced

1 pound green beans, trimmed and snapped in half

Pepper

5 to 7 cups cooked rice or millet

Soak black mushrooms until soft (this takes about 1 hour) and cut into strips. (Fresh mushrooms are simply washed and sliced.) In a large pot, brown tempeh with oil, ginger, and burdock root for about 10 minutes; stir frequently so mixture doesn't burn or stick to the pot. Add soy sauce, water, wine, lotus root and/or water chestnuts, bamboo shoots, and carrots. Simmer over medium heat until carrots are tender and cooked through. Add green beans and mushrooms, and simmer until they are tender. Season with pepper. Serve over rice or millet with a slice of papaya on the side. This dish stores well in the refrigerator, and small portions can be heated and served later.

Jungle Cake

MAKES UP TO 15 PIECES (UNLESS YOUR MONKEYS ARE REALLY HUNGRY)

Now that you are a mom, it's time to add some wonderful treats to your repertoire. As your baby grows into a person (it won't take long), he or she will desire sweets. Mother's milk is sweet and people never seem to outgrow the love of sweetness. Your job is to teach your precious child to eat vegetables and grains, and also to provide a nutritious sweet treat once in a while. After all, celebration is essential to good health. This cake is my family's birthday favorite.

1 cup butter or margarine, softened

1 cup raw sugar

4 eggs

2 teaspoons vanilla

3 ⅓ cups whole-wheat flour

2 teaspoons baking soda

½ teaspoon salt

½ cup quick-cooking rolled oats

1 cup nuts, chopped (Cashews or macadamia nuts are nicest, but walnuts, pecans, or almonds work fine.)

1 cup sour cream

2 cups fresh fruit, mashed (A mix of banana, papaya, and mango is wonderful. If only one or two of these fruits are available, that works fine. Fresh or canned crushed pineapple, drained, may be substituted for any or all of the fruit.)

Preheat oven to 325°. Cream butter with sugar, eggs, and vanilla until smooth. In a separate bowl, sift flour with soda and salt. Add flour and all remaining ingredients to creamed mixture. Pour into a 9 by 13-inch pan that has been greased lightly and dusted with flour. Bake for about 1 hour or until toothpick inserted into center comes out clean.

Coconut-Cream Cheese Frosting

If you are using the passion fruit, which adds a tart, exotic flavor to this frosting, slice it open and use meat and seeds.

- 1 (8-ounce) package cream cheese
- 2 ounces sour cream
- 2 tablespoons honey
- ½ teaspoon vanilla
- ½ cup grated unsweetened coconut, dried or fresh
- 1 fresh lilikoi (passion fruit), if available

Cream all ingredients together. Frost cake when cooled, if the monkeys can wait that long.

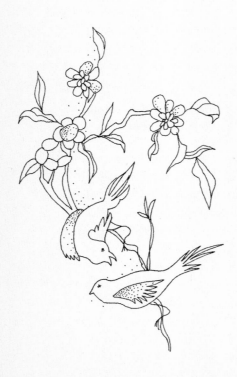

Ginger Tea Cake

MAKES 9 PIECES

This dessert is not too sweet and it's quick to make. Besides being a treat, the cake contains ginger and cinnamon, which relieve intestinal gas, aid digestion, and act as mild pain relievers. Blackstrap molasses is an excellent source of iron and vitamin B_6, and the whole-wheat flour is rich in nutrients we need daily.

½ cup boiling water

¼ pound butter

1 inch ginger, freshly grated, or 1 tablespoon ground ginger

½ cup blackstrap molasses

½ cup brown or raw sugar

1 egg, beaten

1 ½ cups whole-wheat flour

1 teaspoon baking powder

¼ teaspoon salt

1 tablespoon cinnamon

Preheat oven to 350°. Mix boiling water with butter and ginger. Stir in remaining ingredients. Beat until smooth. Bake in a buttered 8 by 8-inch pan for approximately 35 minutes, or until a toothpick inserted in the center comes out clean. Best if served warm with tea.

WOMEN'S ESSENTIAL DAILY NUTRITIONAL NEEDS (AGES 23–50)

NUTRIENT	PURPOSE	NONPREGNANT
calories	life's fuel	2,000 cal.
protein	tissue growth, healing, brain development, milk production	46 g
vitamin A	cell growth, eyes, skin, bones, immune system, mucous membranes, reproductive tissues	4,000 I.U.**
vitamin C	supports all body systems	60 mg
vitamin D	absorption and assimilation of calcium	200–300 I.U.
vitamin E	cell structure maintenance, healthy pregnancy and baby	12 I.U.
folic acid	cell division, manufacturing red blood cells	.4 mg
niacin	to utilize food's energy, skin, cells, nervous system, intestinal health	13 mg
riboflavin (B_2)	body tissue function	1.2 mg
thiamin (B_1)	metabolism of carbohydrates	1.1 mg
vitamin B_6	protein, fat, and carbohydrate metabolism	2 mg
vitamin B_{12}	red blood cell production, nervous system's functioning	3 mcg
calcium	bones and teeth, muscle integrity, blood clotting, heart regularity, nerve and enzyme functioning	1,000 mg
phosphorus	strength of bones and teeth, tissue repair, enzyme activity	800 mg
iodine	thyroid functioning, hormone production	150 mcg
iron	oxygenation of blood, general vitality	18 mg
magnesium	protein and enzyme functioning, body temperature control, muscle contraction, nerve functioning	300 mg
zinc	healing, growth, appetite, digestion, protein synthesis	15 mg

*This caloric intake is the U.S. Recommended Daily Allowance; breastfeeding experts, however, say lactating women require between 3,000 and 5,500 calories each day. This wide range takes into consideration the individual mother/child nutritional circumstances, which vary greatly.

**International units

PREGNANT	LACTATING	GOOD SOURCES
2,300 cal.	2,500 cal.*	all foods—choose wisely
76 g	66 g	lean meats, fish, eggs, tofu, tempeh, legumes combined with whole grains
5,000 I.U.	6,000 I.U.	fish liver oil, liver, most vegetables, eggs, dairy products
80 mg	100 mg	citrus and tropical fruits, many vegetables, whole grains, sprouted seeds
400 I.U.	400 I.U.	sunlight, fortified dairy products, fish liver oil, saltwater fish
15 I.U.	16 I.U.	wheat germ, soybeans, corn, wheat germ and cottonseed oils, nuts and nut butters, whole grains, eggs
.8 mg	.6 mg	liver, leafy green vegetables, nuts, asparagus, lima beans, whole grains, oranges
15 mg	18 mg	poultry, fish, mushrooms, nuts, whole grains, legumes, dairy products
1.5 mg	1.7 mg	liver, dairy products, whole grains, leafy green vegetables, beans, peas
1.5 mg	1.6 mg	peas, liver, yeast, wheat germ, avocados, citrus and tropical fruits, whole grains, nuts, seeds, beans
2.6 mg	2.5 mg	blackstrap molasses, brewer's yeast, brown rice, wheat germ, bran, bananas
4 mcg	4 mcg	all meats (especially organ), fish, dairy products
1,300 mg	1,500 mg	milk, cheese, leafy green vegetables, legumes, almonds, tofu, tempeh, sesame seed products, fish
1,200 mg	1,200 mg	meat, fish, poultry, eggs, dairy products, bran, whole grains, legumes
175 mcg	200 mcg	seaweed, seafoods, vegetables grown in soil with high iodine content, iodized salt
48–78 mg	48–78 mg	organ meats, blackstrap molasses, green vegetables, poultry, fish, nuts, whole grains
450 mg	450 mg	wheat germ, bran, whole grains, nuts, leafy green vegetables
20 mg	25 mg	oysters, wheat germ, meat, poultry, fish, legumes, eggs, popcorn, whole grains

SOURCES: Laurel Robertson, Carol Flinders, and Brian Ruppenthal, *The New Laurel's Kitchen* (Berkeley, CA: Ten Speed Press, 1986); Susan Lark, *The Menopause Self-Help Book* (Berkeley, CA: Celestial Arts, 1990); Arlene Eisenberg, *What to Eat When You're Expecting* (New York: Workman Publishing, 1986).

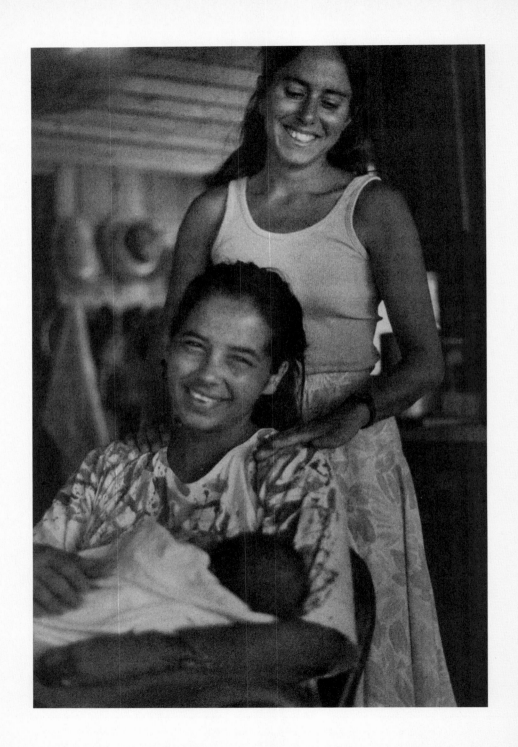

CHAPTER 13

Healing Touch

In our culture, massage is shrouded in mystery. You may think of it as a ritualized form of touching practiced only by those who have gained access to special knowledge. A massage from a professional masseuse is a treat; practice has honed her skills. But massage requires no formal training. Massage can be touching, plain and simple, or it can involve special techniques. Why not enjoy its pleasures and benefits at home?

Numerous books and classes can help guide you, but the art of touching can be learned only through hands-on experience. You should massage yourself. Rub any tense or sore spots you may have as you warm up or cool down from the body toners in part two; it's an excellent addition to any daily routine. You can massage your baby and other children, partner, and friends. They'll tell you what they like and what feels good. Touching is fun, relaxing, and good for body and soul.

Touching is communication, the wordless way to say, "I love you just as you are." You give your baby this gift each time you hold him or her. Every touch is a small healing, a mini-massage.

In the United States in the past, touch as a way to show affection was condemned by those who embraced puritan ethics. Clothing became binding, and drab in color. Bodies were neither seen nor touched. Even touch between married couples was controlled. Laws were passed to limit touching to only that which was deemed necessary to reproduction. Cultural restraints in both the East and West discouraged intimate human contact. Shows of friendly affection became impolite and even eye contact was viewed negatively. Touching became taboo and massage became a lost art.

The strict moral codes of early puritan America continued to influence our culture and by the 1930s and 1940s, a world torn by war, revolution, and hardship forgot how to be playful, forgot how to touch. In the 1950s, tenderness was still out of fashion; this provided the background for American doctors to advise women not to breastfeed and not to pick up their babies when they cried! We now know the importance of responding to a baby's cries, which are the primary means an infant has to communicate "I'm wet" or "I'm hungry," or perhaps most often, "I'm lonely...hold me." By the 1960s, babies of the "touch not" period spoke out for social change, including the right to show affection.

Today we are enjoying a revival of intimacy, but those of us born during a time of limited intimacy may still be uncomfortable touching or being touched. If as a baby your cries were not answered, you learned not to ask for love. But love is your birthright. Everyone deserves to be touched. You may ask to be shown love through touching, or you may give it. It's all right to be uncomfortable with touching until you break through that feeling and can enjoy intimacy.

Pioneers in the field of intimacy have renewed our faith in accepting what feels good. Ashley Montagu in his book *Touching: The Human Significance of the Skin* (New York: Harper & Row, 1986) details our need for almost constant human contact. Babies and adults are healthier and happier when they are touched and touching.

Physician and author Frederick Leboyer teaches that from the moment of birth humans need to be touched gently. Babies should not be hung upside down, spanked, and then separated from mother and father for many hours in the hospital. Leboyer's *Birth without Violence* (New York: Knopf, 1975) has changed the way hospitals all over the world handle babies. Western medical institutions at first criticized Leboyer's suggestions en masse, but now standard medical practice has incorporated his simple wisdom and babies are treated with gentleness.

In countries less affected by the rapid changes technology has brought about, massage has survived as cultural tradition. Leboyer found that for centuries mothers in India have massaged their babies. *Loving Hands* (New York: Knopf, 1976) is his beautiful and inspiring portrait of the traditional art of Indian baby massage. The photographs he includes make it clear that both mother and baby are relaxed and glowing from the massage.

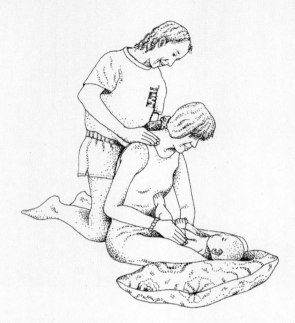

Lomi Lomi massage is still practiced in Hawaii as part of daily baby care in some homes. Mothers and grandmothers consider it an essential aspect of their role as nurturer and healer.

In the Philippines, grandmothers are often the neighborhood healers and midwives. With their age, they have earned the privilege to touch. My own grandmother was skilled in the art of deep therapeutic massage. If you still have your grandmother, massage her. Let her touch you and touch your baby. You never know, there may be wisdom and magic in her hands.

Laying on Your Hands

Massage can be the lightest touch, or it can go deep to stimulate tissues below the surface of the skin. Both types are therapeutic. A light massage begins to heal the spirit, while a deep massage releases tension locked into the muscles, healing old injuries and aches and pains. Massage stimulates the deep muscles and organs and rejuvenates the cells (see chapter 14, Women's Health Wisdom from the East).

Always begin a massage softly. When the muscles and tendons begin to yield to the touch, go deeper. Follow the contour of the muscles. Smooth out lumps and kinks with even pressure that is tempered with gentleness. *Never cause pain.*

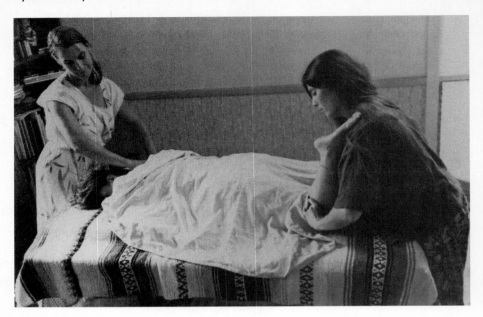

Don't work too long or hard on sore or injured spots as muscles can spasm. Respect the skin by keeping your fingernails trimmed and by applying enough massage oil to prevent abrasions.

When you give or get a complete body massage, don't forget the toes, feet, ankles, shins, calves, knees, thighs, hips, buttocks, abdomen, waist, breasts, chest, shoulders, arms, elbows, wrists, hands, fingers, neck, ears, head, and face. The entire body loves to be touched.

Massage can be platonic or sexual. Your state of mind and intent of hand will determine the nature of the touching you are enjoying. In either case, touching is therapeutic. Touch your partner, let your partner touch you. Your baby will love sharing the time you spend together. The baby may add his helping hand to the massage. Of course he may pull hair or get bored. Most likely as the two of you relax, the baby will relax too. Go ahead and breastfeed your baby in the middle of your massage if he gets hungry or cranky. He may fall asleep, giving Mom and Dad some quiet time to go into another room and allow their touching to become lovemaking.

After Your Massage

Modern times go along with modern concerns. Even the soap we wash up with may be full of unnatural, unhealthy ingredients. Cosmetics, antiperspirants, even shampoos are also to be questioned. This becomes a real concern when we consider the vulnerability of a new mother and a new baby. Naturally we want to protect their skin and overall health. For the entire family, the following simple recipe makes a perfect soap and shampoo. It even cuts the oil after a massage without harming the skin.

Priya & Pradheep's Green Gram Soap

½ pound mung beans (dry, available in health-food stores and Oriental markets)

In a grinder or a strong-powered blender, grind the mung beans into a fine powder. (Mung flour, called "Green Gram," is sometimes available; it is the same thing as finely ground mung beans.) Store in a container of your choice, conveniently in the bathroom. When you want to wash up or shampoo your hair, simply scoop a teaspoon full into your hand, add enough water to make a paste, and suds away.

Massaging Your Baby

Massage is play and babies love to play. While being massaged, infants sometimes lie still and at other times squirm. Because massages are relaxing, your baby may urinate or have a bowel movement during the massage. (It's a good idea to keep a towel or diaper under her.) Massages are especially good for colicky, tense, or constipated babies. As babies get older and more independent, they crawl and roll around during massages. A mother may become frustrated and think that her baby doesn't like being rubbed, when in fact, the baby enjoys it and is adding to the action in his own way. It is fine if his massages turn into games of "chasing monsters." Pleasure and bonding are taking place.

Massage during Pregnancy and Postpartum

Pregnant and breastfeeding women should know that massage releases toxins from stress, environmental pollutants, and junk food that have been locked in body tissues. Massage can cause emotions to become unstuck, and it is not uncommon to have a good cry during or after a massage. Deeper massage releases deeper stress and toxins from the body.

Sal's Massage Oil

When you massage someone deeply, use oil or lotion to prevent injury to the skin. Here is an easy recipe for making your own massage oil from ingredients you may already have in your kitchen. The oils you use should be of the same quality as those you eat, because you are taking them into your body through your skin.

¾ cup safflower or peanut oil (cold pressed)

⅛ cup olive oil

⅛ cup aloe vera gel

Pour the ingredients into a squirt bottle (an empty shampoo bottle works fine). Shake well. Add a few drops of scented oil if you like. Flowers can also be added for scent. Fresh jasmine flowers work well, but use only a few because their scent is very strong. The flowers may be left in the oil or removed. One massage therapist I know adds a gardenia blossom to her oil, but she cautions it must be removed after a day or two or the scent becomes overpowering. Rose petals make a delicately scented oil; lavender smells nostalgic. When adding lavender or rose to the oil, allow it to sit for three to five days and then strain out the petals.

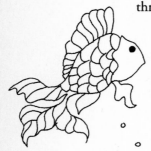

The aloe vera gives this preparation an indefinite shelf life. (Aloe vera may stain some people's skin. Test it on a small patch before giving a massage. Use old sheets and towels.) You don't need to refrigerate the mixture, which is good, as you wouldn't want to squirt oil straight from the icebox on anyone.

Massage for pregnant and postpartum women should be done gently. If a pregnant woman experiences discomfort, so does her baby. A breastfeeding mother can pass toxins to her baby through her milk. Begin with a light, ten-minute massage and increase the length by ten minutes with each massage. For your maximum comfort and benefit, go easy. Eventually deeper massages lasting up to one hour can be enjoyed.

Later, when you are more accustomed to being massaged and your baby is older and no longer entirely dependent upon your milk to meet his nutritional needs, you can try a professional deep massage. If you go to a masseuse, go to someone who is recommended by your doctor or midwife, someone experienced in working with pregnant and postpartum women. As quickly as possible after having a deep massage, drink plenty of water to flush out the toxins that may have been stirred up.

If you want to do further reading about massage, I highly recommend the following two books:

Loving Hands: The Traditional Art of Baby Massage by Frederick Leboyer (New York: Newmarket Press, 1997).

Massage Book by George Downing and Anne Kent Rush (New York: Random House/Bookworks, 1972).

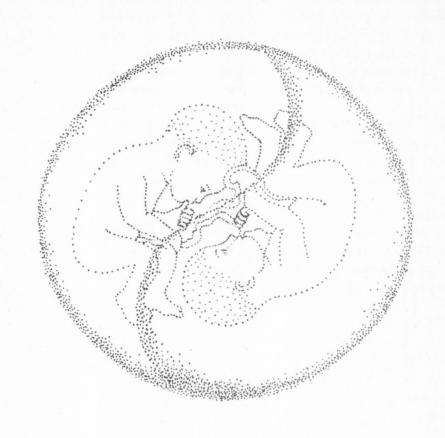

CHAPTER 14

Women's Health Wisdom
from the East:
Internal Massage Exercises

Centuries ago in China, Taoists developed internal exercises to promote the art of self-healing and longevity. Internal exercises are designed to energize the body by improving the functioning of internal organs and all of the body's systems. When each system—circulatory, respiratory, and nervous—is performing correctly, the body is considered balanced; no system or organ must overwork to compensate for another part of the body that is less than efficient. Imbalance causes strain on the body. For example, if your digestion is off, your immune system must work harder to ward off disease. The goal of internal massage exercises is to energize, transform, and, ultimately, give one the flavor of the immortal potential of the body by balancing its systems (see chapter 15, The Ayurvedic Lifestyle).

The Female Deer, Crane, and Turtle exercises are especially beneficial for women after childbirth, and all three can be safely performed immediately postpartum (although many women may find it more comfortable to wait until the lochia has stopped flowing before they do the Female Deer). The animals whose names these exercises bear are noted for their longevity. Practice of internal massage nourishes your organs and revitalizes individual cells by bringing blood and removing wastes without depleting your energy, the unfortunate side effect of many modern Western fitness programs. Dr. Stephen Chang* in the introduction

---

* The internal massage exercises in this chapter are shared with the kind permission of Dr. Stephen T. Chang, an honored Chinese herbologist and acupuncturist. I highly recommend his books, including *The Book of Internal Exercises* (San Francisco: Strawberry Hill Press, 1978), *The Tao of Balanced Diet: Secrets of a Thin and Healthy Body* (San Francisco: Tao Publishing, 1987), *The Tao of Sexology* (San Francisco: Tao Publishing, 1985), and *The Complete Book of Acupuncture* (Berkeley, CA: Celestial Arts, 1976).

to his *Book of Internal Exercises* cautions that excessive conventional exercise programs may produce an attractive figure, but they often do so by depleting the
vital organs' energy. This causes illness and premature aging.

As a mother, you value your precious energy highly; you and your family
depend on it. It is no wonder that many women feel they must give up conventional external exercise when they become mothers. They want to conserve the
energy that, instinctively, they know must be directed toward their children's
needs. Yet it is not necessary or healthy for you to give up all exercise. Design
your movement and exercise program so it is a natural part of your daily activities, and so it increases your energy and ability to perform your exalted role as
mother.

The ancient Chinese designed these internal exercises to prevent disease and
promote health in a hardworking society. Internal massage has proved to be very
effective in reducing excess weight. In combination with the body toners in part
two, they are perfect for the postpartum woman.

The Female Deer Exercise

*The deer is swift, lean, and alert. The Female Deer Exercise is particularly helpful for
the postnatal woman. Most women who try this exercise incorporate it into their daily
routine because it feels so good and takes only a few minutes to do. The benefits from
this internal massage are that it balances the entire body and increases your energy
level, which is very important to sleep-deprived new mothers. In addition, it increases
circulation in the breasts, which helps lactation, and increases circulation to the
vagina, speeding the healing after childbirth. The muscles of the pelvic floor are
strengthened too. Do the Female Deer Exercise, upon rising and before going to bed,
each day for the rest of your life.*

STARTING POSITION

Sit cross-legged on the floor or a bed. One heel is pressed against the opening of
your vagina. Apply steady, firm pressure to your clitoris with the heel. (If you are
not yet limber enough to do this, place a hard round object, like an apple,
between your foot and vagina.)

ACTION TO PREVENT LUMPS

- Vigorously rub your hands together thirty-six times. You will feel the healing
  energy of your body in your palms as heat.
- Place your hands on your breasts, transferring the heat.

- Massage your breasts in an outward circular motion (moving your hands *down* the outer breast and *up* the inner breast). Do this thirty-six times. This outward circular massaging, called "dispersion" by Dr. Chang, helps prevent lumps.
- Do as many kegels (see page 132) as you can do comfortably. Tighten and hold the muscles of your yoni and anus. You can do the kegels at the same time you massage your breasts or after you finish.

ACTION TO STIMULATE CIRCULATION
- Vigorously rub your hands together thirty-six times.
- Place your hands on your breasts, transferring the heat.
- To stimulate the circulation in your breasts, massage them in an inward motion (hands moving *up* the outer breasts and *down* the inner breasts). Repeat this circular massage thirty-six times. According to Dr. Chang, women who have continued to do this massage over a period of time have enlarged their breasts.
- Do as many kegels as you can do comfortably.

ADDITIONAL ACTION
The following two motions provide a mini-massage for the limbs and bring the focus of energy to the heart. Repeat each of these as many times as you like.
- With your entire hand, stroke your arms firmly, first one and then the other. Move from fingertips to elbow to shoulder to heart.
- With the palms of your hands, firmly stroke your inner thighs, from the knees to the crotch, and continue up to the heart.

NOTE: Do not do the Female Deer Exercise during pregnancy, when the body rebalances on its own. At this time, increased stimulation is not needed and the body does best when left to its own wisdom. The Female Deer Exercise is recommended during menstruation only if it feels good to you. Some women's breasts become tender and they are uncomfortable with the increased stimulation.

The Crane Exercise

In China, the crane is known not only for longevity, but for grace and beauty as well. This exercise lets you massage away your tummy. What you are doing in the Crane Exercise is directing your healing energy to an area where many of your vital organs are located. If constipation has been a problem, you will find this internal massage extremely helpful and should notice improvement in the efficiency of your digestive organs within a week or so.

Visualize the energy from your hand melting into your abdomen, sweeping your organs, and revitalizing each cell. It helps very much to send love into your body as you practice the Crane Exercise.

STARTING POSITION
Lie on your back, either flat or in CRP (see page 130), keeping your lower back pressed into the floor.

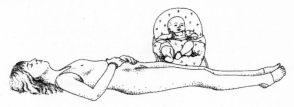

ACTION
- Vigorously rub your palms together thirty-six times.
- Place your warm palms on your lower abdomen.
- Inhale slowly, distending your lower abdomen so it puffs out like a balloon. Do not allow your chest to expand.
- Exhale slowly, pressing your hands into your body lightly. Imagine *all* of the air leaving your lungs. Your abdomen will become bowl-like.
- Repeat twelve times.

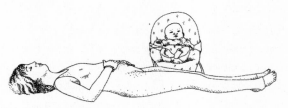

ADDITIONAL ACTION
This additional action helps keep body wastes from stagnating in your bowels, a common complaint during pregnancy and postpartum. You want to feel light like a crane, not bogged down by poor elimination.

- Vigorously rub your palms together thirty-six times.
- Place the palm of your strongest hand (right if you are right-handed, left if you are left-handed) on your navel.
- Massage your tummy with a circular motion (moving up your right side and down your left). Rub in small circles at first. Gradually increase the size of the

circles until you are massaging the upper, lower, and outer edges of your abdomen. Rub slowly, using gentle pressure.

- Reverse direction of circle and move from the outer reaches of your abdomen toward your navel.
- Take the opportunity to do kegels while you massage your abdomen.
- Repeat as often as you like.

The Turtle Exercise

The turtle is known for longevity, strength, and sense of peacefulness. This exercise has been used in China to slow down the individual's experience of time; gaining control over the nervous system in this way slows the aging process. By stretching the spine and neck, this exercise brings energy and strength while removing stiffness and tension. You may do the Turtle Exercise any time you feel tension in your body.

STARTING POSITION

The Turtle Exercise may be done either standing or sitting, with eyes closed gently or while looking at your sweet baby.

ACTION

- Inhale slowly as you let your chin fall to your chest. At the same time feel the back of your head stretch skyward. Let your shoulders drop down and relax.
- Exhale slowly, letting your head roll backward. (Imagine the back of your head touching the back of your neck.) Your chin will point upward. Let your shoulders be drawn up toward your ears, mimicking the tortoise, and let the tension go out of them.
- Repeat the Turtle Exercise twelve times. Do not force your movements; do them smoothly like a turtle.

Combining the Three Internal Exercises

After you have mastered each individual internal exercise, combine them.

- Sit as in the Female Deer Exercise, putting pressure on your clitoris with your heel. Your yoni and anal muscles are contracted.
- Breathe as in Crane Exercise, with your hands on your stomach.
- Move your head as in the Turtle Exercise.

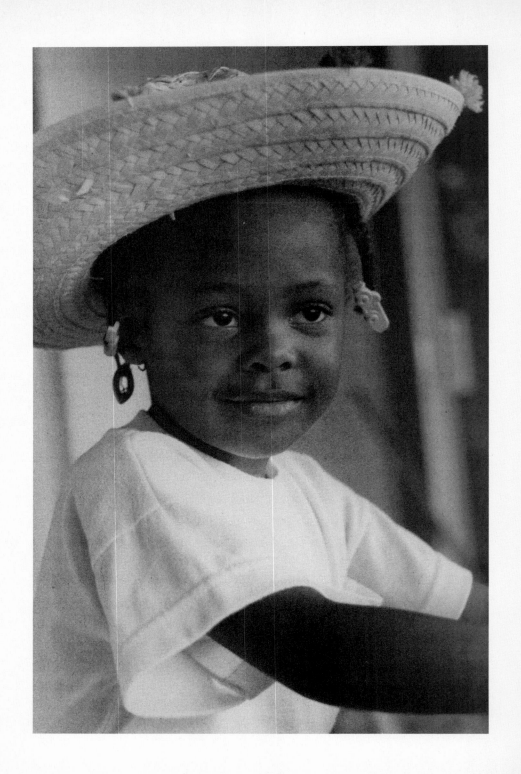

CHAPTER 15

The Ayurvedic Lifestyle

Ayurveda is the science of life that has been practiced in India for over five thousand years and is still used today. It covers every aspect of life: spirituality, physiology, and psychology. The body, the mind, consciousness, and the environment are all concerns of Ayurveda. Ayurveda includes a system of medicine that focuses on preventing illness. It is fortunate that interest in Ayurveda has emerged in the West at a time when it is essential to build and protect a strong immune system.

Unlike medicine in the West, in ancient India Ayurvedic medicine was a household concept and was practiced skillfully at home. Just as birthing was traditionally accomplished in the home where it could unfold naturally, medicine was once a function of family life. Today, though clinics and doctors of Ayurvedic medicine do exist, in India health care falls primarily in the laps of mothers.

Daily routine, massage, diet, and knowledge of Ayurvedic herbal remedies are the holistic storehouse Indian women use against disease. Surely American families, living in a country where conditions are simply more healthy, can adopt this knowledge to maintain optimal health.

Ayurveda has parallels in traditional Chinese medicine. The goal of both Oriental and Ayurvedic medicine is not just maintaining health, but enhancing the joy of living in a human body and promoting longevity. Ayurveda gives us the flavor of the immortal potential of our bodies.

This chapter is designed to provide a basic understanding of Ayurveda, a practice that will give you more control over your family's health care. Routine and diet geared specifically toward postpartum women are covered also.

Ayurveda and Longevity

In our times there is much concern with immunity to disease. Ayurveda not only focuses on building a strong immune system (this is known as *bala,* enhancing life) but also sets its sights on longevity and, ultimately, immortality.

When wishing to promote greater health and longevity, you must consider three main points.

First, heredity. Some people are born with strong bodies. Their systems naturally seem to avert disease and discomfort. They are, in fact, predisposed to good health. Others fall prey to illness easily. The individual constitution is of great concern in Ayurveda. Knowing what you have to work with is the starting point; the goal is good health and longevity.

Second, time, or *kala,* the interplay of the individual's age and the seasons. All creation is connected and cyclical. In infancy, we are vulnerable; we grow strong in youth; in old age, we are vulnerable again. Young children overcome sickness more easily than elderly people. Broken bones mend easily in children, while for adults, the healing of a broken bone can be a long process.

And third, acquisition. Ayurveda teaches methods that, when followed, allow our bodies to obtain their own good health. You need not regret your inherited health or the effects of time. You have the power, in your own healing hands, to evolve your own perfect health.

Ojas and Transcendence

At the foundation of your immune system is *ojas; soma* is the consciousness of ojas. Ojas is the body's "vital essence," the glue of the universe, the quiet essence of your digestive system.

All living things have and can give ojas. For example, a corn plant, which begins life as a delicate green blade that emerges from a seed, draws the vital energy from the five elements of nature. (Ayurveda teaches that everything is composed of five basic elements. In addition to the four elements familiar to Western readers—fire, water, earth, and air—there is ether, which appeared from the subtle vibrations of acum, and is manifested in all living things.) The corn plant is able to transmute the essence of the five elements into a form that humans can eat, a form that allows us to gain strength. This is love manifest in nature. Through love, all life on our planet is sustained.

Doctors Lad and Frawley, in their book *The Yoga of Herbs* (Wilmot, WI: Lotus Light Publications, 1986), say that "ojas is the energy and love contained in a living system." In herbology, the ojas of a plant can be used to heal. However, to be effective, the herbal remedy must be prepared with love. *Love is the bedrock of wellness.* In *Love, Medicine and Miracles* (New York: Harper Trade Books, 1986), Dr. Bernie S. Siegel cites a direct correlation between love and a patient's ability to heal. The married cancer patients he treats have a higher recovery rate than those who are unmarried. They have a greater capacity for fighting off disease. His studies also show that single, elderly people who have a pet live longer. In effect, love and companionship strengthen the immune system.

In the body, love establishes harmony by soothing and increasing the ojas. According to Ayurveda, ojas is the finest expression, the seed, of the maternal essence of the physiology. The most powerful rejuvenator of the heart, mind, body, and spirit is pure awareness or transcendence, which is manifested in love. Perhaps this explains why a mother often remains in perfect health when colds and flus are going around. The intense love and caring she gives while healing her family increases her own strength and endurance.

Ojas is manufactured in the human body when digestion is optimal. Our bodies are more efficient at producing ojas when we meditate or pray, because when we are involved in those practices, we achieve a state of pure awareness.* Health and happiness are by-products of an unbound mind. By allowing your awareness to become receptive through meditation or prayer, you set up the conditions for healing to occur. The person who meditates becomes the healer and the healed, just as a mother is both the nurturer and the nurtured one. In the words of Maharishi Mahesh Yogi, "All love is directed towards the self."

*There are transcendental meditation centers in most major cities in the United States, Canada, and Europe (some may also be found in Third World countries). For more information and instruction in meditation, look in your local phone directory. Many types of meditation are available to be learned, such as Zen meditation through local Zen centers. Japa meditation may be learned without charge from the Divine Mother Mata Amritanandamayi. Check her Web site (www.Ammachi.org) to discover when she'll be visiting your area.

Understanding the Three Doshas

Ayurveda teaches that all creation, including the human constitution, is composed from the five elements of nature: ether, air, fire, water, and earth. Which elements and the degree to which they are present is unique to each individual but fall into three general groupings, or *doshas: vata, pitta,* and *kapha.* Each of the doshas is a combination of two of the five elements of nature. Usually a person is not entirely one or another dosha, but a combination of all three doshas, often with one or two that predominate. A person's constitution, influenced by astrological as well as genetic factors, is determined at conception. In order to achieve prime physical, emotional, and mental health, an individual must discover their distinctive makeup, or *prakriti,* so they can live in a way that promotes health and longevity.

To maintain optimal health and heal Ayurvedically, it is necessary to gain a basic understanding of the doshas and the simple system of balance they describe. Balance, or harmony, is Ayurveda's goal. Imbalance, or *vikriti,* is the basis of disease. Poor diet, stress (either physical or emotional), or change of season can set the stage for disease by causing imbalance in the body and aggravating the doshas. The doshas can be compared to pools that are constantly being filled by the pressures of biological function. To stay healthy, a person must "continually purify the physiology before excesses of the doshas overflow the container and symptoms of illness or imbalance appear." Disease that is rooted in one part of the body can cause symptoms in another area. For example, too much *pitta* often causes problems in the upper digestive tract, but the common external symptom is a skin rash. Treating the rash alone will not cure the imbalance that caused it; one must diagnose the digestive condition and treat the problem at its root.

VATA
Vata is the dosha that results from the combination of the elements air and ether. Vata governs the nervous system and movement; thus people in whom this dosha is predominant tend to move quickly and to be impatient. They are very creative and very active, but they tire easily. People with a vata constitution are generally thin, and either unusually tall or short. Joints are prominent because there is little muscular development. Their skin, hair, and eyes are usually dry.

Vata types learn fast and forget fast. They sleep less than people of other doshas and fitfully. Predominantly vata people are subtle in wit and action, ethereal in appearance, and somewhat frail both physically and emotionally.

PITTA
Pitta is associated with the combination of the elements fire and water. Hot, light, strong, and intense describe the person with a pitta constitution. A person with this constitution is jealous and quick to anger. Often they are extremely intelligent and excellent speakers, making them good leaders once they've tamed their tempers.

Physical characteristics of people who are predominantly pitta include medium height and weight, and moderate skin and hair coloring. They tend to have many moles or freckles. Their metabolism and digestion are strong, causing them to desire large quantities of food and drink, and they tend to crave sweets. Pitta individuals sleep well for moderate periods, six to eight hours, and awaken refreshed and ready to go.

KAPHA

The elements of earth and water produce kapha. Movement of kapha people is slow and deliberate. Generally individuals with this constitution have well-developed muscles though they are prone to carry extra weight, even when they eat very little, because their digestion is slow. They sleep soundly, loving to go to bed early and sleep in late. Their skin is thick, pale, soft, and clear; the eyes of kapha individuals are large and beautiful.

Healthy and peace loving, these people sometimes tend toward greed and attachment. The intelligence of kapha individuals is sometimes underestimated as they are not quick wits; however, their method of taking in information slowly gives them a solid long-term memory. Kapha people fall in love slowly, weighing all aspects and angles of a relationship before making an emotional commitment. Once in love, a predominantly kapha person stays in love.

Determining Your Prakriti

You can review your characteristics (physical, emotional, and mental) to discover which dosha(s) are predominant in your prakriti. (Ayurvedic experts are adept at determining a person's prakriti just by taking their pulse.) To find your prakriti, fill out the following questionnaire by selecting the characteristics that fit you most closely. The seven possible prakritis are Vata, Pitta, Kapha, Vata-Pitta, Pitta-Kapha, Vata-Kapha and Vata-Pitta-Kapha.

TRIDOSHA QUESTIONNAIRE
Test Instructions
1. For each category (1–25) on the questionnaire, select the one choice that most closely approximates your individual constitution, either:
- Kapha (water-type)
- Pitta (fire-type)
- Vata (air-type)

Then put a check in the appropriate box. For example, if your response to the first question is *endomorph,* check box 1, column K.

2. When you have finished answering all 25 questions, add the number of check marks in each category and enter the sum in the subtotal boxes.

3. To obtain a percentage ratio of the three elements in your personal constitution,

CONSTITUTIONAL CHARACTERISTIC	K *KAPHA*
1. Body (frame)	☐ Endomorph: broad shoulder/hips
2. Weight	☐ Heavy
3. Endurance/Strength	☐ Good
4. Skin texture	☐ Pale, oily, white, moist
5. Skin aging	☐ Smooth, few wrinkles
6. Hair lubrication	☐ Oily
7. Hair color	☐ Medium to dark brown, medium blonde
8. Hair texture	☐ Straight, thick
9. Digestion/hunger	☐ Moderate, no excessive hunger
10. Teeth	☐ Large, white, resistant to decay
11. Eyes	☐ Large, blue or brown
12. Elimination	☐ Heavy, slow
13. Sex drive	☐ Cyclical, infrequent
14. Physical activity	☐ Avoids exercise, lethargic
15. Mental activity	☐ Calm, steady
16. Voice/speech	☐ Harmonious, low-pitched, singing, slow, monotone
17. Taste/food preference	☐ Dry, low fat, light, sweet, pungent
18. Sleep	☐ Easy, deep
19. Memory	☐ Long-term memory
20. Financial behavior	☐ Saves money regularly
21. Emotional reaction to stress	☐ Indifference, complacency, withdrawal
22. Dreams	☐ Water, river, ocean, lake, erotic
23. Mental predisposition	☐ Stable/logical
24. Resting radial pulse/quality (self-diagnostic)	☐ Slow, moves like swan
25. Radial pulse/quantity of beats per minute (self-diagnostic)	☐ 60–70 beats per minute

_____ Subtotal K

× 4 = ____%

GRAND TOTAL _____ (express as a percentage)

multiply the number of answers in each subtotal box by 4. If you answered all 25 questions, the three percentage figures should add up to 100, and you will have an approximate picture of your unique constitutional type as determined at conception.

4. Conclusion: Usually one element will predominate—that is, will be a larger

P PITTA	V VATA
☐ Mesomorph: medium frame	☐ Ectomorph: narrow hips/shoulders
☐ Neither too thin nor too stout	☐ Slender—tendons show
☐ Moderate	☐ Little
☐ Soft, oily, fair, pink, delicate, red	☐ Dry, rough, cool, darker complexion
☐ Freckles, moles, pigmentation	☐ Dry, flaky, cracked
☐ Medium	☐ Dry
☐ Light brown, red, light blonde	☐ Dark brown to black
☐ Wavy, fine	☐ Curly
☐ Sharp hunger	☐ Irregular or heavy diet, but remains thin
☐ Yellowish, moderate size	☐ Crooked, large, protruding
☐ Green, gray, hazel	☐ Small, black
☐ Moderate	☐ Tends toward constipation
☐ Moderate	☐ Frequent
☐ Likes regular exercise	☐ Restless, active
☐ Intelligent, aggressive	☐ Restless, active
☐ Medium-pitched, sharp, laughing, shouting	☐ High-pitched, weeping, vibrato, dissonant
☐ Sweet, medium, light, warm, bitter, astringent	☐ Sweet, oily, soupy, heavy, salty
☐ Medium, sound	☐ Short, insomnia
☐ Good, but not prolonged	☐ Short-term memory
☐ Saves, but spends on luxury items	☐ Spends money quickly
☐ Anger, jealousy	☐ Fear, anxiety
☐ Struggle, fire, anger, violence, war	☐ Fear, flying, running, jumping
☐ Judging/artistic	☐ Questioning/theoretician
☐ Moderate, jumps like frog	☐ Thready, slithers like snake
☐ 70–80 beats per minute	☐ 80–100+ beats per minute
_____ **Subtotal P**	_____ **Subtotal V**
✕ 4 = _____ %	✕ 4 = _____ %

© Copyright 1984, by Sattva Foundation

percentage of the total. In Ayurvedic medicine, this is considered the main constitutional type for diagnosis and treatment of the individual.

Working with Your Prakriti

Disease vikriti occurs when there is an unnatural accumulation of one or more of the three doshas that is appropriate for one's particular body type. In other words, vikriti is imbalance. Once you know your prakriti, Ayurveda outlines ways to keep your body in balance. Diet, herbs, level of physical activity, the weather, and even menstruation and pregnancy are a few of the factors that can aggravate and increase the doshas. By adjusting for these factors, you can bring your body back into balance and regain your health (and, ideally, since the focus of Ayurveda is prevention, you can promote your well-being and longevity).

For example, a person can counteract the effects of the weather on their particular prakriti by adjusting their diet. Just as many of us have one dominant dosha in our birth constitution, each season is associated with a dosha. Fall and the dry, cold, windy months of winter are vata. The wet, cool months of late winter and early spring are kapha, and late spring and summer are pitta season. A perfect guideline for choosing foods that pacify the effects of weather on our bodies is to eat foods that are in season. Mother Earth gives us what we need, when we need it.

Eating in-season foods is particularly important when the individual's dominant dosha corresponds to the season's dosha. To counteract the pitta-aggravating effects of a hot summer, pitta people would be wise to eat cooling foods such as tofu, basmati rice, coconut, cool drinks, cucumber, and leafy greens to name a few. These individuals should avoid animal flesh; hot, salty, and spicy foods; and cultured dairy products. In the fall, vata-predominant people should take special care to bundle up and to eat plenty of warm, grounding foods like beets, sweet potatoes, and carrots. To feel their best in the late winter months, kapha individuals must remain active and avoid heavy, oily foods like beef and pork. They can enjoy hearty vegetable soups made with millet.

The Art and Science of Eating

Diet is primary. People have to eat. Your prakriti determines your optimal diet. What is good for one person is not necessarily good for another. Once you have determined your prakriti, you can design an eating style, custom fitted for your constitution.

Thirty years ago there was much attention paid to the effects of vibrations. "Good vibes" became a household phrase, and it still should be. Food is affected by vibrations. The environment that surrounds the growth of the seed from which a vegetable comes, the farmer who grows it, the person who picks it, the store at which it is purchased (even the method of earning the money that buys the food), the cook, and the kitchen all affect the food.

Good vibes equal good health. "You are what you eat" is a basic tenet of Ayurveda. As much as possible, choose the vibration of the food you feed your family. The quality of your life will be impressed upon the food you prepare and eat; likewise, the quality of the food you take will impress upon your health. You can follow these suggestions for improving the vibes of the foods you and your family eat.

- Buy fresh, organic produce or grow a garden using no pesticides.
- Have fun in your garden and involve your children, mate, friends, and neighbors.
- Avoid canned foods.
- Shop in a clean, health-conscious store.
- Only purchase packaged foods produced by honest, environmentally conscious companies that do not exploit other species or humans.

THE RASAS

In Ayurveda there are six *rasas,* or tastes. You should enjoy all six tastes at each meal, but your individual prakriti will determine which you should favor and which rasas to limit. Some foods are predominantly one rasa but also have qualities of another rasa. Foods with more than one rasa are listed below under their predominant rasa with the secondary rasa in parentheses. Each rasa has either a heating or a cooling effect on the body. (You will notice that the sweet rasa, in general, has a cooling effect, but some foods are sweet and heating, or sweet and astringent but heating. These are subrasas.) The six rasas are

1. *Sweet (cooling)* mangos, kiwifruit (sour), melons, pears (mildly), berries, cherries, red and purple grapes, dates, dry figs, prunes, raisins, wheat, basmati rice, sweet potatoes, white potatoes (salty and astringent), red potatoes (astringent), carrots (bitter and astringent), green beans (astringent), peas (astringent), okra (astringent), squash (astringent), pumpkin (astringent), butter, milk (human and cow), goat milk (astringent), honey, sugarcane products, peppermint, licorice

Sweet (heating) oranges (sour), peaches (astringent), apricots (astringent), brown rice, nuts and seeds (many are also astringent), buckwheat (astringent), corn (astringent), oats (astringent), rye (astringent), chicken (astringent), rabbit (astringent), lamb (astringent), pork (astringent), beef, fish

2. *Bitter (cooling)* leafy greens, cabbage, celery, rhubarb, cauliflower, broccoli, spinach, parsley, cilantro (coriander), coffee, fresh turmeric root

3. *Astringent (cooling)* lentils, chanas, eggplant, many beans, barley (sweet), pomegranates, unripe banana, turmeric, goldenseal, myrrh

4. *Sour (heating)* lemons, limes, grapefruit, pineapple (sweet), green grapes, plums, persimmons, cranberries, tamarind, olives, cheese, yogurt, rosehips, hibiscus

5. *Salty (heating)* tamari soy sauce, table salt, seaweeds, all salty foods

6. *Pungent (heating)* hot spices (black pepper, ginger, cumin, cayenne pepper), onion, garlic, chilies, asafoetida, mushrooms (salty)

CUSTOMIZING YOUR DIET*

Vata people should favor foods that are sweet, sour, and salty. In addition to this, your foods should be warm, well cooked, and unctuous (oily). Vata should avoid large amounts of astringent (except dahls, dishes made with dried peas or beans) and bitter foods. You can take heavy foods, like root vegetables, as your constitution is associated with air and space. Use your diet to ground you. Always eat breakfast and eat several small meals throughout the day rather than three large meals.

Pitta-type people do best to favor sweet, bitter, and astringent tastes. Also eat food that is cool. Limit your intake of foods that are sour as well as foods that are very salty. As the pitta constitution is associated with fire and water and you have a tendency to eat large amounts, your foods should have a cooling effect. Pungent foods, especially garlic, onion, hot peppers, and radishes, can cause the pitta individual's temper to flare. Always eat breakfast.

If you are predominantly kapha in constitution, you must favor pungent, bitter, and astringent tastes. Avoid oily, heavy, and cold foods. Sweet, sour, and salty tastes should be taken in moderation. You will require smaller quantities of food as your constitution, associated with earth and water, causes you to digest food slowly. Avoid eating before 10 A.M. and after sunset, and make lunch your largest meal.

The general suggestions that follow and the dosha food guideline charts must be adjusted for specific dosha predominance, general state of health, digestion, food allergies, season, and availability.

FOOD GUIDELINES FOR VATA DOSHA

FOOD GROUPS	SUGGESTED FOODS
Vegetables (favor cooked vegetables over raw, and especially root vegetables; serve raw vegetables with oil)	beets, carrots, yams, sweet potatoes, garlic, radishes, daikon, green beans, okra, zucchini, asparagus, cucumbers, red cabbage, leafy greens, lettuce, parsley, spinach, sprouts
Fruits (avoid dried fruits)	apricots, ripe bananas, berries, cherries, fresh figs, red or purple grapes, mangos, melons, pineapple, oranges, papaya, peaches, plums, avocados, kiwifruit
Grains (eat these grains well cooked)	oats (cooked only), short-grain brown rice, basmati rice, wheat
Animal Protein	fish, fowl (only white meat), beef, eggs (fried or scrambled)
Legumes	mung beans, tofu, lentils
Nuts and Seeds	small amounts of all nuts and seeds (except peanuts); blanched almonds are best
Dairy	moderate quantities of all dairy products

- Avoid white sugar; moderate amounts of all other sweeteners are fine.
- All spices are good.
- All oils are good, especially sesame oil.

FOOD GUIDELINES FOR PITTA DOSHA

FOOD GROUPS	SUGGESTED FOODS
Vegetables (favor sweet and bitter vegetables)	broccoli, asparagus, cabbage, potatoes, cucumbers, squash, brussel sprouts, cauliflower, celery, green beans, leafy greens, artichokes, avocados, lettuce, okra, peas, parsley, sweet peppers, sprouts
Fruits	apples, oranges (sweet only), pineapple (very ripe), red and purple grapes, avocados, figs, prunes, raisins, pomegranates, plums (only sweet and ripe), melons, mangos, cherries, pears, coconut, bananas
Grains	barley, basmati rice, oats (cooked only), wheat
Animal Protein	fowl, eggs, rabbit, shrimp (in very small amounts)
Legumes	soybeans and products made from them (like tofu) are especially good; all legumes except lentils
Nuts and Seeds	sunflower and pumpkin seeds only; no nuts other than coconut
Dairy	butter (unsalted), ghee, cottage cheese, milk

- Avoid honey and molasses.
- Use no spices except cinnamon, saffron, coriander, mint, cumin, cardamom, fennel, turmeric, black pepper (small amount), and ginger.
- Avoid cultured dairy products such as buttermilk, cheese, yogurt, and sour cream.
- Avoid corn oil; use olive, coconut, sunflower, or soy oil.

- Sweeten with raw honey only (avoid all other sweets).
- All spices are good.
- Avoid salt.
- Avoid oils except small amounts of almond, corn, safflower, mustard, and sunflower.

FOOD GUIDELINES FOR KAPHA DOSHA

FOOD GROUPS	SUGGESTED FOODS
Vegetables (favor raw vegetables with bitter and pungent tastes)	lettuce, sprouts, leafy greens, parsley, asparagus, artichokes, squash, garlic, potatoes, carrots, cauliflower, okra, beets, cabbage, chilies, radishes, peppers, spinach, chard, bok choy, celery, broccoli, brussel sprouts, eggplant, peas
Fruits	apples, apricots, berries, cherries, dry figs, kiwifruit, persimmons, cranberries, pomegranates, prunes, raisins, pears, peaches, mangos
Grains	raw oats, barley, corn, millet, basmati rice (in small amounts), rye, buckwheat
Animal Protein (eat in moderation)	turkey or chicken (dark meat), rabbit, shrimp, eggs (never cooked in oil)
Legumes	all legumes except dark lentils (the red are okay), kidney, soy, and mung beans
Nuts and Seeds (avoid all nuts)	sunflower seeds, pumpkin seeds
Dairy	ghee and goat milk only

THE YOGA OF COOKING AND EATING

According to Ayurveda, when you eat a meal you also ingest the thoughts of the cook. It is important to keep this in your heart and mind when you prepare and eat food. Another essential is that the kitchen be clean, calm, quiet, pleasant, and pure. The proper method of taking food requires clean hands, a clean dining environment, and a clean heart. Begin each meal with a moment of prayer. Join hands to focus the family's silence. Bless the food, the cook, and the eaters. Pray that everyone on the Earth will have enough to eat. This prepares your heart, mind, and body to enjoy God's gift of food.

The eating in earnest should begin with the rice or grain. This fuels the *agni,* or digestion, as rice is cooling to the doshas. This can be flavored with ghee (see Food for the Gods, below), which lights the fire of agni. Dahl or a soupy bean dish should follow as this will pacify vata. Lemon can be added to rice and dahl for taste and digestion. For increased stamina, you can now eat bread, which is a heavy strengthening food. In India chapati, unleavened skillet bread, is eaten daily. Vegetables are an essential part of any good meal, and after or with the bread is the best time to eat them. Now you are ready to drink a small amount of either water or juice (cut to half strength with water). Do not drink milk with meals. At this point a sweet food may be taken. Green salads and/or sour pickles should be eaten next to aid salivation. Again you may take a sweet or heavy food; this provides energy and nutritional value and more liquid to mix the food in the stomach. After meals always clean your mouth and teeth by gargling and swishing with water. You can chew cardamom seeds, cloves, or fennel seeds for digestion and to freshen breath.

FOOD FOR THE GODS

Ghee (clarified butter), honey, and milk are called "food for the gods." A nightly cup of warm milk with ghee and honey is known to increase strength. This drink is particularly good for promoting healing of tissues damaged or stressed during birthing, and postpartum women should take it often. In addition, the nutritive power of herbs is greatly increased when mixed with milk, honey, and ghee. (Drink milk with sweets, cereals, or toasted breads. It is recommended that you not take milk with meals. You may have milk twenty minutes or more after a meal.) Milk should be gently boiled and when it is boiling is the best time to add any herbs you may be taking. Cool milk until just warm, then add honey and ghee to your milk as it cools in the cup. Honey should never be heated or used in baking because it can be toxic. Remember also, never give honey to infants under one year of age. Until children reach this age, botulism spores found in some honey can put your child's life at risk. This wonderful drink pacifies vata and encourages a good night's sleep.

Ghee aids digestion, and it also is said to strengthen ojas, the essence and subtle quality of all body tissues that is the foundation of strength, clear perception, stamina, and longevity. (See page 204 for more discussion of ojas.) In the last month of pregnancy, ojas is passed from the mother to the fetus. This is one reason premature infants have difficulty surviving. Mother's milk provides the baby with ojas and by aiding digestion sets the stage for the child to make his own ojas. Like all living things, babies make ojas from the moment life quickens in their bodies. Mother's milk facilitates their capacity to do this.

Ghee, being a primary food for enhancing ojas in the body, should be a staple in every household. It is easy to make and should be made in large batches so you have plenty on hand. Simply heat one pound or more of butter (raw, unsalted is best) over low heat for about fifteen minutes. It will have a nice aroma and a golden color. Slowly pour this liquid as well as the foam that's on top into a jar, discard the sediment at the bottom of the pan, and you have ghee. Ghee can be used in milk, in cooking, or by itself as a medicine. Store ghee in a jar with a tight-fitting lid. You don't need to refrigerate. Because ghee is so good, you will finish it before it could possibly spoil; however, discard ghee if it begins to taste "old."

Milk with ghee and honey is not only nutritious, it is nurturing. Ayurveda says that imbalance is the cause of "dis-ease." Balance or imbalance begins on the emotional level, so to nurture ourselves and others is basic to health and well-being. Milk is the infant's first food. It is widely known that the optimum food for babies is their mother's milk because it balances the doshas and provides ojas. Human milk is sweet and unctuous. For adults or older children, when we add honey and ghee (sweet and unctuous) to cow's or goat's milk we are creating the taste of mother, the feeling of mother. Whenever you or someone you love is emotionally upset, a warm cup of milk, honey, and ghee will work miracles. Who amongst us does not need the love and nurturing of a mother? This is the food of the child in all of us, the food of gods.

Ayurveda for Postpartum Women

The fundamental advice of Ayurveda for new mothers is to rest. Rest. Rest. Rest. Beneficial changes in the body can most readily be made during the first weeks postpartum because you are so open, but care must be taken to avoid fatigue and exposure to disease while you are this vulnerable. Your focus is uplifted due to the arrival of your baby so recently from God. This is a time of total loving. Keep in mind that what you give yourself, you've automatically given your baby. Maharishi Mahesh Yogi, who brought transcendental meditation to the West, says the postpartum period is a time to develop unity consciousness. This state occurs when the individual perceives everything as God and God as everything, including the self. When the universe is seen as having unity in diversity, health and higher states of being are gained.

Vata dosha has been predominant during pregnancy and still is now that you have given birth. Slowly, over weeks and months, as your hormones rebalance, your body will return to its pre-pregnancy dosha. After postpartum, predominantly pitta and kapha women return to their pre-pregnancy doshas and must follow the food guidelines (see pages 213–14) for those doshas. A kapha woman tends to keep the weight gained during pregnancy unless she carefully follows guidelines for her dosha. A pitta woman will often have more trouble with PMS and a hotter temper toward her children if she does not maintain balance.

During pregnancy, you may have felt spaced out, overly sensitive, restless; you may have been prone to headaches and insomnia; you may have had cravings;

your digestion may have been inefficient, causing constipation—all of these conditions can be caused by overabundance of vata. Both mother and baby are closer to the ethereal elements of ether and air during pregnancy, parturition, and postpartum, so vata naturally predominates. As vata is the least dense of the three doshas, only a gentle nudge toward health is needed to promote healing. By following the simple guidelines below during the postpartum period, you set up the conditions to balance the three doshas.

- Rest. Stay at home for the first twenty-two days minimum postpartum. Forty-two days is better.
- Stay near your baby.
- Do only things that make you happy.
- Avoid all heavy work, lifting nothing heavier than your baby.
- Avoid excessive talking by keeping visitors to a minimum.
- Get a daily, light body massage with sesame or coconut oil, and massage baby daily after the umbilical stump has healed. If no one is around to massage you, simply rub your own skin.
- Shower daily; don't take long tub baths. Shallow sitz baths are recommended for healing perineal tears and stitches.
- Put off lovemaking until you stop bleeding completely, and longer if you feel so inclined. When you do resume sexual activity, go easily. Your uterus is a sacred temple where so recently your baby, a Buddha, lived. Your yoni is the gateway where only love must enter.
- Both mother and baby should stay out of the wind because wind aggravates vata dosha. Cover your baby's head.
- Eat light meals and eat whenever you're hungry. It's better to eat many light meals throughout the day than to load up on food during a couple of meals. Make sure you start the day off with breakfast. Do not try to lose weight because dieting causes imbalances and ill health. Get friends and family members to cook for you as much as possible. Eat foods suggested for vata individuals (see page 213).

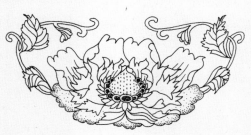

Ancient Recipes for New Mothers

Prasadam, blessed foods and drinks, are the gifts of God's mercy. Offered here are a few simple recipes that you can customize to suit your tastes, prakriti, and health goals.

Rice

Rice, particularly basmati rice, strengthens the body and is easy to digest. Rinse the rice a minimum of three times to clean it. To cook rice, use 2 parts water to 1 part rice. Bring it to a boil in a pot with a tight-fitting lid. Lower the heat as much as possible and simmer for 10 to 20 minutes. Don't stir the rice while it cooks. Be careful that you don't burn the rice; cooking time depends upon the quality and quantity of the rice you are cooking. For example, freshly harvested rice, sometimes labeled "new crop," does not require as long a cooking time. Watch for the steam coming off the pot to subside; when it does the rice will be done. Eventually your intuition will be your best guide when it comes to cooking a perfect pot of rice.

Coconut Rice

SERVES 2 TO 4

This sweet side dish gives strength to new mothers and pleases their families. Coconut pacifies pitta disorders (like PMS) and is soothing for mothers who have the blues, and the gram massala aids digestion.

   3 tablespoons ghee (page 215)

   1 teaspoon gram massala (page 224)

   1 teaspoon black mustard seed

   ½ cup shredded unsweetened coconut

   2 to 3 cups cooked rice

   1 tablespoon sweetener (if you use honey, do not cook it and add it last)

Heat ghee over medium heat in a large frying pan. Add spices and coconut, brown. Stir in rice and sweetener. Serve immediately.

Morning Rice

....

SERVES 4 OR MORE

New mothers need something warm, nourishing, and easy to digest to start their day. This is a very traditional Ayurvedic morning meal or midmorning snack. Almonds provide protein.

- 1 cup organic brown rice

- 4 cups pure water (may need more)

- 1 cinnamon stick

- 1 teaspoon cardamom

- ½ teaspoon dried ground ginger

- 2 cups organic milk

- ½ cup organic sugar

- ½ cup blanched almonds, coarsely ground

- ¼ cup organic raisins

- ¼ teaspoon saffron threads

In your blender, grind brown rice until it has the consistency of course sand. Bring water to boil, lower heat, add spices. Add ground rice, while stirring with a whisk. Simmer uncovered (enjoy the aroma) for about 30 minutes. Stir often; don't let it stick to bottom of pot.

In a separate bowl, mix milk, sugar, ground blanched almonds (may be ground in your blender), raisins, and saffron threads.

When rice mixture is well cooked, add milk mixture, continue to stir, and simmer for 10 more minutes. Morning rice should be the consistency of thick gravy. Serve warm.

Lemon Rice

SERVES 2 TO 4

Rice is recommended for soothing vata. Lemon and the other spices in this recipe will aid digestion. Ghee helps strengthen new mothers and is also good for pacifying vata.

2 to 3 tablespoons ghee (page 215)

½ teaspoon turmeric

½ teaspoon cumin or black mustard seed

½ teaspoon coriander seeds

2 to 3 tablespoons lemon juice

2 to 3 cups cooked rice

Salt

Heat ghee over medium heat in a large frying pan. Add spices and let them pop without burning. Add lemon juice and rice. Season with salt. Stir well and serve.

Alesia's Life-Saving Date Shake

SERVES 1 HUNGRY NEW MOTHER OR 2 REGULAR FOLKS

2 cups organic milk

¼ teaspoon ghee (page 215)

5 to 6 drops food grade rosewater (available in Oriental and health-food stores)

1 Medjool date (other dates may be used; if smaller, use 2 dates)

¼ cup raisins

1 pinch dried powdered ginger

1 pinch dried powdered cardamom

1 pinch dried powdered cinnamon

In a saucepan, slowly boil milk with ghee, rosewater, date, and raisins. Let cool; you want it warm, not scalding hot. Add spices. Pour all into blender. Blend until smooth. Enjoy.

Aam or Mango Lassi

SERVES 1 TO 2 SERVINGS

"I have never met anyone who could not drink lassi."—Dr. B. D. Triguna

Lassi is taken by itself or sipped after a meal. (It is not wise to drink lassi while eating.) It is a digestive aid and, as it is so delicious, a mood booster.

- **1 cup organic yogurt**

- **2 cups pure water**

- **1 ripe mango** (peeled and pitted)

- **1 pinch ground dried cardamom**

- **3 to 4 dates,** (optional for those with a sweet tooth! Choose soft ones, remove pits)

- **Rose petals, for garnish** (unsprayed from your garden)

In the blender, combine all of the above ingredients, except rose petals, until smooth and creamy. Serve garnished with rose petals.

Punjiri

MANY SERVINGS

Punjiri is traditionally given to postpartum women in India. It enhances healing and enriches breast milk. It balances and nourishes the body's tissues.

- **1 pound almonds, blanched**

- **½ pound pistachios** (optional)

- **½ pound dried shredded coconut**

- **¼ pound ghee** (page 215)

- **¼ cup organic sugar**

- **2 teaspoons dried ground cardamom**

In a cast-iron skillet, roast nuts in ghee, later add coconut.(If you wish to blanch almonds at home, it is easy to do: Bring to a boil, let cool, pinch/squeeze each almond, skin will slide off.)

In a food processor or powerful blender, grind roasted nuts with sugar and cardamom. Eat 2 tablespoons morning and evening or snack on this whenever you're hungry.

Marjan's Favorite Beets

serves 4 to 6
Calcium-rich beets are spiced so they are easy to digest and so delicious.

6 to 8 small beets, peeled and cut into bite-sized pieces

1 ½ inch fresh gingerroot, peeled and diced

Optional after sixth week postpartum:

2 crushed cloves of garlic or a pinch of hing
(also called asafoetida, available in Oriental/Indian food part of store)

1 tablespoon butter or ghee (page 215)

SAUCE

1 cup orange juice

2 teaspoons organic sugar

2 teaspoons arrowroot powder (may substitute cornstarch)

A generous handful of fresh mint, minced, **or 2 teaspoons dried mint**

Steam beets until tender; put aside.

Sauté ginger (and garlic or hing if used) in butter or ghee, on low heat in a saucepan, for about 1 minute.

Stir together orange juice, sugar, and arrowroot powder until dissolved. Now whisk/stir orange juice mixture into ginger-butter, continue to simmer and whisk/stir until thickened.

Pour over beets and toss with the finely minced mint. Serve hot or cold.

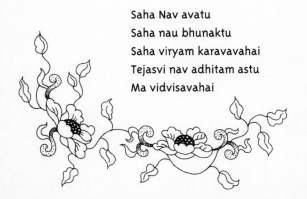

Saha Nav avatu	Let us be together
Saha nau bhunaktu	Let us eat together
Saha viryam karavavahai	Let us be vital together
Tejasvi nav adhitam astu	Let us be radiating truth
Ma vidvisavahai	Radiating the light of life
	Never shall we denounce anyone
	Never entertain negativity.
	Rig Veda

Khichari

SERVES 4 TO 6

Khichari is like fast food. Easy to digest, easy to make. Quinoa, a grain native to Central America, is rich in protein, B vitamins, iron, calcium, and other minerals.

1 cup dahl (use chana, toovar, or matar, also called split-pea dahl)

1 cup organic quinoa (found in health-food stores)

5 cups pure water

1 teaspoon turmeric

Pinch of cinnamon

Pinch of ground dried cardamom

Tiny pinch of organic sugar

Salt

½ teaspoon coriander seeds

1 teaspoon cumin seeds

1 teaspoon fennel seeds

4 tablespoons ghee (page 215)

Wash quinoa and dahl, bring to a boil in a large pot with water. Add turmeric, cinnamon, sugar, cardamom, and salt to taste. Lower heat and simmer about 1 hour, until it is the consistency of gravy (add water if necessary). With a mortar and pestle (or small grinder), crush coriander, cumin, and fennel seeds. In a small saucepan, melt ghee, add crushed seeds, and simmer 1 to 2 minutes. Stir ghee and seed mixture into well-cooked quinoa and dahl. Serve in a deep bowl.

Gram Massala

MAKES ABOUT ½ CUP

Gram massala is the traditional Indian name for mixed spices. This particular mix of spices is my favorite. You may wish to experiment with your own tastes and come up with your own gram massala. During postpartum, use gram massala freely as all spices are good for pacifying vata dosha.

2 tablespoons ground cinnamon (aids digestion)

1 tablespoon ground ginger (a *sattvic* or life-supporting spice, and good for digestion and relieving menstrual cramps)

1 tablespoon ground cardamom (aids digestion, circulation, and respiration)

1 tablespoon ground coriander (good for relieving high pitta disorders like PMS)

1 tablespoon ground nutmeg (helps one absorb nutrients and calms the mind)

¼ teaspoon ground cloves (good for reproductive and lymphatic systems)

Mix all ingredients together and store in a jar with a tight-fitting lid. Use in sweet recipes, chutneys, and to flavor teas.

Yogi Tea

SERVES 4 TO 6

This relaxing tea aids digestion.

6 cups water

2 tablespoons gram massala (see recipe above)

1 cup milk

1 tablespoon honey

Bring water to a boil. Add gram massala and simmer for 10 to 15 minutes. Remove from heat. Add milk and honey. Enjoy. Leftover tea may be refrigerated and served cool.

Curry Powder

MAKES ABOUT 1 CUP

Curry is used to flavor food and to balance doshas. People of kapha constitution may enjoy all spices except salt. Pitta-type people must also avoid salt and take other spices in moderate to small quantities to avoid increasing the dosha and aggravating their tempers. Vata-predominant people will find that spices have a grounding effect on their minds and bodies.

If you have a grinder at home, buy these spices whole and grind them fresh. Otherwise you may purchase them ground and mix them yourself. Do not hesitate to experiment. If you are out of some of the ingredients or find them unavailable, leave them out or substitute others. Do not use asafoetida while pregnant or during high fever, and reduce your intake of turmeric when pregnant.

3 tablespoons ground turmeric (antibacterial; aids digestion [even of junk food] and circulation; said to have the energy of the divine mother)

3 tablespoons ground cumin (alleviates kapha and aids digestion)

1 tablespoon ground coriander (good for pitta constitution; clears up infections of the urinary tract; aids digestion)

1 tablespoon ground ginger (reduces vata and kapha; alleviates gas)

1 tablespoon ground cardamom (lights the fire of *agni*, digestion; clears the lungs as well as the mind; calms the nerves)

1 teaspoon ground black pepper (destroys toxins; said to contain the energy of the sun; lights digestive fires)

1 teaspoon ground asafoetida (this optional Oriental herb aids digestion; prevents flatulence; cleanses intestines of old accumulations)

Mix all ingredients together and store in a jar with a tight-fitting lid.

Vegetable Curry

Any vegetables in season, from the store or your garden, may be used in this recipe. The vegetables I've listed here are just suggestions. The yield will vary depending on what vegetables (and what amounts) you use. All vegetables should be well cooked but still bright in color. The amount of yogurt varies depending on your taste and how many vegetables you cook.

4 to 6 tablespoons ghee (page 215)

1 to 2 tablespoons curry powder (see previous recipe)

1 head broccoli, cut into small flowers, peel and slice the stem, steamed

2 potatoes, diced and steamed

1 large sweet potato, diced and steamed

2 carrots, diced

¼ pound green beans, snapped in half

¼ pound peas

1 or 2 zucchini, sliced

¼ pound okra, whole or sliced

Juice of 1 orange (optional)

½ to 1 cup yogurt

Salt or tamari soy sauce

In a large pot or wok, melt ghee over medium heat. Add curry powder (the amount depends on the quantity of vegetables being prepared and your taste). Toss in vegetables. Keep heat on medium. Stir in the orange juice and yogurt. Season with salt or tamari soy sauce to taste. Serve with basmati rice.

NOTE: Omit white potatoes and broccoli from your diet until after week six postpartum, as they aggravate vata.

Cucumber Raita

SERVES 4

Raita is a traditional side dish similar to salads. This recipe helps balance new mothers because cucumber, which is sweet and astringent, decreases vata. The yogurt is good for digestion and alleviates diarrhea and painful urination. For people suffering from hypertension, cucumber lowers blood pressure.

1 teaspoon cumin seeds

2 cucumbers, diced and peeled

1 ½ cups yogurt

½ teaspoon salt

Roast the cumin seeds in a dry frying pan; when brown, place on a cutting board and crush with a rolling pin. Mix all ingredients together and let sit for half an hour before serving.

Banana Raita

SERVES 4

Serve as a side dish or by itself as a snack. The cardamom helps digest the bananas, and ginger helps digest the yogurt.

2 to 3 ripe bananas

1 ½ cups yogurt

1 teaspoon cardamom

½ teaspoon ground ginger

Slice bananas, mix with yogurt and spices. Let sit a few minutes so the flavors come out.

A Simple Dahl

SERVES 4

Dahl is a traditional protein source in cultures that do not advocate eating meat. This soupy bean dish is a perfect postpartum food. Most legumes are sweet and astringent, helping to pacify vata, stop bleeding, heal wounds, and prevent uterine prolapse when eaten in the early postpartum days. Make sure dahl is very soupy when prepared for new mothers so they can digest it easily.

In East India, dahl made from well-cooked legumes, ghee, salt, and spices is an everyday food. There are many dahl recipes, but this is my favorite. The brown rice makes it a source of complete protein. Dahl may be made with split peas, garbanzo beans, mung beans, or lentils. This recipe calls for lentils but may be changed so you can try the other variations. Just substitute the alternative beans or peas for the lentils.

2 cups lentils (the small salmon-colored lentils cook faster and digest more easily; if unavailable, use mung beans or yellow split peas)

1 cup brown rice

6 to 8 cups water

4 to 6 tablespoons ghee (page 215

2 tablespoons curry powder (page 225)

Salt

Bring lentils, rice, and water to a boil in one pot. After it boils, reduce to low heat and allow pot to simmer until lentils fall apart completely (30 minutes to an hour). Dahl should be thin and soupy, so add more water if needed. Stir in remaining ingredients and serve.

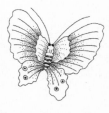

The food is thy blessing
and in thy service
we accept with all gratitude
my lord.

—Maharishi Mahesh Yogi

Chutney

SERVES 4

Chutney is said to increase bliss. What new mother could refuse more bliss? The role chutney plays is to promote digestion and make the meal more beautiful. Apples, mangos, and pears work well in chutney. Don't try bananas as they are not well suited for chutney, but if you have a peach or apricot tree these fruits work wonderfully. Add a handful of raisins or chopped walnuts. Use your imagination.

> **4 to 6 pieces of in-season fruit,** cut into bite-sized pieces
>
> **1 to 2 tablespoons gram massala** (see recipe, page 224)
>
> **¼ cup ghee** (page 215) **or butter**
>
> **½ cup honey**

In a large pot, cook fruit with the spice in a minimal amount of water. Fruit should be soft and cooked thoroughly. Remove from heat, add ghee and honey. Serve as a savory with meals. Store in the refrigerator; it will keep for about 1 week.

Hom

SERVES 2

Hom, or hot almond milk, is a wonderful snack any time of the day, providing energy and improving ojas, the subtle essence of the body.

> **20 to 25 almonds**
>
> **2 cups milk**
>
> **1 teaspoon honey**
>
> **Pinch *each* of cardamom and black pepper**

Soak almonds overnight, and remove their skins in the morning. Warm milk over low heat. Do not boil. Pour into blender with almonds, honey, and spices. Blend at high setting until frothy.

Ayurvedic Herbs for Postpartum Women

The following herbs are traditionally used in both Ayurvedic and Chinese medicine. I have chosen just these few for their powerful partnership in healing and rejuvenating the female reproductive system and balancing our emotions. They are becoming increasingly available in the West. You will be able to purchase them as a powder or tincture (most convenient and potent form) in most health-food stores. Many communities now have herb shops where you may find even rare Oriental herbs, as well as advice on their use and preparation.

Always go carefully. Herbs are powerful medicine, a little goes a long way, and it is possible to take toxic amounts. Consult a doctor of Chinese or Ayurvedic medicine about your condition. Also get a copy of Dr. David Frawley and Dr. Vasant Lad's *The Yoga of Herbs* (Wilmot, WI: Lotus Light Publications, 1986).

GOKSHURA

The fruit of this herb stops bleeding, nourishes the reproductive system, and is known to help postpartum women regain energy. It is also a strong aphrodisiac. Because it rejuvenates pitta and pacifies vatta, gokshura (or caltrops as it is known in the West) is considered a sedative. You can take 250 mg to 1 gram in tea or in warm milk with honey and ghee. If you suffer from back pains, add ground ginger to the milk decoction.

GOTU KOLA

Ayurveda's primary rejuvenative herb is the gotu kola plant's leaves. In India, gotu kola is called "Brahmi" because it brings knowledge of Brahman. Besides increasing intelligence, it strengthens the immune system and purifies the blood. Gotu kola heals skin disorders by improving the digestion, the root cause of problems with skin. Because this herb pacifies vata and reduces kapha, it is good for mothers recovering from birthing. It also balances pitta, helping with high-pitta menstrual symptoms. Gotu kola aids circulation and fortifies the nervous system. Take 250 to 500 milligrams in warm milk with ghee and honey, or prepare with boiled water as you would any herb tea. Yogis take gotu kola tea with honey before meditation to enhance experiences of refined states of consciousness.

JASMINE

Women suffering from postpartum blues will feel their spirits lifted if they add a few dried jasmine flowers to their tea (do not boil the flowers). These fragrant flowers strengthen the lymphatic system and cleanse the uterus. Because jasmine flowers promote compassion and passion in women, they are especially beneficial when one suffers from emotional roughness. They should not be taken by women suffering from chills as their effect is cooling.

MYRRH
The resin of myrrh is known for its ability to reverse the aging process by detoxifying the body and aiding the growth of new, healthy tissue. Women who either have excessive menstrual bleeding or fail to menstruate will benefit from taking two 00-size capsules of powdered myrrh two or three times a day. Myrrh causes old blood to be shed from the uterus and also helps dispel stagnant emotions. Women with symptoms of high vata or kapha benefit most from taking myrrh. If you suffer from high pitta (see questionnaire on pages 207–10 to determine your prakriti), you should not take myrrh.

REHMANNIA
Rehmannia is a tonic for the uterus. Many of the most common postpartum discomforts (back pain, lack of vitality, sexual debility, hair loss, irregular menstruation, and weak kidneys to name a few) can be treated with this wonderful cooling and rejuvenating herb. Though vata individuals generally should steer clear of cooling herbs, rehmannia is an exception. Simmer five to ten grams in a pint of water, with cinnamon to aid digestion and make it taste very nice, for thirty minutes. The rehmannia root is sold by weight in irregular, black, leatherlike pieces. You may want to simply bite off chunks and eat it (if so, you may take up to one ounce this way).

ROSE
Traditionally and medicinally, the rose is the flower of devotion and love. Picture in your mind's eye a rose as an opening heart. This revered flower restores health while purifying the blood. An emmenagogue, which means that it promotes regular menstruation, the rose is very cooling and alleviates high-pitta disorders like PMS. It also helps heal sores in the mouth. Combine rose with shatavari for an excellent means of regulating menstruation. Six to eight petals may be warmed with milk and honey to fight constipation.

SANDALWOOD
The wood and oil of this sacred tree have a calming effect on the body as well as on the restless mind. An antibacterial and anti-inflammatory herb, sandalwood is cooling and reduces fever. Use the powder, mixed with water to form a paste, or

the oil externally on sores or on the forehead to reduce fever and PMS symptoms. This wonderful medicine that balances pitta is a blessing in every home. Sandalwood incense is a good aid for meditation because when it is burned, intelligence and devotion are stimulated.

SHATAVARI

Among the hundreds of healing herbs available, both Eastern and Western, shatavari is the Ayurvedic herb of choice for most disorders of the female reproductive system (as ashwagandha is for men). This root, which soothes and calms vata and decreases pitta, is such a powerful rejuvenator and toner for women that it is said to give one the capacity to have a hundred husbands! Shatavari heals inflamed tissues, increases milk production, and increases fertility. It is also good for treating common diarrhea and dysentery. Because the herb supplies many essential female hormones, shatavari is excellent for women who have high-vata or high-pitta menstrual symptoms, are going through menopause, or have had hysterectomies. Shatavari has the added charm of increasing one's capacity for love and devotion. Prepare up to three grams of shatavari powder in a cup of warm milk with honey and ghee. Enjoy daily.

TURMERIC

This sacred yellow root is antibacterial, antifungal, and has anti-inflammatory properties. When high-protein foods are cooked with turmeric, they become easy to digest. To ease pain, swelling, tears, and/or stitches in the perineum after childbirth, make a sitz bath with turmeric, salt, and warm water. Mix turmeric powder with ghee and apply to cracked nipples for effective healing.

These few basic herbs along with the Western herbs recommended in chapter 11, Herbs for the Postpartum Woman, are enough to supply your basic home herbal pharmacy. (To obtain a catalog or purchase Ayurvedic herbs and products by mail order, write or call Lotus Light, P.O. Box 2, Wilmot, Wisconsin 53192, 414/862-2395.) There are many Ayurvedic herbs that I have not mentioned. The ones I did outline are my personal favorites for postpartum women. Herbs heal the subtle (spiritual and emotional) as well as the physical body. It is fascinating to me that the herbs that heal the reproductive organs are also aphrodisiacs. Ones that increase milk flow and supply female hormones also increase feelings of love and devotion. Those that soothe the brain and nervous system also increase intelligence and promote higher awareness. You may have fun reading more on

Ayurvedic herbology and finding your own favorites. To begin your reading, let me recommend the following books:

The Yoga of Herbs: An Ayurvedic Guide to Herbal Medicine by Vasant Lad and David Frawley (Wilmot, WI: Lotus Light Publications, 1986)

Wise Woman Herbal for the Childbearing Year by Susun S. Weed (Woodstock, NY: Ash Tree, 1986)

Ayurvedic Tips for the Menstrual Cycle

Women are so fortunate to have the opportunity to purify with each moon. Ayurveda advises us to take full advantage of this precious cleansing. But in the West, our lifestyles do not allow menstruating women to get the rest and peace they need in order to benefit from the body's natural cycles. Thus many women suffer from premenstrual stress, which is a common precursor to full-blown premenstrual syndrome. This is because they literally are not doing their periods right.

A common cause of premenstrual syndrome is the accumulation of toxins that were not released by the body during previous menstrual cycles. Excess doshas are eliminated during the period. In the beginning of menses, which is characterized by mucus secretion, excess kapha is expelled. In the middle, bright red phase, excess pitta is eliminated. In the end, brown menses, excess vata is shed.

As a woman, your reproductive system is pitta in nature. Pitta is associated with blood. Disorders such as menstrual irregularity (particularly early onset), uterine infection, increased bleeding, and premenstrual syndrome (PMS) are high-pitta conditions. They can be treated with cooling herbs and foods, and by cooling your living conditions, which may be as simple as opening more windows.

Delayed or absent menstruation and painful cramping of the uterus and/or legs can be due to high vata. In this case, the woman may be treated with heating foods and herbs. During her period, she should also bundle up and stay out of the wind.

If you are breastfeeding, it may take up to a year or longer for your period to return regularly. Most women begin to menstruate again about the time the baby starts to eat solid foods.

PREPARING FOR YOUR MOON TIME

Prepare for a healthy "moon time" before your period begins. In the week before you begin to flow, eat lightly and take relaxing baths and wash your hair. Clean your home. Do your shopping. Generally prepare to rest during menstruation by putting your life in order. Do this as leisurely as you can so you do not strain yourself. If you suffer from PMS, drink one or two ounces of liquid ghee per day and take up to one ounce of aloe vera orally to pacify pitta. Ginger tea lessens vata and may be taken if you tend to have late or painful periods. A sesame oil enema, or *basti,* before your period helps pacify vata, decreasing pain during menses. Do not give yourself a basti if you currently have a vaginal infection or are prone to them. Oil increases kapha, and vaginal infections are caused by excess kapha. (If you find you still experience cramping and pain, a hot water bottle on your stomach works wonders.)

DURING YOUR MOON

In Bali, the Hindu Dharma women call their menstruation *datang bulan,* which means "the moon is here." Once your bleeding has begun, you experience a very strong subdosha called *vata apana.* During vata apana, vata moves downward. When a woman is overtired or strains herself physically while menstruating, the movement of her vata is forced upward. This reversal causes impurities to stay in the body, irritating pitta, which creates profound effects on the mind and emotions, causing symptoms typical of PMS or PPD (see page 262). Rest, especially in the first two to three days of your period, is essential. At this time, also keep a positive attitude about the natural functions of your body.

Failure to take good care of your body, mind, and spirit before and during your menses causes impurities to stay locked in the body until the next cycle. Cramps, emotional instability, excessive bleeding or failure to bleed, and hot flashes are all causes by fatigue and stress forcing vata upward.

These basic rules clear the pathway to a healthy menses.

- Rest the first two to three days of your period.
- Eat lightly (especially no chocolate or cheese) both before and during your period.
- Engage in only uplifting activities.
- No heavy work or lifting.
- Reduce talking and visiting.
- No oil massages (called *abhyanga,* which are not recommended during pregnancy). Oil may be applied as a moisturizer; however, vigorous massage moves vata up, and vata should be moving down now.
- Shower daily but avoid tub baths.
- Do not shampoo your hair.
- No intercourse until bleeding stops because it moves vata up.
- Avoid tampons; use pads that allow blood to flow out.

AFTER YOUR MOON TIME

After you have stopped bleeding completely, you may massage head and body with warm sesame oil (leave on hair for two hours if possible), then shower and wash hair. If you tend to have PMS and/or excessive bleeding and heat in the body, you suffer from high pitta. In this case, instead of sesame oil use warm coconut oil, which cools the system, for head and body massage. Abhyanga, oil massage, balances doshas and restores health, which is important to do before you jump back into activity after menstruating.

You may also wish to do a sesame oil enema after your period, especially if you have not taken proper rest. Improper rest during menses causes toxins that should flow out with menstrual blood to remain in the body. An enema helps dislodge accumulated toxic substances in the colon. Again, if you have or are prone to suffer from vaginal infections (a high-kapha condition), do not do an oil enema (see page 234).

If you do not suffer from excess kapha, after you shower soak a sterile gauze pad in sesame oil. Roll into the shape and size of a tampon and insert it into your yoni and leave gauze in for two hours. The oil suppository gently dislodges stagnant blood and discharge from the uterus and vagina and helps it drain out of the body. If you are going to bed, you may leave it in overnight.

A Prayer for Your Period
Thank you for our blood, Mother
Our cycle of fertility.
Thank you for our men, Mother
The seeds of our children.
Thank you for our milk, Mother
Which nourishes great spirits.

Daily Routine for the Entire Month

"A mother's work is never done" is all too true. Be patient with yourself and your little ones. Mothers who plan to stay home and care for their babies full time and mothers on maternity leave may use this framework to structure their days. This daily routine is not a strict set of rules, but just one more tool you may use to improve the quality of your daily life. Your routine or daily plans must always stay flexible to take the changing needs of your baby into consideration. The highest activity is taking care of children, so enjoy and evolve.

MORNING

- Wake up early (this will come quite naturally as babies are early risers).
- Drink a cup of warm water.
- Urinate and have a bowel movement.
- When baby wakes, attend to his or her immediate needs (cuddling, food, change of diaper).
- Give yourself and your baby a mini oil massage (chapter 13, Healing Touch).
- Brush teeth and clean tongue.
- Shower or bathe.
- Put on comfortable, clean clothing.
- Meditate or take a few minutes of silence or prayer.
- Stretch, ease into moving your body.
- Eat a light breakfast.
- Now begin the activity of your day. In the early days postpartum, this will mainly be caring for your baby and other children. New mothers and babies will benefit greatly by being close to the earth. This is a good time to be in your flower or vegetable garden. Weather permitting, put your baby in a basket, protected from the sun, and take her along with you. You will soon find time just for you to read, study, or pursue your creative occupation.
- Take plenty of liquid during the day, especially if you are breastfeeding. Don't forget your herb teas and milk decoctions.

AFTERNOON

- Eat a balanced lunch according to your prakriti (see page 210) and suited to the season. Eat enough to reach three-fourths of your food capacity.
- Enjoy an uplifting activity; some physical activity—dancing, gardening, body toning—will keep one from becoming too inactive. (Conclude exercise at least half an hour before meals or wait one hour after eating.)
- Practice afternoon meditation or prayer.
- Enjoy a light snack.

EVENING

- Eat supper (don't forget to bless the food).
- Take a short (ten to fifteen minutes), pleasant walk.
- Read or listen to music, play with children, or any other pleasant activity.
- Get to bed early.

PART IV

Mothering:

An Openhearted

Lifestyle

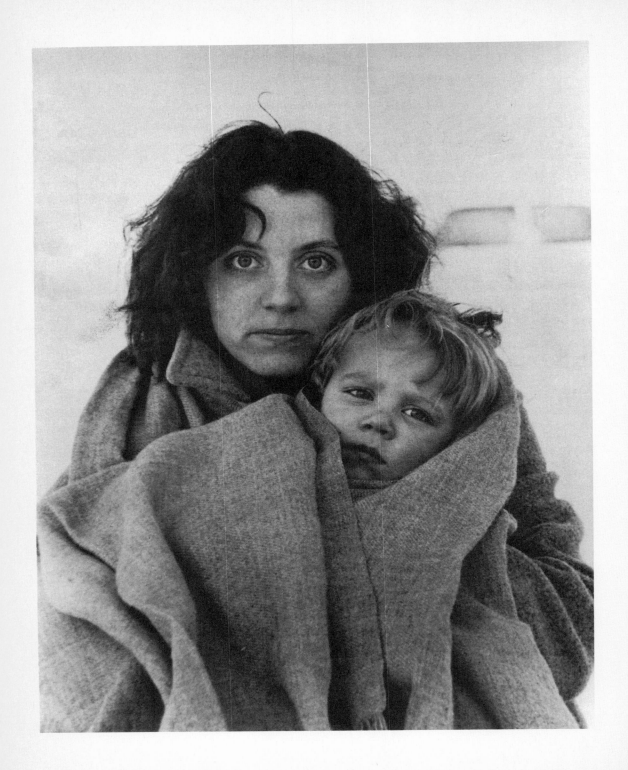

CHAPTER 16

Issues of the Heart

The postnatal period may be the most trying time of your life, emotionally as well as physically. Your body, with all its amazing parts; your mind, with its complexity of thought; your spirit, which is both individual and universal, are expanded to meet the demands of your precious new child. This tremendous openness can bring you home to the center of who you are. But the route is neither short nor easy. To weather it, you must focus not only on your baby but also on your changing self-image.

You have a partner in this journey of growth; your baby, who was with you constantly, nudging you from within during the nine long months of waiting, has joined you in the world. The journey you may have thought would be over once you gave birth is only beginning. It is no wonder so many women feel their children are also their teachers; Erica Jong wrote a poem called "The Buddha in the Womb" about her developing child.

If your baby is not in your arms because of prolonged illness, the decision to relinquish him or her for adoption, death, or any one of the many challengers that can unfold, your journey is even more difficult. Your need for skillful nurturing is more profound. Allow yourself to be postpartum. Remember, once you have been pregnant, regardless of the outcome, you are a mother. In many ancient cultures, by virtue of being a mother you enjoy ascended status.

Every postpartum woman feels her heart being tested. Your heart may feel as if it is bursting, leaving each fragment larger and stronger than the whole once was. You may cry more than you are accustomed to; you will also smile and laugh more. Small things will move you, like the curve of your baby's mouth, overhearing a conversation between a father and his infant, or an older sibling's drawings for "the baby."

You are delicate. You are passionate. You are strong. You need to be nurtured tenderly just as your child does. Here I wish to touch on some of the issues of the heart, the range of emotions you may feel, and the many aspects of your relationship to yourself, your family, and the world that changes as you enter (for the first time or once again) the precious role of mother.

Bonding

Traditionally defined, bonding is the establishment of the mother/child and father/child relationship immediately following birth. But our culture is just beginning to accept what many Eastern cultures have believed for centuries: the bonding process begins before birth. Birth is an important, but not the initial, step in establishing the connection between the infant and mother, father, siblings, and extended family members. Joseph Chilton Pearce, author of *Magical Child* (New York: Bantam Books, 1981) and *The Crack in the Cosmic Egg* (New York: Crown Books, 1988), further extends the concept of bonding and describes it as "the connection forged between mind and heart." He claims it is this connection that facilitates humans' spiritual evolution.

In recent years, progress has been made to protect the important bonding process. Hospitals are increasingly sympathetic to the desire of parents and infants to be together during and after the birth. Fathers are now allowed in the delivery room, where they belong. Upon request, rooming-in is possible at most hospitals in the United States. When a mother asks that her baby room-in, her child is allowed to stay with her in her room, day and night. However, the majority of hospitals still keep babies isolated in the nursery for many hours immediately following birth. Perhaps in the future hospitals will do away with this policy that is harmful to the bonding process.

Bonding is not limited to what takes place between the parents and infant but involves the baby's relationships with brothers, sisters, extended family, all the world outside the womb, and God, nature, or Spirit. For this reason it is becoming more common to include siblings at home births. Most hospitals still exclude children from the delivery room. I have seen many children at home births, and the experience was always positive when they have been taught not to fear birth and had a loving adult to hold them. For both parents and children, sharing this event is a fascinating experience that will never be forgotten. Children are good helpers at births, and they like to be involved. Some midwives give a soft cotton

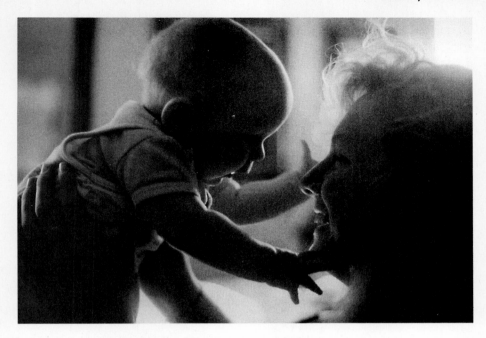

receiving blanket to each child and ask the children to keep them under their shirts. The blankets are at body temperature when the baby is born, and the siblings have provided the baby with his or her first warmth outside the womb. Brothers and sisters should be allowed to hold the baby soon after the birth.

Bonding is an ongoing process that begins in the uterus and continues throughout life. Ashley Montagu in *Life before Birth* (New York: Signet Books, 1965, o.p.) cites the significant effect of prenatal influences on the baby. Mothers who receive good nutrition and who have stable emotions during pregnancy tend to produce healthy, happy babies who bond with their families, can relax, eat well, and sleep soundly. Mothers who had unhappy pregnancies and did not get the nutrients they needed are more likely to give birth to unhealthy babies who have trouble bonding.

Bonding almost always occurs easily, which is fortunate because human infants' survival depends upon this attachment. When either the mother or the baby has difficulty bonding, the most common barrier is stress. For baby, the factors that create stress are loud sounds, bright lights, the cold, separation from parents, and pain such as that caused by some hospital procedures like injections and circumcision. Anesthesia given to the mother during the birth passes to the baby through the umbilicus and makes the baby limp and groggy, hardly a condition conducive to bonding.

Dr. Frederick Leboyer's much acclaimed and controversial study *Birth without Violence* (New York: Knopf, 1975) has brought attention to the importance of maintaining a stress-free environment immediately after the birth so that bonding can take place. Leboyer advocates dimming the lights, keeping the room warm, and eliminating loud sounds. For mother, stress can be due to a difficult pregnancy and birth, money, relationships, her treatment in the hospital, and many other reasons. Somehow, regardless of her situation, the overwhelming feeling of love takes over and sooner or later most mothers bond with their babies.

It is reassuring to hear Elisabeth Kübler-Ross, renowned psychiatrist and pioneer in the field of human emotions and healing, say that "human beings are 100 percent repairable." Even babies who have difficult births or are separated from their mothers for one reason or another are able to bond. Adopted children bond to the parents who choose to raise them; and when they are reunited, even decades later, with their birth mothers, many adopted children feel they rebond with their biological mothers, as if a thread were maintained across the miles and through the years.

Throughout life the bonding process is repeated and extended from the sweetness of the mother's lap and the immediate family to friendships and love relationships. I accept the common Hindu belief that we learn our basic lessons about love from our mothers during the first few months of life. Many people have discovered during psychotherapy, rebirthing, and other forms of self-examination that the barriers to intimacy they experience in relationships were actually erected in the womb and reinforced during infancy. Because bonding is a lifelong process, these obstacles can be overcome and each of us can be healed. What a rewarding gift for a new mother, to know that her nurturing sets the lifelong pattern of how her child gives and receives love.

Bonding is at once a spiritual and a sensuous function. You've felt it in your heart; you've seen it in your baby's eyes. All the senses of everyone concerned work and play together to bond.

Smell takes messages directly to the nervous system. Babies are extremely sensitive to odors. It is important to not confuse your baby about your natural scent by using perfumes or heavily perfumed soaps, deodorants, or other products for the first few weeks after birth. Likewise, avoid using soaps and perfumed powders on your baby. His nose and sensitive skin will appreciate it. The Filipino and Thai cultures kiss by sniffing. In America, it is not uncommon to see a new mother "gobble up" her baby with her nose. Indeed, babies smell wonderful.

Touch is a crucial bonding tool. Animals lick their young. We cuddle. Skin-to-skin contact is best. If you are worried that your baby is cold, avoid the temptation to bundle her up with too many layers of clothing. Your body warmth and a minimum of cotton clothing is the best protection from cold in temperate weather circumstances.

Taste plays an important role in the bonding process. You taste good. Your milk is sweet, your skin is slightly salty. Your baby learns this through her contact with you. You may find the temptation to take your baby's foot in your mouth undeniable. Babies taste good too.

In the past it was commonly believed that babies could not see. It is now known that babies see, and they see very well. The best news that researchers have found is that the image babies love to look at most is the adoring face of a loved one! So go ahead and gaze at your baby. You are his favorite form of entertainment. Colors are important to babies too. Rudolf Steiner, German philosopher and the founder of Waldorf education, says babies and small children need to be surrounded by pastels. Perhaps when you were pregnant and feeling the nesting instinct, you decorated your home with beautiful colors. Your efforts are being rewarded by the pleasure your baby gets from looking at these calming colors.

New babies have extremely sensitive hearing. Listen to your environment and weed out noise pollution. Exposing him to loud music or sounds is not recommended. Be watchful that people who hold your baby do not talk directly into her ears in loud conversational tones. I can't count how many times I've seen well-meaning friends or relatives hold a baby up to their faces, then turn just enough to position the baby's ear directly in front of their mouths, and yell, "Isn't she cute?!"

The sound of your voice is soothing to your baby—he could recognize it even before he was born. Even if you don't like your own singing, your baby loves it. Sing to him, talk to him. Fill your home with pleasurable sound. Go outside and listen to the sounds of children playing and birds singing.

In India, it is believed that the events of a person's life, from the present back to birth, pass before the eyes as one leaves this world. Sound is said to be the last sense to leave humans at the time of death. Therefore it is recommended that the first sound the baby hears is the father's or mother's voice saying one of the names of God. This ensures that the person's last earthly experience will be the name of God.

The sixth sense, which has been termed ESP or psychic phenomenon, is called intuition by mothers. There seems to be a deep, unexplainable connection between parents and children; perhaps it is the by-product of physical and spiritual bonding. How is it that a mother knows when her baby needs her? Why does a woman's milk often let down precisely when her child becomes hungry or cries? This sometimes happens even when the mother and child are miles apart! Parents have described beautiful dreams about their children in detail only to have them come true months or even years later. If anything will convince you that something in addition to the physical world exists, bonding will.

Welcome Ceremonies

At some point after you and your baby are settled at home, you may wish to have a welcome ceremony. This ritual serves to welcome the baby into the world. It also welcomes you back into your community, now that you are wiser and are to be respected for your new role. Many of your friends have eagerly awaited the

A Sample Baby Blessing

This is an example of a baby blessing used at a welcoming ceremony. It is lovingly offered by Reverend Jayne Sturgeon who lives in Springfield, Oregon. You may want to use it to help you come up with your own blessing for your baby.

"Welcome, Baby. You have been awaited and are cherished by all of us. Thank you for joining us on this plane of awareness and sharing with us your perceptions and insights, your lessons and challenges, and your creativity and appreciations. You will enrich our lives with your smiles and tears, and you will teach us new ways to express love and happiness. We make a pledge to support you with all that we know."

(Give a rose bush to the mother and say her name.) "I give you this rose as a symbol of earth in its abundance. Your gift to your baby throughout her life will manifest in her every experience of this plane. May you enjoy her as you do this rose—her budding and unfolding, the pruning of her stalks, and the joy of her blossoming."

(Give a candle to the father and say his name.) "I give you this candle and ask you to light it in your own way as a symbol of the path you will illuminate for opportunity to cuddle your baby and greet you as a wise woman who by giving birth has been reborn.

In Hawaii, we sometimes gather our friends and family together for a baby blessing. Flower leis are always shared. The mother is given a *lei po'o,* a crown of flowers for her head, for she is the queen of the day. Each friend brings some food and an offering—a poem, prayer, song, dance, a massage, a gift, and always plenty of hugs.

A baby blessing can take any form. Go ahead and get involved in the planning of your blessing. Ask your friends to do all the legwork, but let them know what you want to do on this special day.

your child. (Pause for lighting.) May you keep the light and lightness for her life, allowing her to walk the path her own way, waiting patiently if she stumbles, standing still if she varies from the path so that she may return and find you there, pacing her as she runs, and guiding by example as you walk the path with her."

(Give a helium-filled balloon to the godfather and say his name.) "I give you this balloon. Hold it as you will hold your godchild's hand as she learns to walk and to dream, and before the day is done, release it into the air to travel its flight without attachment. So, too, when this baby has outgrown the need for your support and assistance, let her go to fly without hindrance."

(Give a crystal to the godmother and say her name.) "I give you this crystal as a tool to focus your awareness on the inner realm, to learn and share any lesson that will help this child develop as an individual, to grow in intuition and perception. Learn this child as you learn the crystal. Use it on her behalf and when her own perceptions grow to maturity, pass it on to her, for her own use."

(Sprinkle water on the baby's body and lips, say the baby's name.) "I give you water. May it bathe and sustain you on this plane and may your stream of life lead you on an interesting journey and back to the ocean of oneness from whence you came."

In many religious traditions, baby blessings are baptisms, which join together the extended family and serve to renew love and the commitments of love. Just because your family may not be religious, it does not mean you are not spiritual. We live in a time of great questioning of religious values and experience. The arrival of your child is the perfect time to begin establishing your own special spiritual practices and rituals.

In Bali, every baby is welcomed into the human family by her village community on the 105th day of life. This ritual, called "Nyambutan," marks the day the baby's feet touch the Mother Earth for the first time. With elaborate offerings of food and fragrant flowers, the baby is ransomed from the spirit world to live and grow in the physical world. After the ceremony, it's time to share food and fun. The welcoming day is a good time to take pictures. Your child will someday love having a photo of "Auntie Christine" or "Uncle Greg" holding him when he was a baby. At the close of the day, friends and family should make sure there is no cleanup left for you to do. As the baby's mother, this has been your special day, your day to be pampered and honored.

When all is quiet and friends and family have left, you may wish to take a few minutes to write a letter to your baby. Tell him how you feel on this day. Tell him how precious and loved he is. Someday, when you are having trouble paying for his braces or he is having growing pains, you can bring out this letter and share with your child just how precious he has always been to you.

The New Father

It is extremely important that your child's father be attentive to your physical, spiritual, and emotional needs, especially immediately after the birth and during the early weeks postpartum. Your memories of your partner from the delicate postpartum bonding period may become your sweetest. You will be bonding to your lover as well as to your baby.

Unfortunately, too often new mothers feel abandoned by their partners. This happens when the baby's father does not interrupt his daily routine to give special attention to you and the baby. His lack of attention may stem from feeling overwhelmed. He may be focusing too much upon the financial burdens of being a family man. These burdens may be imagined as well as real. For many generations, our culture has put undue pressure on young families to show they are responsible through hard work and financial gain. If this is the case with you and your partner, it may be time to reevaluate your priorities and decide just how important quality time spent with the baby and each other is; no price can be put on this time. He may need to be reminded how much you need his emotional support.

You may feel that your partner's life is relatively unchanged while yours is completely different since you had your baby. Share these changes with him, ask that he "be there" for you. He is your partner, not a stranger on the fringe of your new life. And remember, the quality of your relationship with him directly affects your baby.

A NOTE FOR FATHERS

Did you plan this baby? Or were you surprised by his or her advent into your life? Whether or not you pictured yourself in the role of father, you've put a baby on this earth. Congratulations.

Over the course of your partner's pregnancy, you watched the physical changes overtake her life. You may have, at times, felt yourself an outsider. If you

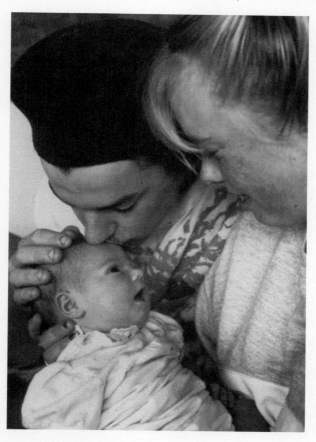

were present at the birth, you witnessed just how intense her partnership with creation is. In birthing this baby, she became a link in an unbroken chain of women, reaching back to the first. Do you remember the conception? It was then, while making love, that you too became a creator. You are not an outsider.

With the conception of this baby, your job just began. Every bit of nurturing you gave your partner while she was pregnant had a direct positive effect on your developing child. Now as you hold him or her in your arms, you may wonder just how your life will change and what you can do to help your child and your partner.

You may be overwhelmed by the mix of strong, and sometimes conflicting, emotions that you feel. For example, though you were awed by the wonder of birth, you may feel guilty, as if you caused your partner pain. You may feel intense love and a deep sense of connection with your child and at the same time find yourself jealous of the baby because much of your partner's attention must be directed toward his or her care.

Here is a thought list for postpartum fathers. You may wish to add to it as your own experience grows.

About My Partner
- She does not blame me for the pain she experienced during the birth.
- She has plenty of time and love for both me and our new baby.
- She needs rest and good food and drink, and she needs my help to get them.
- She needs my help and emotional support to be happy and to do her job of mothering well.
- She is still my lover; it's okay to be turned on by her. However, it serves us both if I am patient, not demanding sex during her delicate postpartum period. She is still turned on by me, and I can ask her to guide us back into fulfilling lovemaking when she is ready.
- She still needs romance: flowers for no reason, the unexpected kiss, a love note.

About My Baby
- Even if my child is breastfeeding, he or she needs me as much as my partner.
- I can nurture this child in many ways: cuddling frequently, changing diapers, getting up with him or her at night (even when I'm too tired), singing to my baby, giving baths, taking him or her for walks.
- I can tell this little person how I feel. I may not get an answer, but he or she will hear.

- I am not bad if I am jealous of my baby. Many fathers experience jealousy toward their babies. This will pass.
- My new role as father and the responsibility I feel to support this family sometimes make me want to run, but I want to be here with my partner to see this baby grow up. I can handle these feelings.
- When I am tired and impatient, I take loving breaths and wait for these feelings to pass.
- Nothing I accomplish in the world can compare to the profound pleasure of spending time with my family.
- Even if I am not able to live with my child, I can still nurture and support him or her.
- My expectations of "father" need not interfere with the way I father this child.
- Being a good husband and a good father is being a good man.

Lovemaking

You may wonder if you'll ever again have time for sex. New babies keep you very busy, but love will find a way. It is important to wait until you have stopped bleeding completely before resuming sexual activity. Bleeding indicates that your cervix is still somewhat open. If you make love too soon, your uterus is vulnerable to bacteria that can be introduced during intercourse. Also allow time for the vaginal wall muscles to regain their strength and elasticity. Doing yoni exercises (see page 132) will speed up this process. Be certain any tiny skids, rips, or tears in or around your yoni have healed. If you had an episiotomy or a large tear, you will have to give yourself more time to heal.

Most doctors recommend that you wait at least six weeks before you make love. This is also the general rule in many cultures; it helps protect the newly postpartum woman from possible infection and discomfort. If you wish to make love very soon after birthing, first ask yourself if you are ready, emotionally and physically, to be sexual again. Then ask your midwife or doctor to take a look inside your vagina. If he or she sees that you are well healed, you'll get a go-ahead.

If you feel discomfort, it may be too soon for you to resume intercourse. You can make love without penetration. When you feel ready again, try having intercourse gently, taking plenty of time and experimenting with different positions. You need not rush into sexual activity after giving birth. When it feels right, you'll know you're ready. If discomfort or pain during lovemaking does not pass within a reasonable amount of time, two or more weeks, talk to your health-care giver.

Natural lubricants such as coconut oil or cocoa butter may be helpful because your body may not secrete as much mucus during sexual activity as you are accustomed to. To order Lover's Helper, an all-natural lubricant, contact Beverly's Gardens (see Reading and Resources). Don't worry if you are not as moist, and reassure your partner that it does not mean that you are not turned on. It is natural for breastfeeding mothers to be quite dry. Also, don't be alarmed if your

Ariel...A Father Sorting through the Confusion of Postpartum

It's a paradox for me. I thought I could be nurturing long-term, but my male part wants to provide. This brings up deep emotions from inside of me. Both sides of myself are looking at each other. One side is saying, "Hey, man, this is not your stuff. You're supposed to go out and make a living." I never had this before, this compulsion to be totally male in a socially acceptable sense. It's not what I want. I see that the either/or male society is not working, but it's difficult to break out of the roles in our heads.

It's very different to nurture. I feel my impulse is to bail out, to go out and fill the bank account. My heart says, "No, that's not what you started out to do." But it's what I feel. Ama wants the sharing, I think, more than the big bank account, just like I really want this sharing too. It is as if there's a major separation that happens when you have a child: mother nurturing, father providing.

It's a very delicate subject. It's yin and yang, a balancing act. Having experienced, in the past, many different ways of being in relationships, I thought I understood the balance. Now yin and yang with a child, that's something different. It's like both sides of the coin and also the edge of the coin. It's mixed up and it's not easy. Sometimes it gives me the postpartum blues.

It's as if having a child has made the male/female roles more clear. After Joël was one month old, I told Ama she had to let me have Joël in some way too. I was afraid I was not able to nurture him, like her, because I don't have tits. I was on the outside, looking in; knocking at the door, not knowing how to come into this intimacy. I'm not jealous, just looking from the outside at this mystery. So I walked with Joël every morning for breasts leak during lovemaking. This is a natural response to sexual stimulation and can be pleasurable for both partners.

You or your mate may be a bit shy at first. This is normal. One father said that he missed his wife's big belly and that he felt like he was having an affair with a skinny lady! You have both been through a major life passage. The birth of this child may leave the father in awe of your powerful ability to bring forth life. If

two to three, sometimes four, hours. I showed him the flowers and the horses. I showed him the trees. I held him right next to my heart. I did this, but seeing him breastfeeding and how he looked at her was something else.

So I can see how starting from this point, from the outside, it's easy for a man to stay out. This way he delegates the emotional role to the mother. It's the major mistake of our society, but it's very difficult to correct. It takes commitment, determination, endurance, and daily acceptance to put everything in balance.

Babies need caring and patience and so many things daily, for years. I see so many men who just give up. Daily I see it, so I find myself thinking, "Let me out." Now that I feel I got in, I want out. It's too dangerous. There's no me anymore. A man should know who he is and…I think Ama needs this, that I know. It's difficult to be both male and female, to be both assertive and open.

Nevertheless, I am doing it. Joël calls Ama and I both Mama and Daddy. It's funny, we have mixed the roles. The way Ama and I try to approach having a child is to nurture this guy. It's not easy, but I can see the fruits of our effort coming. Ama's patience and determination, my endurance to bear what I'm looking at. I see the light at the end of the tunnel, for a while I didn't see it, the light, just the tunnel. I had no idea raising a child would be like this. The idea to grow a child is one thing, the reality is another.

The other day a friend said, "Where is Joël? He is your hero, isn't he?" It went so deep. It's very true. I'm not running away from here—I'm not going anywhere.

this is his first baby, he is seeing you in a fresh way, as a sort of heroine. And you may have learned to love your mate in a deeper way now that you've had a child together. This increased feeling of devotion for one another may cause you both to feel bashful. Enjoy and play with this feeling of sweetness.

Many women who wrote to me said they did not want to make love for a long time (up to a year or more) following childbirth. They experienced pain and resentment surrounding the act of intercourse because they felt pressured by their husbands to perform the same sexual scripts they played before the pregnancy and birth roles that did not take into account these major life passages. Some of them felt obligated to satisfy their husbands. Others communicated their feelings to their partners who, for the most part, were understanding. If you feel you want to put off lovemaking for a while, this is your right. Trust that your sexual desires will resurface in good time and remain open to tenderness.

"I asked my midwife to examine me before I resumed sexual activity about three and a half weeks after my baby was born. She gave me a green light because my vaginal tissues were well healed. Nevertheless, when I did make love it was uncomfortable. We stopped and waited a few more days. The next time we tried, it was pleasurable. A few weeks later I felt little or no desire to be sexual. Maybe it was fatigue. Maybe it was hormones—I'm breastfeeding. My partner and I don't make love as much as he would like to these days. When we do, it's very tender. Sometimes I make love with my husband as a gift, when I don't really feel excited; this was my midwife's suggestion. Once we get going, I enjoy it too."

Jennifer

Single Mothers

"A mother alone is like a little bird who sits with her young on a dry twig. She always knows that the branch will crumble at any moment and her family will fly. She must, because of the nature of her life, always trust in the divine to catch her; she will not fall as her faith is in spirit not in the material world. This spiritual well she digs her grandchildren, and all the generations to come, will drink from. Her spiritual path is assured."

Mata Amritanandamayi

Many women today are choosing to become single mothers. They are consciously deciding not to wait until the right relationship or situation manifests to have children. Also, through divorce or the death of their mate, many women become single after they have had children. Whether a woman is a single mother by choice or circumstance, she travels a difficult road.

If you are a single mother, you have the full measure of joy and rewards enjoyed by women who have partners. Most likely you also are under increased financial stress, get far less support and nurturing, have less help around the house, and also get less sleep. On top of all of that, you may feel somewhat of an outcast in a society still geared toward the traditional, two-parent family.

Because you are giving constant loving attention to your baby, you need to be held (if you have more children, this need is greatly intensified). You need to be reassured. You need help—all on a daily basis. You may ask for help and receive some, but you feel the weight of your bottom-line responsibility.

Fortunately single mothers are banding together to help one another. Seek out other women who are sensitive to your problems and willing to share your trials and triumphs. Networking with other single mothers can bring great relief. The number of single mothers in America is increasing sharply. Perhaps community support and services for one-parent families will also increase. As things are today, single women with children must rely on each other for help in the home, child care, cooperative food purchasing, shared shelter, emotional support, and much more. Women are women's best and most available resource.

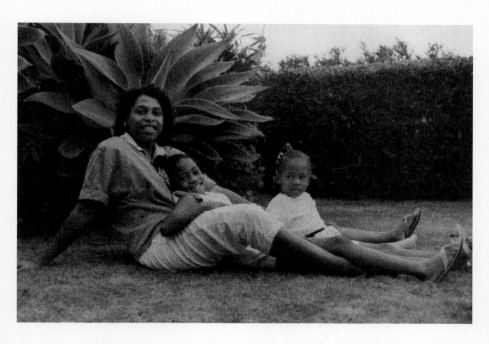

Ask your family to be truly supportive and nonjudgmental. They may have to let go of their vision of what families "should be" if they are to honor the family you have created.

You may worry about the quality of life you are able to give your children. Most single mothers do. If you have a son, you may wonder how he will find male role models, though there is no proof that male role models are necessary to raise healthy-minded adult males. Regardless whether you have sons or daughters, you may wish to look to your own father, brothers, and male friends to provide male companionship for your offspring.

There will be days when you feel you simply cannot cope. It may sound corny, but tomorrow is indeed another long, hard, but beautiful day. When life feels too tough, *elect* to feel peace instead of difficulty (it is often merely a matter of choosing). *Love Is Letting Go of Fear* (Berkeley, CA: Celestial Arts, 1979) by Gerald Jampolsky may help a single mother cope with her feelings of uncertainty and inspire in her an openness to trusting and loving.

Returning to Work

If you are planning to return to work after you have your baby, like many women it is likely that you plan to take a maternity leave of six to eight weeks. This may have seemed like a considerable amount of time before you had your baby, but as you adjust to your new role of mother you may be quickly discovering just how short a leave this is. For some mothers, the date they intend to return to work, even to a job they love, looms darkly in the too rapidly approaching future. First-time mothers cannot prepare themselves for the intense connection they will feel for their babies after giving birth and the intense pangs of separation they will experience upon being apart from their infants during the time they are at work.

Some women are able to extend their maternity leave by using vacation time, sick days, or taking an unpaid leave of absence. This extra time allows a mother to recuperate more fully physically, bond more closely with her baby, and, if she is nursing, to work out a routine that combines breastfeeding with bottle-feeding, either formula or expressed breast milk (see pages 94–97), for the feedings when she will not be present.

Though it is very common for mothers to return to work shortly after giving birth, many women carry with them the additional burden of judgment. You must always remember that you and other working mothers are good mothers who love your children. The decision to work outside the home is made in the light of many life circumstances known only to each woman and those close to her. Regardless of the reasons for returning to work, it is never easy to leave a young baby in another's care, but knowing that you have dependable, high-quality child care is a major factor that helps ease the transition. To function effectively at your job, you must trust completely that your baby is well nourished and given loving nurturing.

I recently bought carpet from a sales manager who had with her at work her three-year-old and six-month-old sons. I delighted in these boys' attempts to get all of mom's attention away from the customers. She was not having an easy time and explained wearily that she had recently discovered that her baby-sitter had been spanking her baby. She decided to take the boys to work with her until she could find the kind of day care she wanted for her children. She was fortunate that she was able to work this out with her employer, the owner—her father. Most working mothers do not have this flexibility built into their lives so they must be careful when selecting child care.

Remember, your baby will take in all that he or she hears and sees, and the day care you choose will have a profound impact. When choosing child care, it is important to follow your instincts. If you do not have a good feeling, even though you cannot say why, about the individual or center you are considering, do not entrust your child's care to them. Look farther. Make sure you screen the candidates carefully. Do they have first-aid training? How will they respond in an emergency situation? Do they have a license? Do they have references? Ask them for a medical release form. If they balk, look farther. If it is an agency that places nannies or a child-care center, are their employees bonded and licensed? Once you have chosen child care and have begun leaving your baby with them, make drop-in visits. These visits may be the only way you have to confirm that your choice was right. The following are some of the child-care options available to mothers.

- *Members of your family.* Your mother, father, sister, brother, or an aunt may prove to be the most caring person to watch your children if they live nearby and are willing.
- *Professional nannies.* For those families who can afford this option, a nanny who shares the parents' values and has good references is a godsend. Even if you go through an agency that screens its nannies, make sure you do your own thorough screening.
- *Private baby-sitting in the caregiver's home.* If you are checking into this option, make sure the house and yard are clean and safe for babies and small children. If there are animals in the neighborhood, what are their temperaments? Find

out who else will be there during the day, either to visit or to help care for the children. Are the other parents using this sitter satisfied? How long have they used this person's services? How many and what are the ages of the other children being watched? Will the children be exposed to television—how much and which programs? What will the children be given to eat? What happens if the baby-sitter becomes ill—what backup care will be available?

- *Privately owned and operated day-care centers.* Spend a good deal of time at the center before you leave your baby with them. I've seen day-care centers that are wonderful but have also seen some that are terrible. Make sure you check out the facility thoroughly and feel confident that this is where you want your baby to stay. What is the ratio of children to caregivers? Observe whether the caregivers are loving or indifferent in their interactions with the children. Are the babies' diapers changed promptly? How do the children relate to each other? What is the general level of health (are there a lot of runny noses)? What are the children fed? Are the building and grounds safe and clean? What kinds of activities will your child participate in? What is the general noise level?

- *Company owned and operated day-care facilities.* An option becoming more prevalent, this service is offered by employers to increase employee satisfaction and, therefore, employee efficiency. These facilities are often excellent and staffed with caring professionals. However, often they do not take children who are still in diapers, leaving the new mother in search of interim child care.

- *Job sharing with another mother or your baby's father.* This partnership allows each person to work part time while the other cares for the children. Your income may be only half of what it would be if you worked full time and you may not be entitled to full benefits, but you save the expense of child care and are able to spend more time with your baby. This option is limited to those whose employers are flexible and open to this concept.

Most mothers who return to jobs are able to work out the emotional issues as well as the logistic bugs and soon develop a balanced routine between career and home life. A simple piece of advice that has helped many new mothers is to place a good photograph of you *with* your baby where you can look at it throughout the workday. Talk to your coworkers about your birth and share your joy of having a new baby.

When you return to work, you will want to have a support network that will take up the slack for you in a pinch. Being called away from work at times to attend to an emergency involving your child is inevitable. Fortunately these emergencies are rarely more than an upset tummy or a bloody nose. Plan ahead.

Ask relatives and friends who don't work or who have different schedules than you if they will help out when one of these minor crises occurs. Have one or two coworkers that you can depend on lined up to take over for you if a serious situation that you must deal with personally does arise.

Remember that you are still postpartum and for weeks, even months, should pamper yourself. Rest is essential to enable you to juggle your job and your role as mother. Rest, rest, rest whenever you can. Ask your baby's father to share equally in the household chores.

If you take on the persona of superwoman, juggling too many balls too fast, you're apt to drop one if you don't slow down. If you feel working full time is too much for you, consider dropping back to part time. The financial compromise will be a bargain when you consider that the health and well-being of you, your baby, and your entire family hang in the balance.

Jealousy

According to psychiatrist Elisabeth Kübler-Ross, jealousy is a natural human emotion. If continually denied, it mushrooms into envy. Jealousy can actually be beneficial, but we have come to think of it in only negative terms because we often use jealousy synonymously with the word envy. Jealousy helps us learn. A child becomes jealous of another's ability to swim, so she strives until she too has the pleasure of swimming. Envy is characterized by ill will toward another because of their advantages or possessions. If your older children cannot fulfill their natural desire to have some of your attention and yet see the baby getting it, they will become envious.

Anyone can be jealous of the new baby. Siblings, fathers, pets, even the mother. Don't dismiss a family member's strong feelings. Talk about them and find ways to work through them.

To decrease sibling jealousy, create a special time when you focus your attention on each of your older children. This can be as simple as talking to them as you brush their hair. You may want to ask your closest friend to bring a small gift for an older child when she comes to visit. Many people will bring gifts for the baby, so let this friend help you remind your other children that they are remembered and still very special. Later, when the household becomes more settled, break the routine by taking one of the big brothers or sisters out for a special lunch or to a movie with Mom. Play with your children. In the summer, get someone to hold your baby so you can get into the water with your other children instead of sitting on the side and just watching all day. This may help prevent them from acting out their jealousy and allow your family to avoid disharmony. Also, give each of your children a chance to bond with the new baby. Encourage the brothers and sisters to spend individual, special time holding the baby. This shared caring will help siblings feel closer to the new member of their family.

Loneliness

Every woman who has had a child feels just how profoundly her life has changed— babies rock our boats! Yet even during this joyous, whirlwind period, many women find this is the loneliest time of their lives.

During your pregnancy, you very likely received special care and attention from your mate, family, doctor or midwife, doula, coworkers, and friends. Now that the birth is over, you may feel abandoned. Plus, a tiny, dependent person needs your care.

In cultures with extended families, this isolation did not occur often. Large families living under one roof meant that grandparents, aunties, uncles, and older siblings and cousins pitched in to help with the new addition. A mother may have had no privacy but had plenty of help and company.

Why have we not structured our modern society to alleviate postpartum loneliness and isolation? Our culture minimizes the importance of a strong family life. Fathers generally work outside of the home. Often mothers must also generate income to support the financial needs of her family by working full or part time. Children above the age of five or six often participate in public education or attend private schools. This means that a mother and infant may spend their days alone in a neighborhood that is abandoned early each morning and reinhabited each evening by people who feel too rushed to do much more than wave. (A grass-roots movement is afoot to reduce the isolation of our present society. Some of the solutions people have created to break out of the current structure are cottage industries, home schooling, and small family farms. Creating a lifestyle different from the norm takes courage and commitment but has many rewards.)

One solution to the loneliness you may be feeling is to extend your family. Ask your grandmother or an elderly person from your neighborhood to visit. Older people often suffer from loneliness too. They'll have wonderful tips and tricks about mothering to share with you. Your sisters, brothers, and friends won't mind your asking for help and time. Ask your mate to give extra nurturing. Seek out other mothers; they are lonely too. Many women have met other mothers by putting notes on bulletin boards where other new mothers are likely to go, by joining dance or exercise classes for postpartum women, or by going to the children's story hours at local libraries. Go to places where mothers frequently take their children and open up to others who may be lonely. You will find dear friends to share your joy and help to shoulder your burdens.

Postpartum Blues

After birthing, the tremendous physical, hormonal, emotional, spiritual, and psychological changes of postpartum will make your heart feel tender. At the time you gave birth, you lost your placenta, which accounts for a steep drop in serum estrogen and progesterone, two of the hormones provided by the placenta to maintain pregnancy. Within twenty-four hours of birthing, the levels of these hormones fall to a tiny fraction of what your body has become accustomed to. Therefore, do not be surprised by the tears that may seem to come often. The smallest smile from your baby's lips may make you burst out crying. Your partner rushing off to work may be perceived by you as a brush-off. This could make you sad and bring you to tears.

Because mothering an infant is a round-the-clock job, you may feel exhausted. Fatigue will make your emotions even more raw. Try not to judge the tears. Let them wash like healing waters over your heart. The spiritual seeds you planted during pregnancy have sprouted. They need watering now. As these seedlings grow into strong trees, the flood of tears will slow to a trickle. However, don't expect to be just the same as you were before you had a baby. You were pregnant for nine months; you'll be postpartum for the rest of your life. This is good news. Your changes are all part of a divine plan, which makes strong and sensitive mothers for the next generation. Along with the birth of every child comes the rebirth of the mother. Transitory "postpartum blues" affects from five hundred to eight hundred women per thousand births. This is from 50 to 80 percent of all new mothers. The onset is usually one to three days postpartum.[1]

We cannot ignore the fact that most women become "blue" when their milk comes in. The third day postpartum is characterized by hormonal changes. In many countries midwives say, "When the tears flow, the milk will flow." Thus the "blues" are actually a very normal physical, mental-emotional, spiritual, behavioral response to having a baby. Most women are "blue" in the immediate postpartum. The rocky emotions will find stability as your hormones settle down. The tenderness of heart you feel may never go away. You'll always be more sensitive; this makes you a better mother.

Adjusting to your new baby is both exciting and exhausting. It's a huge undertaking. While your heart and mind adjust to your new role as mother, your body is going through immense changes. Take all of this into consideration when you feel emotional.

Symptoms of Postpartum "Blues" May Include Any of the Following: [2]
- Lack of sleep*
- No energy*
  (*The above two are also just part of having a new baby.)
- Food cravings or loss of appetite
- Feeling tired even after sleep
- Anxiety, excessive worry
- Confusion, nervousness
- Concern over your physical changes
- Feeling "I'm not myself, this isn't me"
- Lack of confidence
- Sadness
- Feeling overwhelmed
- Crying more than usual
- Hyperactivity or excitability
- Oversensitivity
- Feeling easily hurt
- Irritability
- Lack of feeling or overconcern for the baby

  If the above feelings extend beyond what you feel is a reasonable amount of time, and if the severity increases with time, start talking about it; share with anyone who will not judge you.

Homeopathic remedies, Bach Flower remedies, and herbs have helped many women soothe the "blues." Shatavari and rehmannia, two Ayurvedic herbs (see pages 231 and 232) that are high in female hormones, calm the emotions while they tone the uterus. Ingesting the placenta as some women do in other cultures helps restore some of these lost hormones and nutrients. Naturopathic physicians, doctors of Chinese medicine, herbalists, and many midwives can provide you with a remedy.

Herbs for Coping with the "Blues"...
- Licorice root—helps balance one's hormones
- Red raspberry leaf—increases calcium, which is calming—tones the uterus

- Rosemary—increases milk flow and elevates calcium
- Skullcap—soothing, strengthening, calming—elevates calcium

These herbs are easily available at health-foods store and apothecaries.

Steep in water to make tea, sip frequently. (See page 151, Herbs for the Postpartum Woman.)

Watch your diet. Low blood sugar has been associated with the "blues." Eating well and feeling well go hand in hand. Beware of sugary treats that give you a fast lift but then cause your emotions to crash when blood sugar dips to overcompensate for the sugar rush.

Regarding transitory postpartum "blues," remember that as your body stabilizes and regains its pre-pregnancy chemistry, your emotions will too. Don't be alarmed if you are weepy, cranky, moody or just plain downhearted until this process is complete. Your moods may swing from elation to depression. Remind yourself and your family that you need lots of compassion now. Don't browbeat yourself because you think you should be on cloud nine instead of down in the dumps.

There is an old wives' tale that Mary, mother of Jesus, often wore blue. Perhaps blue is the color that best embodies the bittersweet experience of mothering. A

Coping with Postpartum "Blues"

- Make sure you get enough rest.
- Do something for yourself each day.
- Look at your diet. Are you getting what you need nutritionally?
- Eliminate caffeine, sugar, and excess salt.
- Eat three main meals per day *and* three small meals in between.
- Eat high-protein snacks to fight fatigue and depression.
- Get together with a friend or loved one each day. Avoid isolation.
- Seek the support of other women who have had the "blues."
- Exercise, even a little, daily. Stretch, try yoga, walk, dance; the body toners in this book are wonderful.
- Relax, meditate, pray, read an inspirational book, breathe.
- Enjoy the out-of-doors. Dig in your garden, smell the flowers.
- Let some things go. It isn't a crime to leave dishes in the sink or laundry in the basket.
- If things get out of hand or you feel unable to cope, seek professional help. There is nothing to be ashamed of.

woman knows that she brings her child into a world that is both beautiful and imperfect.

Postpartum Depression

Somewhere between thirty to two hundred postpartum women per thousand births suffer from postpartum depression (PPD). That is an estimated 3 to 20 percent of birthing women. For those who have had PPD, reoccurrence after subsequent births is 10 to 35 percent.

The onset of depression may occur at anytime after delivery. The symptoms of PPD may last from a few weeks to several months. For about 4 percent of women suffering from PPD, symptoms persist for as long as one year.[3]

There is great need for further research in postpartum depression and its causes. By accessing the Web site for Postpartum Support International (www.postpartum.net), one can find much helpful information including an article called "An Introduction to Postpartum Illness" by Lawrence Krukman and Susan Smith.

One cause of PPD, currently the focus of research, concerns the hormonal/biological changes a woman experiences postpartum.[4] This research has been found both problematic and controversial as there are always individual variations in hormone levels. Also, researchers have found only a potential not a direct link between postpartum hormones and depression.[5]

Other causes of PPD may include traumatic childbirth experiences [6] as well as social, economic, and interpersonal factors.[7] There seems to be a ray of hope in the current bio-cultural research in PPD. This holistic approach looks at the biochemical action surrounding birth as well as the family structure, values, beliefs, and rituals surrounding childbearing.[8]

Some anthropologists believe that mothers in non-Western rural cultures with large extended supportive families do not suffer the symptoms of PPD the way women in the West do. In 1998, Lawrence Krukman extended his argument stating that rituals may cushion or prevent PPD. He gave several reasons.[9]

- Rituals channel powerful emotions like fear associated with childbirth.
- Rituals solidify the role of mother.
- Through rituals, responsibilities, attitudes, and techniques for parenting are taught.
- Group participation in rituals rally the physical support and spiritual attention crucial to the new mother.

Thus pregnancy, birth, and postpartum are celebrated in community. This is in shocking contrast to the isolated modern Western "civilized" mother who shoulders the responsibilities of new motherhood in isolation. My own field experience, including six years of midwifery work in Indonesia and one year in the Philippines, leads me to believe that cultures that honor motherhood, support breastfeeding and bonding, and provide families with spiritually uplifting rituals surrounding the occurrence of a new baby have less occurrence of PPD.[10] I can't help but attribute it to the culturally and spiritually rich, family-centered village life. I did however find Balinese and Filipino women suffer from "the blues" with about the same frequency as Western women.

Personal experience and research into the causes and treatment of PPD confirm that every woman is unique. Her circumstances are unique. Her biochemistry is unique. Among women suffering with PPD, there are degrees of severity. It comes and goes along a continuum of reactions.

We women must listen to our bodies. Physical symptoms are related to brain chemistry and our bodies do not give us messages for no reason.

Symptoms of Postpartum Depression May Include: [11]
- Headaches
- Numbness, tingling in the limbs
- Chest pains, heart palpitations
- Hyperventilating
- Despondency or feelings of despair
- Feelings of inadequacy
- Inability to cope
- Hopelessness
- Helplessness
- Impaired concentration or memory
- Loss of normal interests
- Thoughts of suicide
- Bizarre or strange thoughts
- Panic attacks
- Hostile behavior
- New fears or phobias
- Intrusive, bizarre, or strange thoughts
- Nightmares
- Exaggerated guilt that doesn't go away
- Fear of not bonding with baby

- Overconcern for baby
- Feeling "out of control," i.e., not being able to perform the simple tasks
- Having no joy
- Feeling like you are "going crazy"

There is a certain normal "feeling crazy." You may not actually be going crazy, but it's a commonly used term. Remember, mothering is a process of "letting go." Mothers need people who are nonjudgmental to help them evaluate what degree of loss of control one is experiencing. With help from friends and family as well as professional assessment, new mothers challenged with depression can get the assistance necessary to come to terms with PPD.

Over 90 percent of postnatally depressed women sense that something is wrong. Sadly only 20 percent report their symptoms to a health-care provider.

Postpartum Psychosis

Postpartum psychosis is relatively rare, occurring on an average of one to two per thousand births, approximately 1 percent. Onset is sudden and severe, usually within the first month postpartum, though there are cases that set in later; 80 percent of the cases set in within three to fourteen days postpartum.

This is a medical emergency that requires immediate hospitalization and medication. The mother's life and the baby's life are in jeopardy. There is risk of suicide, infanticide, or both.

Symptoms of Postpartum Psychosis May Include: [12]
- Refusal to eat
- Agitation, fatigue
- Inability to stop activity
- Frantic excessive energy, hyperactivity
- Extreme confusion
- Delusions
- Feelings of hopelessness and shame
- Loss of memory
- Incoherence, rapid speech
- Bizarre hallucinations, hearing voices
- Suspiciousness
- Irrational statements
- Alterations in mood
- Preoccupation with trivia

Postpartum psychosis, though rare, is all too real if it is happening to you. Do not be ashamed to seek the help you need. Usually a mother who is experiencing postpartum psychosis does not recognize her illness. It will most likely be your significant others, friends, and family members who become aware that something is not right. It is they who *must* intervene and guide the mother suffering from postpartum psychosis toward the help and treatment she needs. Postpartum psychosis differs from postpartum depression in onset, symptoms, and severity. Both PPD and postpartum psychosis are treatable, and women who suffer from these illnesses need and deserve help from a care provider familiar with postpartum disorders.

DEPRESSION PREVENTION FOR NEW MOTHERS

While you're still pregnant, learn all you can about pregnancy, birth, postpartum, and parenting. Read, attend classes when available, get to know other couples with children.

Rest is essential in the postpartum time; this means you'll need help with all the day-to-day chores. Depend upon your partner, friends, and relatives.

Reach out for wise women in your community; they will gladly help and impart their experience in childbearing.

Let the little things go. Unimportant tasks will only increase your stress.

Absolutely do not move house or relocate soon after your baby is born.

Let yourself go natural. Don't be overconcerned with appearances. The natural look of a glowing mother is far more beautiful than the carefully made-up look.

Take naps, meditate, pray. All these forms of deep rest are essential. You must rest your body and rest your soul too.

Keep it simple. Friends and relatives should be encouraged to keep their visits short. They can help out when they come, i.e., bring a meal, fold laundry, then leave you to your rest. The last thing a new mother needs to do is play hostess.

Talk it over. Discuss your feelings with your husband, women friends, your mom or aunt, whomever you trust to share your worries and concerns.

Trim back unnecessary responsibilities.

Choose to breastfeed; ample prolactin, which is what breastfeeding moms have more of, seems to be a component in maintaining emotional stability in the postpartum.[13] Postpartum researchers L. Kruckman and S. Smith say, "It is reasonable to assume a possible relationship exists between the decline of breastfeeding in the U.S., the rapid decline in prolactin in mothers who do not breast-feed and postpartum depression."[14] This important relationship requires

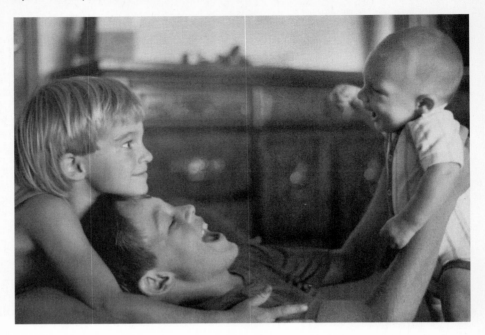

more research. It should be said, however, that breastfeeding does not make a woman immune to PPD.

Rearrange schedules to ensure your rest is respected, and that your baby's natural rhythm of rest and activity is easily followed.

Don't lose yourself. Whatever makes you tick will keep your spirit going strong when times are tough. An artist must make art. I, for one, must write. Some mothers sing, garden, read. The list of creative expressions that mothers excel at is endless. Without getting stressed out, little by little, make some time for that special part of you. By following your star, you teach your child to dream and reach for those dreams.

As early as you can in the pregnancy choose good caregivers—midwives, doctors, chiropractors, acupuncturists, and others who share values with you. Having a network of trustworthy people who can help when you need them can really help families cope during challenging times.

Share the responsibility, share the joy. Letting others—your mate, family, friends—help out with the baby will decrease your stress while increasing happiness for all.

Know your personal and family mental health and stress-trauma history. This includes any alcoholism, substance abuse, eating disorders, sexual abuse, or unresolved grief. If your mother, aunts, or sisters suffered from PMS, depression, and/or PPD, be alert and take the above advice very seriously, as you may be at increased risk for PPD. The body and the brain remember trauma, denial keeps us resilient, but the birth process alters our biochemistry so significantly that old scars can resurface.

The challenges of postpartum are too many to write about. As a new mother, you must heal your body, strengthen your soul, sharpen your mind, manage your time wisely, and juggle the life you had before the baby's arrival with the life you now lead. It's a heck of a lot of work. Generation after generation, women have been doing it.

Take into consideration that never before in "her-story" have postpartum women been so alone. Modern American women face the reality of doing a job that demands one's full attention twenty-four hours a day, seven days a week, without the support of tribe or village or community. The isolation can be devastating. This is why I urge you to reach out and network with other mothers. Because there can be no cash value placed on mothering, people tend to forget how very essential and valuable an at-home mother is.

It is up to us women to redefine the value of motherhood in our individual homes, communities, in our country. We can broaden our political pro-motherhood reach by supporting projects that lower the risk of maternal and infant mortality and protect the integrity of breastfeeding internationally. We are the caregivers for the future generation; in a very real way, it's our world to heal and to change.

One of the miracles of postpartum is this: With every baby, we find ourselves growing wise and growing young, all at once. In an average day, a mother may wear the hat of an expert nutritionist, a singer of children's songs, an accountant, and a bicycle repairperson. Sometimes it's a rocky road, littered with dirty laundry and sleepless nights, broken kites and bumps along the way. Life's windstorms burnish us and teach us to glow.

Joseph Campbell wrote of the "dark side of parenting," suggesting that the birth of our offspring is powerful portent of our own mortality. As parents, we become aware of the fragility of life. Yes, life is precious and fragile, and it is also tough and tenacious. Loving our children teaches us all of this and more than can ever be articulated here. Nothing we did in the way of preparing for childbirth could prepare us for the power of our emotions concerning the baby. When we look for the first time into our baby's eyes, we meet our teacher. We meet our highest and largest and smallest self. We meet the stranger we have always known. We meet the universe in a tiny newborn hand.

Fred...A Husband Coping with His Wife's Postpartum Depression

I had lost my job and we had a baby on the way. Then a couple of weeks after our son was born, Samantha fell apart.

She began to smoke cigarettes in a big way. She was frustrated and angry. I just didn't know what was going on. The cigarette smoking became an issue between us. I didn't handle it well and couldn't back off. This was a big mistake, not backing off from the smoking issue. It was all tied up with my protective feelings for our baby. We would fight. It was an outlet for my own frustration and anger. The combination of financial stress and no sleep—this baby just didn't sleep much—was devastating to both her and me.

This went on for months. Samantha was abusive to me. It made no sense. I was trying to be nurturing, and I took on extra responsibilities. I'd try to be there. I'd try to be kind. I was unable to reach her on any level. I just didn't have the skills. I didn't know how to nurture her. In my personal self-image, I was this wonderful, strong, responsible, supportive guy. I took care of the baby, the house, and got into my job, working at home, all for her. I thought I deserved some kind of medal of merit. All I got was Samantha's anger and rejection. It was a dead-end feeling trying to nurture her.

We knew we needed help, but we'd have to pay for it. All the help we did get, we had to pay for. There were no social services or friends who were really able to reach out for us. We were sinking.

The selfless, unconditional love you give your baby will transform you. All this love when directed at the baby, who is after all the mirror of your heart, will bounce back and nourish you. Love is self-sustaining. Motherhood in short is an everyday miracle, proof that "love conquers all!"

Postpartum is an individual experience, yet there are aspects, flavors that all new mothers share. It is a precious time. Time to reinvent yourself. You are the artist, the canvas. Think of your baby as the paint, and at the end of the day, you two together are the masterpiece.

On top of it all, Samantha hid her depression, and mine, from her closest friends. Had her friends known how deeply troubled we were, they might have helped.

Finally we went in to see a doctor. He showed a spiritual caring. We went in for a regular appointment, and he ended up listening to us for over two hours. He knew we were in crisis. He recognized my part in the drama and gave me a pat on the back. I had needed so much to be heard.

Nobody had an easy solution. Drugs were prescribed for Samantha to help her cope with the suffering. It was total hell for all of us.

We both had big things to learn about our relationship that had gotten mixed in with the postpartum depression. When a couple goes through something like this, people legitimately give lots of attention to the woman. As with any codependent relationship, no one partner is the hub of the problem. Samantha's postpartum depression was not the entire problem.

For other men who may be going through this, get help! You can't get it from your wife. You need support from outside the family because you're having to be supportive all the time within it.

Now, several years later, we're just starting to work through all of it. The scars are there, but we're healing.

Postpartum Support International
Jane Honikman, founder
927 N. Kellogg Avenue
Santa Barbara, CA 93111
(805) 967E/N7636
Fax: (805) 967-0608
E-mail: jhonikman@earthlink.net

or: Sonia Murdock, president
109 Udall Road
West Islip, NY 11795
(631) 422E/N2255
Fax: (631) 422-1643
E-mail: postpartum@aol.com

See Postpartum Support International's Web site (www.postpartum.net) for the most up-to-date information on how to find a postpartum support group in your area, both in the U.S. and abroad.

Recommended reading for women wishing to establish a postpartum support group in their area: *Step by Step* by Jane Honikman. Available directly from Jane for $20.00 including postage (address above).

Miscarriage

"When I was little, before my brothers and sisters were born, my mom had a miscarriage. She told me she lost the baby. The next day I heard a song on the radio that said: 'Taking all I got and now you're leaving...oh, baby, don't go!' I cried and cried. I didn't want to lose our baby."

Déjà, age nine

Miscarriage is common—so common that the percentage of pregnancies that end in miscarriage is not known; perhaps that is why it is too often brushed off as "no big deal." But it is a big deal, physically and emotionally. True, some very early miscarriages go almost unnoticed; yet many miscarriages are felt deeply by the woman and often by her mate and by her children. A woman may feel a deep sense of emptiness, concern that she may never be able to have a child, a nagging feeling of failure, worry that she did not provide healthy genetic material, and the baby was not "perfect." These and countless other emotions may flood through you if you've had a miscarriage. Let loose the tears and release some of these feelings.

Bleeding, even slight bleeding or dark brown discharge, is a warning signal that a threat of miscarriage is present. (The technical term for miscarriages during the first trimester is spontaneous abortion.) Don't panic, but call your health-care giver immediately. Up to 50 percent of women bleed at some point during their pregnancy. Rest in bed for twenty-four hours. Do not engage in intercourse until the threat of possible miscarriage has passed. (Consult your health-care provider for more information.) If no further bleeding or cramping is observed, your pregnancy will probably proceed normally.

If you bleed profusely and have intense cramping, a miscarriage is inevitable. If you expel clots, a fetus, afterbirth, or tissue, save them in a sterile container if possible and bring them to your doctor for testing. In the event of an incomplete miscarriage, you will probably need medical attention to remove the remaining tissue. In some cases, tissue that did not pass out immediately decays and sloughs off naturally. If any tissue remains inside the uterus, you are in danger of developing a bacterial infection or hemorrhaging. Usually the only sign of an incomplete miscarriage is vaginal bleeding that continues for two days or more after clots and/or a fetus has been expelled. You must monitor yourself carefully during a miscarriage. If you suspect you are bleeding too much, cramping too intensely, or if you feel uncertain about your condition, you should see your health-care giver immediately.

An incomplete miscarriage may make it necessary for you to undergo dilation and curettage (D & C). In this procedure, the cervix is dilated and either scraping or suction is used to free the lining of the uterus of any remaining tissue. A D & C, which usually takes fifteen to twenty minutes, can be done under local or general anesthesia.

Prayer for Lydia and David

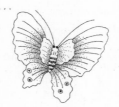

A sunny child is playing in the garden.
She sings, smiles to her mother,
chases the cottontail of the rabbit.
Watch her as she runs dancing
between tulips and the orange trees.

In the house, a flow of blood,
an angel taking a tiny soul
back to the house of her ancestors
along a trail of shooting stars.

Listen, an invisible voice
is singing to you.
My prayer is that she will return.

For now, turn your eyes
to olive trees, blood red roses,
sunflowers blooming in the garden.
Let the universe hold you in her arms.

Diane Frank

In the event of a miscarriage, keep in mind that you are postpartum. A birth has taken place, though you may have been early in your pregnancy. Afterward you do not have the fulfillment of having a child to care for, which is all the more reason you should be well taken care of. It is a time of grieving, a time of healing. Sometimes it is important to have a small funeral or personal ritual for the lost child. Plant some flowers in his or her honor. Light a candle, and offer a prayer or a poem.

After a miscarriage, it is best to wait two or three menstrual cycles before trying to conceive again. If a woman has had three or more consecutive miscarriages, the same problem may have caused them all. There are many reasons for repeated miscarriages—some of them being hormonal insufficiency, nutritional problems, environmental pollution, or cervical dysfunction, when the cervix is not able to hold the baby inside the uterus. Many of these problems can be overcome with your doctor's or midwife's help. Doctors of Chinese medicine and homeopaths are skilled at helping women prevent future miscarriages. Look into visiting one before you attempt to achieve pregnancy again. It will take courage, determination, and lots of support and faith to continue with your childbearing plans if you have suffered multiple disappointments.

> "I've had many miscarriages. Some in the first trimester, others late, even toward the end of pregnancy. I've wept for all my lost babies. Through it all, I kept praying for the big family my husband and I so much wanted. We now have five living children, and seven who are with God. After this last baby girl was born, her daddy went out into the yard and cried. She looked so much like our little daughter, Mikel, who was born too soon."
>
> *Jan*

After a Voluntary Abortion

Voluntary abortions are physically and emotionally difficult. The decision to discontinue a pregnancy is not an easy one. Having an abortion does not mean that you won't be a wonderful parent someday. You probably will never forget the child that you did not have, but you can honor the pregnancy that did not come to fruition by giving excellent care and unconditional love to the children you do choose to bring into this world. It is important for couples to be supportive and gentle with one another when an abortion has occurred. Try not to lay blame. Don't become victims of guilt. Grieving is a very important part of the healing process. Be patient and kind to yourselves. Talk it out, cry it out. If you don't have a partner with whom you can share your grief, ask a friend or family member to support you. When deciding whether to terminate a pregnancy or not, remember…having the baby will indeed change your life forever. Having an abortion will also change your life forever.

Premature Babies

Neither you nor your baby was prepared for birth, but your pregnancy was interrupted and birth took place. You may feel your baby was torn from your body, particularly if you had planned a natural birth. You may be separated from your baby for long periods of time while she receives specialized health services and/or surgery. Your baby's pain is your pain. Coping with your feelings of anger, guilt, depression, shock, and denial will be challenging. How premature your baby is, what his or her unique physical status is, and the availability of quality health services determine the degree of complexity and grief you must face.

You have good reason to remain hopeful. Most premature babies do live. Survival rates range from 80 to 90 percent. Babies born two pounds or under, who had no chance of survival just ten years ago, now have a fifty-fifty chance. You may be concerned about the quality of life your child will enjoy if he is left with handicaps from the early birth, and only time will determine his future condition. Even if your baby does not survive, you may hold in your heart that you have grown and your life has been enriched by becoming a mother.

All of this is a lot to integrate while your body attempts to return to its pre-pregnancy state. Because your pregnancy did not last full term, your body is somewhat confused and you need to take special care to rest and recuperate, even in the face of extreme stress. If your baby cannot suckle and you are pumping your breasts to nourish her, you are faced with a frustrating and sometimes painful, self-sacrificing routine. Yet nourishing your child is something you can do for your baby, and mothers of premature babies often receive a great deal of comfort from doing so. If your baby is in the hospital, perhaps at great risk of dying, you may feel helpless and in the way. Remember, your presence near your child at the hospital is essential. The life force in your love may be his only advantage.

If you have a partner, you and he must accept this family crisis and the fact that it is just beginning. The stress and worry over your baby's health and the financial realities of hospital bills can alienate you from each other unless you stand together, strong in your love. Hold and comfort one another. Some mothers of premature babies are single. If you are single, look for someone who will give you the emotional support you need and help you in your grief. *The Premature Baby Book* (New York: St. Martin's Press, 1983) by Helen Harrison and Ann Kositsky is an excellent guide for parents who must cope with the difficulties of having a premature infant.

If Your Baby Has Died

Here are some rituals you may wish to do now that your baby has died. You may ask the hospital staff for their assistance in enabling you to perform these and other steps that will help you through your grieving.

- Spend private time holding your baby's body.
- Encourage your baby's father to be there with you.
- Kiss your baby.
- Talk to him or her.
- Name your baby.
- Take a picture that you can keep forever.
- Keep anything that you treasure and that can help you cope: the baby's hospital bracelet, clothing, etc.

Special Children and Children Who Have Died

If your baby has health problems, is handicapped in any way, or has died, your life is entirely different from that of many new mothers. Along with the myriad of emotional and physical aspects associated with becoming a mother, you have grief. You may feel utterly alone, betrayed by God. You may feel guilt and be thinking, "If only I had done something differently, my baby might be okay."

You can reach out, seek loving support, but this will not take away the grief entirely. You must allow the tears to flow and the anger to erupt for healing to begin. *Remember the Secret* by Elisabeth Kübler-Ross (Berkeley, CA: Celestial Arts, 1988), which helps children cope with the loss of a sibling or any loved one, has helped many families through this difficult time.

If you have a special child, if your baby is sick or has died, you can receive support by networking with other families who are grieving. The names and addresses of support organizations and books are listed in Reading and

Resources at the back of this book, or visit the Compassionate Friends Web site: http://www.compassionatefriends.org.

Mothers Who Relinquish Their Babies for Adoption

Sometimes a woman must make the heartbreaking decision to relinquish her child for adoption. When this happens, the mother must hold in her heart the knowledge that she has given her child the gift of a body. She has been the instrument through which a life was possible. It takes tremendous love and courage to give life, and then to pass the child to someone else to provide for his or her future.

If you are faced with the decision to relinquish your baby, your feelings will cover a large range. You may fear for your baby's future as well as your own. You will feel judged by many. The far reaches of your spiritual strength will be tested. In *Adoption: A Handful of Hope* (Berkeley, CA: Celestial Arts, 1990), Suzanne Arms reaches out to both birth parents and adoptive parents as well as to adopted children.

When You've Lost Yourself

Many women with children feel at times that they have lost themselves. This does not occur just in the first weeks or months postpartum. Years after becoming a mother, you may suddenly and profoundly feel you've lost your identity, that you don't know who you are except somebody's mother. This doubt can come over a woman even when she is progressing with her life goals. Along with the feeling of loss of self, emotional numbness often pervades.

This is the time to breathe deeply and feel your body. If the tears come, allow them to flow. A heart-to-heart talk with another mother is usually the perfect prescription. Share your feelings; you will find that other mothers feel these things too, and your words and thoughts will lift their hearts as theirs lift yours.

Western culture is obsessed with individuality, which may compound the problem many women face. It may help you to remember that in Eastern cultures, the universal self, which is a kind of selflessness, rather than individuality, is prized. Saint Francis of Assisi wisely said, "[I]t is in dying to self that we are born again to eternal life."

Healing the Past

When you become a mother, you face a new depth of intimacy. All your relationships, including the one you have with yourself, will reflect this depth. With depth comes healing of past emotional wounds. The healing process can be painful sometimes, particularly if you have many bad experiences and emotional scars from the past.

Pregnancy, birth, and postpartum have left you openhearted. So whether you feel ready for it or not, your process of healing may be upon you now. If you were abused as a child, your new role as a parent may bring these memories to the surface. Be patient with yourself. Allow for your own tenderness and vulnerability.

Seek loving and supportive help. Don't be ashamed if at times you cry and feel you cannot cope. Friends, family members, clergy, and professional therapists can be an immense help. If the cost of professional therapy is prohibitive, free Twelve-Step programs exist in virtually every community across the country. To find out more, look for Alcoholics Anonymous (AA) in your phone directory. One need not be an alcoholic or an addict to benefit from the Twelve-Step process. AA also provides extremely low-cost individual therapy services. Victims of child abuse who wish to break the generational cycle may wish to contact Adult Children of Alcoholics (ACA). Victims of abuse may also find support organizations by calling the local crisis lines that are usually listed near the front of phone directories.

Keeping a Postpartum Journal

To put a child on Earth, an immense amount of creative intelligence flowed from the Great Spirit through nature itself into your body, heart, and mind—remaining, now, as an integral part of your own spirit. This energy is yours forever. Like a pocket, deep and filled with magic seeds of creativity and healing, this is the source of unconditional loving from which every wise woman since the beginning of time has drawn her strength.

As a mother, the chores of your everyday life will put your spiritual potential into practice. A wise woman has a master's degree in diapering, a doctorate in daily bread!

By keeping a postpartum journal, you map out and empower your spiritual, emotional, intellectual, and physical well-being. Birthing has opened a door to personal healing, and for many women, keeping a journal takes them through that door.

Choose or create a book with no lines on the pages (this will help free your thoughts). Make it a safe and sacred place into which you pour your feelings. Years ago when I was struggling with my first baby and suffering from a painful bout of clogged milk ducts, my friend Jane, pregnant with her fourth, brought out her "secret" journal and shared it with me over tea and cookies. We laughed ourselves silly—and cried too. I learned of her mistakes and triumphs and of the many little ways she had learned to cope with a life so simple and so profound. As Jane shared her healing process, I began to feel my own heart and body gain strength (and my milk once again flowed from me painlessly). This is the wise woman way, which you can experience too.

Put a favorite photograph of yourself in your postpartum journal. Decorate the pages with your words, your drawings, your dreams. Write loving letters to your baby. Draw yourself as a child, as you are now, and as you will be in old age. Write a story about a day in your life when you are eighty-two. Write about your own mother. (How are you different from her and how are you the same?). Use five words to describe each of your loved ones. (My four-year-old daughter once described a family friend as "praying, sugarcane, bird, lipstick, grass.") Your own words will illuminate the poetry in your closest relationships. Make lists of your life as it is now, of what you are calling into your life, and of what you are leaving behind. Honestly express your expectations—how they've been met and how they can be met. Write how being a mother has changed and challenged you. Write a letter to the man in your life, telling him what kind of woman you are; tell him what kind of lover and father you wish him to be, and tell him what you appreciate and love about him. If you are not with a man, write about the kind of partner you may wish to draw into your life. Draw your dream place and write about it. Draw and write about your animal spirit guide and your guardian angels—invite them to become a vital part of your existence, ask them to protect you and to help you in your mothering role. Write your own poems; fill them with your freshened feelings for the everyday objects in your life like teapots, roses, refrigerators, receiving blankets, dogs. Take notice of how the smallest details have become profound now that you are a mother. Use your postpartum journal to let yourself go! Write about and draw your wildest dreams, and give yourself the power to make them come true.

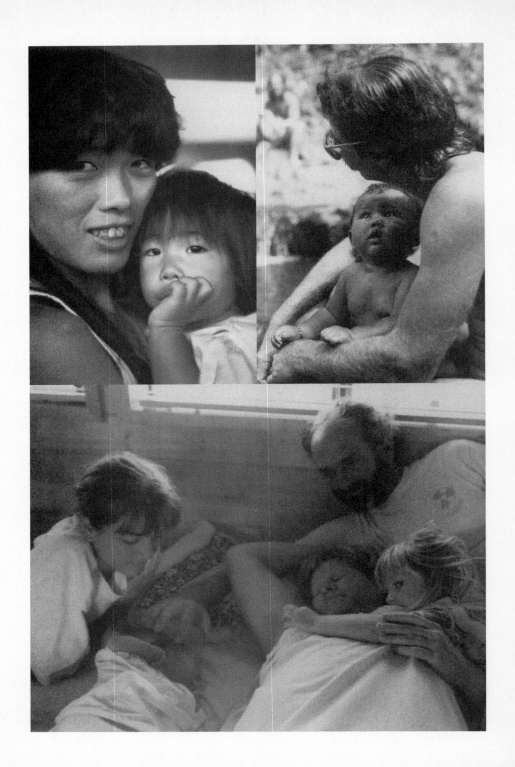

CHAPTER 17

Shared Stories

While writing this book, I was blessed to have the trust of hundreds of postpartum women. Every mother I met or with whom I corresponded had her story. (Each one of you also has a heroine's courage and your own story. Chapters 2 and 18 provide space for you to write it down.) Some of these women were teenagers, some were in their forties, and the others were every age in between. They gave me their honesty. We shared pain and joy.

I offer my heartfelt thanks to the mothers who have given this book life. Here are a few of their stories.

"Love is delicate, and, at the same time, it is most vital and strong. A tiny, tender wave of love rocks the boat of life."

Maharishi Mahesh Yogi

"I lost everything in the post-natal depression."

Erma Bombeck

Jane...Her Firstborn

I remember holding our daughter, precious and small, bringer of great joy to our home, who made us a family. The love I had felt for her as she grew inside me had been so wonderful. I hadn't been able to imagine how much greater it would become when she actually emerged from my womb into this world.

My husband was with us throughout the birth—even though the labor was thirty-six hours long! Right from birth, our daughter slept through the night. At the hospital, we had "rooming-in," so she was always beside me in a little glass-walled basinette. I remember those mornings of our seven-day hospital stay (extra long so I could recuperate from my long labor). I'd wake up early with a tingly feeling in my nipples. I would look over at our baby. She would just be starting to get hungry—her eyes still closed but her lips moving in those sucking motions. I was happy that we were so tuned in to each other—she didn't have to cry; just an easy transition from sleep to breakfast in Mommy's arms.

At home, one experience stands out as a lesson that I'm still learning (seven years and one child later). I was holding our daughter, maybe a few weeks old, and she was fussing. I tried all the "usuals"—she wasn't hungry or wet or being poked by a pin. I was rocking her, walking with her, sitting down and jiggling her, and all the while my mind was racing: "Why was she crying? What was wrong? What could I do?"

Then, like a blessing, the thought, "Go inside," came to mind. Instantly the baby calmed. That one thought of truth—a reminder of the spiritual love and peace that is inside all of us—changed the whole atmosphere. Insecurities and nagging worries couldn't stick around when that center was touched. This experience was vivid and immediate proof of the power of love. So often when babies are upset, we get upset, which of course makes it all last longer. Babies recognize when we go to that "inner sanctuary of peace," and all is well.

Diane...Learning the Importance of Kegels

My second daughter was eighteen months old and I was nearly thirty-five when I experienced my first signs of something "pooching" down from my vagina. It was scary not to understand what was happening with my body. I was away from home and knew I couldn't see my doctor for six more weeks.

Fortunately a close friend referred me to a midwife, Katie, who graciously offered to check me. Since both of my daughters were born in a hospital, this was my first experience with a midwife. From the beginning of our meeting, I felt completely relaxed and so appreciative of her positive, caring nature and thoroughness. She explained that what I was feeling was caused by the weakening of the upper vaginal walls, which allowed my bladder to pooch down.

Her prescription was to do two hundred kegel exercises a day. We talked about aging and the importance of doing kegel exercises. Katie explained that exercising the pelvic floor leads to increased strength, tone, and body awareness. Her favorite anecdote was "Start each day with a pelvic smile."

Barbara...Healing the Damage

The doctor asked me if I wanted to push my baby out or have a cesarean section. So I pushed. I was dilated only eight centimeters. After only two strong pushes, Carly was born. She weighed eight pounds, six ounces, and I guess she had a large head.

It took a really long time to sew me up. My first baby, Jared, was a head and shoulder presentation. I had to push for two and a half hours, but I had nowhere near the damage after he was born. This time I stayed in the hospital for twelve hours after my birth. I was given no help during my stay. The stitches hurt, so I asked for an ice pack. I had to ask for it. The doctor wanted me to stay, but he did not communicate to me that I was in bad shape.

At home I had difficulty pooping and I couldn't sit properly. I didn't get any medical attention until I saw my doctor at my six-week postpartum checkup. He told me I hadn't healed properly and that I'd need to spend a day in the hospital for some repairs. I'm pretty tough, and I didn't want to be separated from my breastfeeding infant. I also had lost faith in this doctor, so I didn't go into the hospital.

Two years later I went to a doctor in Des Moines. He handed me a mirror so I could see my pelvic floor. As I watched, he pulled two muscles out of my anus and said, "These should be connected." I had a third-degree tear and no existing perineum. He told me I would be spending at least seven days in the hospital, and the amazing thing was I had kept myself so clean that I had no infection. Carly's birth had cost $2,400. The repair surgery was $5,000.

After surgery, kegels really helped me. My husband and I couldn't have sex for two months. Three years later, after he left me, he said it had bothered him that I was not "the same down there" after Carly's birth. I was in bad shape right after the birth, but we started right up having sex again within a week. Society sets up sexual expectations in men's minds. These were strong in my husband, and he made me feel guilty if I wouldn't have sex, even after the birth when I wasn't healed right.

For me, one of the best things about postpartum was that my sister and I breastfed each other's babies. That was great. We were born and raised in a very conservative neighborhood. I'm sure lots of people would have thought that our shared breastfeeding was odd, even disgusting. But my sister and I have always been close, so it felt natural. I think more women should look for a special breastfeeding partner. We were able to give each other breaks from our babies, without worrying about feedings.

Tess...Surviving Postpartum Depression

My birth was totally normal. For a few days I was fine, exhilarated to have this baby. By week two or three postpartum, Max was not sleeping much, and I was not sleeping at all! It got progressively worse. By the time Max was one month old, I was full-on depressed.

My symptoms were much like menopause. I had panic attacks, a rapid heart rate. I felt an imminent sense of doom. I feared I'd lose my baby, my perfectly healthy baby. Day and night I had severe nausea. I couldn't exercise. I couldn't eat. I was afraid of getting sicker and sicker and losing touch with my baby. I could not get back on my feet, and I was breastfeeding.

By the third month, I realized I needed professional help. My friends wanted so much to help, but the way I looked frightened them. They were put off as I never had a positive thing to say. It pushed them away, and they knew they simply did not have the skills needed to help me. Thank God I got professional help. I called in help for taking care of the house, which felt weird, like an invasion. My weight dropped to 102 pounds. My doctors wanted me to wean Max; they said I couldn't breastfeed him since I was losing so much weight.

So began the next crisis. Against my better judgment, I weaned Max overnight. I did it immediately, without preparation for myself or my baby. He was only seven months old. It was a big mistake. My relationship with my husband was so strained that nursing Max was the only warm physical contact I had. While I breastfed I felt normal, like part of the human race. Much as I needed that, I couldn't breastfeed if I was to take the medication my doctors wanted me to be on.

For about a year I was on Atavan, a tranquilizer, and Sinnequan, an antidepressant. You know, they tell you how to get on this medication, but nobody teaches you how to get off. Well, with the drugs and therapy, it was still a good year before I began to feel hopeful.

Suddenly my big fear, losing my baby, seemed to be coming true. Max got a lump in his throat. All the doctors had a different direction for me to take. One said operate, another said do nothing, plus every possible kind of advice in between. Here I was, barely able to decide which utensil to eat with, a spoon or a fork; the smallest decision was impossible. All the while I kept thinking how healthy he was until I weaned him. After weaning, he developed digestion problems too. He would throw up if he got upset, or even if he was happy. For a full year, Max threw up at least once a day.

Meanwhile my husband lost his bread-and-butter writer's job. We had no sense of security. My house became overrun with centipedes. "Oh my God, what's next," I thought. If any one thing had been different, if Doug hadn't lost his job, if my mother could've come, if I had had more of a support system, maybe I could have handled the depression without weaning Max and going on drugs. I don't know.

Fortunately the lump in my baby's throat turned out to be something that was not life threatening. By now I was angry at God. I had to look at why I had so much anxiety, such a fear of loss.

I was an adopted child. For the first seven days of my life I stayed in the hospital, waiting for a mother to come and take me home, waiting for someone to love me. Thankfully I was given to a wonderful set of parents. I couldn't help but think that I still carry around that feeling of being abandoned, even by God. When I was six months pregnant, my best friend died. She was the light of the world, then bango—she was gone.

So I had reasons for fearing loss. Also there was financial and personal stress in my life. It was not until Max was two or so that I began to rebuild my own spirituality.

Then I had about a year of feeling fine. I got off the drugs. Max was well. Before too long all the problems my husband and I had before the pregnancy resurfaced. I'm getting up at 4 A.M. every morning now, four years after the birth, with anxiety attacks again. Doug and I have a lot to work on, and we're getting through it.

Postpartum depression was not having the perspective that "this will pass," because it just didn't feel like it would. The turning point came through a therapist named Diane, a Science of Life practitioner. She taught me a five-step technique that restored my sense of hope. I learned to identify God in my life, to relate God to me, to accept my future good. I learned to give thanks and to let go. I guess I was tested. It's been four years, and I'm still looking for answers.

Nece…Swimming and Having Time for Me

Having my two children was, and is, my most inspiring and uplifting experience. I feel fortunate; both were normal, easy pregnancies and births. I was blessed to have them at home with the love and support of my sweet husband and strong yet gentle midwives.

When pregnant with my first child, I gained the usual amount of weight. I had swelling and bladder discomfort. My postpartum recovery was gradual. I was up and around the next day, very elated to be a mom. However, as it often is for first-time mothers, I was the only one around to take care of her. I could have used more help. The baby was fussy, bringing much frustration for me. The extra five to ten pounds remaining after the birth stayed on my body, which added to the depression.

When my daughter was eighteen months old, I discovered aerobic exercise. I continued exercising daily when I was expecting my second child. Gradually, toward the end of my pregnancy, I allowed my pace to slow. During that time, I took up swimming. I learned to love it and now I much prefer it over running or dance exercise. The water took the stress off my entire body, even when I was heavy with child.

Swimming is also excellent exercise for mothers after they have the baby. Because mothers are constantly holding their children, getting in the water is so pleasurable. It frees your arms and makes you stronger at the same time.

I found that after the baby had established a sleeping schedule, I could set an alarm and get up about an hour earlier than the rest of the family. In this time I would write, meditate, exercise, and do all the things I thought I'd have to give up when I became a mother. For me, having "my time" is very important.

Having kids is a great discipline and joy. It has made me whole. I manage to work out of my home, take care of two children, and exercise regularly. This could not happen without the support of my wonderful husband. The more productive I am around the baby, the more he seems to understand that I need to work, and he occupies himself, right by my side.

Rita...Learning to Love My Baby

Who is this perfect little creature that came forth from me? Her birth was a great spring day. I had planted in the garden earlier that day with my two-year-old son Justin, the love of my life. I was sure there was room in my heart for another.

I never anticipated the emotions that I experienced after my daughter's birth. I felt a crack in the bond between us was growing wider, and I couldn't heal it. The days of relentless giving. The hours of filling her seemingly insatiable needs. The unending demands on my tired body. I knew love could heal the crack, but I didn't have that feeling. Mothers are expected to love their babies, but I felt dry, unloving. I felt robbed of a feeling I assumed I'd have.

Baby Gina had so many needs. Her older brother had been pure pleasure for me. But no matter how much I gave to the baby, it wasn't enough. Sometimes I would not look at her when I breastfed. Her cries didn't call to my heart the way her brother's did. I just wanted to sleep for more than two hours before she woke me.

Now I understand how parents can become abusive. At least I had control over my actions.

Then she'd act so sweet and be so smart. She'd soak up everything around her like a sponge. I wonder how much of my sadness she soaked up?

Her baby book was empty. I had time to write in her brother's book, but I couldn't bring myself to open Gina's. A couple of months ago, almost a year and a half after Gina's birth, while the two children slept, I did get out her baby book. I just felt the need to do this. "First smile, first step, first tooth," I could hardly read the words and see the blank spaces, through my tears. In very tiny letters I wrote "i love you." Then larger, "I Love You. I LOVE YOU."

Chris…Learning to Trust Her Intuition

When I became pregnant, there were plenty of people around to give me advice about everything under the sun that dealt with childbirth. But no one ever talked to me about what to expect after the birth.

I guess, somehow, I figured once the baby was out, the tummy became as flat as ever. I took for granted that I would go back to normal, emotionally and physically, relatively soon. Well, the extra weight didn't just mysteriously disappear in the night, and my emotions were up and down for a while. I was heavy and had the "baby blues."

Nevertheless, what I learned is that life *does* return to normal. With a little attention to my physical and emotional bodies, both got back into shape. All was not lost because I had a baby! The most valuable lesson I learned was to *love myself, no matter what.*

I no longer felt that no one would understand my doubts, fears, and all the incredible highs and lows. I now know that all women experience these things, and knowing that helps. I learned to trust myself, my very own feelings and intuition. That is a tough one because of all the well-meaning advice and opinions of others. Remembering to always accept and love myself for my ups and downs gave me strength and courage.

In this same way, I loved my body, as overweight as it was. Well, maybe more accurately, I loved *me* for loving my body as it was. I felt very important and right about giving myself time, and giving my babies each a full year of nursing, before doing something about my excess weight. I didn't torment myself because I wasn't my toned and shapely self.

This first year postpartum was important. It became my greatest gift to the children. I ate. I continued to eat well. I produced great milk—milk to make the children strong and healthy. I gave my best. I feel good about myself for that.

Pamela...On Going Back to Work

Six weeks after I had my baby, I returned to my law practice, never dreaming it would be so difficult. Other women in my office seemed content to have a baby and return to work after a short maternity leave. They are good mothers too. They love their babies, and returning to work is right for them.

I felt good about the woman I'd hired to care for Amanda. It was for only eight hours a day—after work, there would be plenty of quality time for us.

I decided not to wean my baby. There was no way I could have predicted the agony of being separated from her, or of having my breasts swell up. The physical pain was a constant reminder. The picture of the tiny vulnerable baby on my desk haunted me. Was she mine? What if something happened to her and I was not there? How could my husband, Jon, have gone back to work so painlessly after taking only four days off?

I had trouble concentrating. I called home and spoke with the nanny hourly. By the end of the day, it was difficult to wait a full hour before making that phone call.

My secretary has raised three sons. She watched me until she felt I'd had enough, then said, "Why don't you go home?" I fell into tears and told her how hard I'd worked to get through law school, how the practice was everything, how responsible I had to be. She laughed, "Look at me. I've got plenty of time to work outside the home. But I wouldn't have missed changing one diaper or bandaging one knee when my boys were small. When it's time for you to return to the world, you'll know it. Today you know it's not time."

I went home. Amanda is three now, and I work a bit here and there. I think about going back to work full time. Jon carries a greater financial load now, and I think he'd really like a maternity leave of his own. Then he sees the immensity of my job here at home. He's beginning to appreciate my mothering role. I figure I'll be a lawyer for the rest of my life. Amanda will only be a child for a few precious years.

Marilyn...Two in a Row

The minute Norman, my firstborn, had a bite of food other than breast milk, I got pregnant! I hadn't had a period or anything, but I knew I was pregnant.

By the time I was three months pregnant, Norman was ten months old. I was feeling drained from the pregnancy and the added burden of breastfeeding, so I weaned Norman.

Gary, my husband, and I took the childbirth preparation class again, even though we'd just done it. In those days, the hospital wouldn't let the father in the delivery room unless he had gone through the class.

When Norman was born, I was working full time. I took three days off and went right back to work, taking my baby along. When I had Paul, I wasn't working, and that was real nice, especially now that I had two babies.

Paul was a bigger baby and a more difficult delivery. It was hard sometimes because Norman was still so young and wanted to be picked up all the time too. So here I was, almost thirty-three years old, juggling a high-need baby and a newborn. I don't know how I could have done it without a baby frontpack. When Paul was able to sit up, I got a twin stroller and that helped out.

I'm glad it happened like this, one right after another, even with all the challenges. At our age, if we had had time to think about it, we probably wouldn't have had two children. Gary and his brother were ten years apart. He says he'd never do it like that; it's too lonely for a child.

After the first two years, it got much easier. I'm glad they're both boys; they can share so much. Of course Paul was really frustrated trying to keep up with his older brother. When Norman could run, Paul could only crawl. Now, at ages eight and nine, they go out for different sports, but play with the same toys and have the same friends.

Danya...Birthing at Forty
In a cabin by a stream, almost twenty miles from town, I had Chandi. She must have had the most beautiful start in life, sleeping peacefully with the sound of the stream singing. I gave birth outside under the stars in a hot tub. Tina, my midwife, and Rick, my husband, along with other friends and my two sons, eight and five years old, were there.

When Chandi was born, I was forty. I was expecting to come right back into my pre-pregnancy body as I did when I had my other children. It was shocking how different it was this time. I felt extremely weak. This weakness made me feel very relaxed. So I tuned into the baby and tried not to think too much about my body.

I had a prolapsed uterus. It was a scary feeling, like everything was falling out. Chandi was big, ten and a half pounds, which was a lot for me being forty years old. I knew I had to do kegels, so I did them every time I thought about it. I did kegels and deep breathing about twenty times a day.

I ate some of my placenta every day. There was a lot of it. Rick made it into a stroganoff with mushrooms, sour cream, onions, and garlic. It was absolutely the best thing I had ever tasted and gave me an incredible amount of energy. It got me going, but then I would do too much, like work in the garden, and then I'd be exhausted.

I was in a dream world. Kai and Durien, my older kids, seemed so angelic. Rick was there all the time. He stayed home with me, doing the cooking, washing, grocery shopping. He ran the house, and I didn't even have to get in the car for about three weeks.

I felt like I was between ecstasy and nervous collapse. I was feeling loss.

I did cry a lot. It was not focused on sadness or happiness, just emotional release. It felt like a cleansing. I didn't feel like socializing. I wanted to keep myself centered in my little family unit. People were sensitive to this. When they did come, they would stay for just a short time.

I did yoga during pregnancy, thinking my energy would come back faster when it was over. I was doing all I could do, yet I was surprised to be so weak. Being forty, I was more relaxed about getting my girlish figure back. It took me three years to get all my energy back and about four years to get my body back to how it was before I was pregnant.

Listening to a lot of classical music, especially Bach and Mozart, helped me a lot in the first few weeks postpartum. It helped align myself with my own mastery. With my other children, I felt the divine presence so strongly in them. This time, perhaps because this baby is a girl, we mirror each other, at times. I feel the presence of Mary, mother of Jesus, in me and around me.

Beverly...Giving Up Natalie and Having Two Sets of Twins

I was eighteen years old when I had my first baby. I let my parents convince me that I was too young and gave her up for adoption. I remember my postpartum with her as being all about loss. I felt pretty good until my third day, when a nurse snuck me in for a few seconds to see my baby from a distance. That's how I found out she was a girl. Then I went into five days of deep depression. As soon as I left the hospital, I had sex with my boyfriend to make myself feel better.

Natalie was seventeen the next time I saw her. I don't advocate closed adoption. If you've given up a baby, find that child. He or she needs to know your story and to know it wasn't because they weren't loved; even twenty or thirty years after the adoption they need to know.

With Mike and Abbey, my first set of twins, I was euphoric, really on cloud nine after their birth. I didn't sleep for seven days. I gave birth on Sunday and literally did not sleep or feel tired until Saturday night! I didn't know I was having twins, so I was in awe. They were so tiny, just over four pounds each. They were beautiful. Mike had white-blond hair, like a baby duck. Abbey's skin was dark, and her hair was all black ringlets stuck to her head. There they were—together. I was twenty-seven and at my peak. Postpartum was bliss, a different state of consciousness.

At age thirty-three, I had another set of twins. It was a lot harder on me. I got so big. They were both seven pounds at birth. I was already big when I was only one month pregnant. I had headaches. For two weeks before the babies were born, I had a terrible burning, itching sensation in my hands and feet. Every day it would start at 5 P.M. and it didn't let up until about 5 A.M. I was so happy it stopped when I gave birth.

I stayed in the hospital for as long as I could. I knew what the reality would be when I got home: two small children and two new babies.

By day three, my breasts got giant. They were so full I'd actually wake the babies up so they could nurse and relieve some of the pressure.

Bill, the father of my babies, didn't allow the feeling of bliss in our house. I don't remember being depressed or blue. There were no real low feelings, no highs either. Just lots of work.

I was chairbound. I mean I actually sat in this one chair with a baby on each side of me, all the time. I ate, slept, and existed in that chair. I breastfed constantly. I had rented out my body for nine months. Then I became a milk machine. That was the year Mike and Abbey learned to make their own sandwiches. They were six years old.

Each of my postpartum stories is different. With my first baby, I had everything to be depressed about, and I was. When Mike and Abbey came, there was the shock of being a single mother with twins. I was in no way ready for two babies, but there was so much bliss. With the second set of twins, I was more prepared. I knew there were two babies coming. I won't pretend it's been easy for me, but being a mother is what I do. I try to do it well.

Jan...Learning to Trust the Process

"Be tandy little one...dare to be strong and courageous. That is the road. Venture anything. Be brave enough to dare to be loved."

Sherwood Anderson

Shortly after David and I were married seventeen years ago, I got pregnant without any premeditation. Our innocence was bliss. We didn't know what we were getting into. After four and a half months, there was heavy bleeding. I gave birth to a stillborn son. The emotions were so strong yet we suppressed them. Somehow we came to know that life goes on. After our son's birth and death, David and I realized that children were to be an important part of our life together. This is my life's lesson; it came through hardships.

Three months later, we were pregnant again. This pregnancy ended in two months, yet I never doubted that we would be parents.

Within three more months, I was pregnant for the third time. Conception is the easy part for us. This baby thrived well into the sixth month. I woke one morning with a bloody mucus show. I talked to my neighbor, went to the doctor, and by two o'clock in the afternoon I had another stillborn son. We still had faith in our ability to have children, yet, emotionally, this had been a very difficult birth for me.

The birth took place while I was totally anesthetized. Later, I *begged* to see my baby. The nurses and the doctors said, "You don't want to see 'that.'" There were no malformations, but even if there had been, we should have met. For months afterward, I dreamed of this baby, of holding him, of having his picture on our nightstand. Always the same dream, again and again. I'm still working on this one. We buried him on a hillside. I haven't yet buried my hopes and dreams for him. I never saw him. I never held him. He has a name, Chad David.

But life goes on.

Six months later…conception. One more time, we were thrilled. Afraid for ourselves, but again full of hope—this would be the one to fill our aching arms. The baby grew inside me, kicking and telling me, "All was well."

We had complete faith in our doctor. I was eight months pregnant. While having a series of Braxton-Hicks contractions [false labor], I was admitted to the hospital and had contractions through the night. In the morning the doctor came in. He broke my bag of waters and put me on Pitocin to induce labor…why, I don't know. After forty-eight hours of a totally drugged and anesthetized labor and birth, my daughter was pried from my body with forceps.

She was not put on my belly; our eyes never met. She was torn from me and I from her. Her four-and-a-half-pound body was whisked away to the nursery to be "better cared for." Certainly a mother didn't know what was best for her baby.

David was "not allowed" to be with us. He was "not allowed" to help the ones he loved most. Years later we realized his desires were not so unusual. Ignorance and blind trust in hospital procedure stood between us and our baby.

Our daughter seemed fine. She was small but her Apgar score was between eight and nine, which is very good. I saw her through the nursery windows. The hospital staff felt "it best that we not touch her." Suddenly, when she was ten hours old, her health deteriorated rapidly. She lived for two more hours. We were told she succumbed to hyaline membrane disease [premature lungs]. I have no doubt her death was a mistake. She was forced to be born too early, torn from my body and taken away, never to return to my arms. Never to leave my heart.

Her spirit lingers on. For a long time, I heard her baby cries. Her cries matured to "Mama," calling me in the night. She has come to me, she is growing in heaven, surrounded by children. We have an angel of our own. When I last saw her, she let me know that she misses me too.

Life goes on.

The next few years brought changes. We left our military lifestyle. Changed our surroundings. Had another miscarriage.

Through the divine plan, we found ourselves back in our home state with family and friends. And we were pregnant again!

This time, with the support of a conscientious doctor, we delivered *naturally*. Times had changed and David was at my side. A beautiful, perfect daughter was put immediately in my arms. Our eyes met. She suckled at my breast. Over and over again, I cried, "It's Mikel, it's Mikel!" Mikel was the name of her sister who had died. It is her name too.

This was the beginning of a new era; we were a family. Even when it hurt the most, in my heart I knew I'd be a mother. It was learning to trust the process of life unfolding. After twelve pregnancies, births, and deaths, David and I have five children. They are wonderful, growing and thriving in every way. We have experienced together all the emotions of humankind. We've had hopes and fears. We've laughed, we've cried. Most of all, we've loved. And may we never forget how special each and every child of this earth is.

My message is "be tandy." Learn everything you can. Read books, talk to people, listen. Actively take responsibility for your life and the lives of your children. Know that it is your parental duty to make educated choices. May you never regret.

Debby...Recovering from Premature Births

My first baby, Marstin, was premature. He weighed only three pounds, twelve ounces at birth. When I first saw him, he was making mewing sounds. He was busy sucking a bottle that was as big as he was. This baby was so full of life. I never worried about him.

During my second pregnancy, I was being careful not to go into labor early. We were living in Switzerland at that time. In the seventh month, during the middle of the night, I felt the baby kicking. My bag of water broke.

At the hospital, I was given medication for four days to stop the contractions. This didn't work. I still wanted to birth naturally, so I asked them to allow me to do the Bradley method of childbirth. My labor was very long, and the doctors seemed tuned into death, not life. Then I was given Pitocin. After that, the contractions were so intense, I was arching in pain.

When David was finally born, the doctor said, "Too small," and threw him down on a table. But he lived. When I first saw, him he had pieces of gauze stuck to him and was wrapped in aluminum. Three and a half pounds. Screaming. There was a problem with my placenta still being attached. The infant intensive care people from Bern (sixteen miles away) arrived like angels to help little David. He was whisked away.

I was very sick for ten days. I could not sit or walk. I had high fever and pain in the "area." I did not take antibiotics. Two weeks later, I still felt sick and knew there was a piece of placenta stuck in my uterus. The doctor did not believe me. Two months after the birth, when David was actually due, I had contractions and delivered a big chunk of placenta.

I had not stuck up for myself in the hospital. Alex, my husband, was not there for me emotionally. My five-year-old, Marstin, was upset. I was totally separated from David. I was extremely isolated. I had no visitors except one friend, Lynn. Her visits meant a lot to me. I remembered when I was twelve years old and got my first period, I said, "The devil got me today." When I was thirteen, I lost my mother. Alex and I had been distant for a long time before this baby. I've been alone all my life.

David's tiny lungs burst, he had only a ten percent chance of making it. Alex was going to the hospital a lot. Though he could not seem to support my emotional needs, he was blessed to be able to care for David. He laid his hands on our son and chased the darkness from the baby's lungs with light. A healing. David's almost fourteen now. He's big and strong.

With both premature babies, I was still able to keep my milk going so I could breastfeed. In these times, I was challenged to learn how to nurture myself emotionally. I did it.

Judy...Mothers Who Adopt Experience Postpartum
Five years after adopting our daughter and three years after adopting our son, I'm just coming out of the fog; it's all starting to fit together. We feel blessed beyond belief.

There's no way anybody can prepare you for the highs and lows of parenting. It's a world of absolutes. I'd say I suffered from postpartum fatigue, though I did not carry these children through pregnancy. I wonder how women who give birth cope. After two or three sleepless nights, I had to take a can of beer to bed to get back to sleep.

Our daughter came to us from Korea. She was two and a half when we adopted her. We had just a picture of her and her baby brother with number cards around their necks. The night we made the decision to adopt them both, we got a phone call telling us the baby boy had suffered crib death. It hurt.

Our real test came when, on twelve hours' notice, we were given a newborn baby boy! Seven o'clock on a Thursday, night we got a call. The next morning I was bringing home a son. When this kind of thing happens, you just don't say no.

The first week with a new baby everybody fusses over you. The next week, everybody goes away. One friend gave me the gift of sleep. She came over in the middle of the day and sent me off to bed. I went right out. I'll never forget that.

Before the children, I had been fully employed. Going from being employed and social to acting on my decision to stay home was a leap. I didn't know much about children. I remember taping my son's umbilical cord back on because, according to the book I'd read, it fell off forty-eight hours too soon!

I had anxiety about losing my son. How could anybody give up this baby? Surely she'll change her mind, I thought, and, I'm so lucky. Which leads me to a bizarre feeling that my luck came through someone else's misfortune. My happiness had to come from someone's loss. It saddens me. At times, I get angry at my children's birth parents. Then I rejoice that the children have a safe place here with us.

Jewell...Cesarean Recovery

When the doctor said, "We're going to do a cesarean section," I felt defeated. My husband was actually relieved. He didn't want to be part of the birthing at all. I told the staff, "Okay" (as if I were asked!), but I had to be awake to see my baby. After much adversity, they agreed, and my nine-pound son Jermaene was born. He was yelling his protests even before he was out of the uterus. I cried for joy, but the staff wouldn't let me see him until the next day. I was told he was fine, but procedure was thus and so. For six days, I had terrible gas pains and headaches. Finally we left the hospital.

My well-wishing friends and family wore me out. Each time my husband left for work, the tears flowed. I felt so abandoned. My mother-in-law's answer to my "sadness" was to "stop breastfeeding so you can get away."

"All is fine. You can use the same diaphragm you already have," the chief of obstetrics said at my six-week checkup. A year later, I was pregnant and couldn't believe it! My marriage was very difficult and we decided to terminate that pregnancy. The Planned Parenthood center told me diaphragms should always be refitted if a woman dilates at all. I hope this information will be valuable to other mothers who have had surgical births.

Five years and a new husband later, at the age of thirty-four, pregnancy! I was told I couldn't have a vaginal birth because my records weren't accessible. I'm still reminding myself to get off my case for giving up my power to the doctors. I went to several OB/GYNs. I couldn't convince any of them to allow me to try a vaginal delivery, even in the operating room as a precaution.

My friends weren't very supportive this time. "You already have a baby. It's harder when you're past thirty…what about birth defects?" My husband expressed concern about my being a new mother again and having gray hair. I was concerned about the chemicals in the hair dye I'd used for nine years affecting the fetus, and he was worrying about how I appeared!

I was not allowed to go into labor this time, so we selected May 1 for my second son's birthday. This time the doctor described all that was happening, and my husband held my hand. At 5:55 P.M. I got to touch my baby, Dion.

More intense gas pains followed this birth and no relief from the hospital staff.

Something I'd like to mention being faced with is the decision of whether to have a tubal ligation on delivery day. My papers were signed and the decision had been made ahead of time, but it was still the last chance to change my mind. The doctor said it's easier to do at the same time—it isn't easier emotionally.

My stomach looked like a deflated balloon after the cesarean births! I grieved over my darkened saggy tummy for years. Having been a model, Miss Swimsuit, and then Miss New York State, I was very aware of my appearance. I bought into the pressure put on women to always be trim. I let *no one,* including my husband and girlfriends, see my saggy balloon. For almost two years I had much counseling and attended women's workshops, where I learned to accept others' imperfections, but not my own.

Finally, when my youngest son was two years old, I stopped nursing and had a tummy tuck and breast lift. Everything "tightened up," but the scarring was so bad it had to be redone. I'm still self-conscious with my scars, $1,500 later.

Beth…A Mother Alone

I never planned to be a single mother. Jim and I were married and very much in love when I got pregnant. I'm still not clear on the reasons he left. He was wonderful to me during my pregnancy. He would massage me and talk to "his" baby. I thought we had an ideal relationship.

When Ivan was born, Jim was my hero. He put himself in charge of the birth. I felt so lucky to have Jim and, now, Jim's son.

Not long afterward, Jim became distant. He would complain a lot about how the baby and I kept him up at night. I was so happy in my new role, breastfeeding mother, that I paid little or no attention to Jim's complaints. We almost never made love.

He made an easy transition out of our little family. For me, the transition was not easy. I cried so much. I still cry. For a while, I thought it would be wise to wean my seven-month-old son. I feared my milk was getting bad from all my emotions. Losing Jim was the most traumatic thing I've ever experienced. Having Ivan has been the most blissful.

So here I was, torn between the heaven of having this precious baby and the hell of going it alone. To make things even more difficult, Jim skipped town and has not sent me any child support. We didn't discuss this much. I simply assumed he cared and would support his child.

I'm very strong. I'm also deeply happy about being a mom. I wouldn't change the fact that I had a baby. I'm going to make it, for this little guy, and mostly for me.

Laura...Birth and Death

I didn't know anything about death and I had never given birth. When I was eight months pregnant with Hari, his father, Andre, died.

I couldn't admit to myself that Andre was dying of cancer. I guess I had to protect myself. Even on the last day, I didn't believe it. He knew he was going to die, but I didn't. Why couldn't he wait until Hari was born? It's funny, but I was consoled by the thought that Andre was going to come back, to be Hari, his son. Now I know that it doesn't matter if Hari is Andre. He is, in a sense, and it does not matter.

I don't know how I got through that month: waiting for my baby to be born, funeral and legal arrangements, his family—I had to do everything. Andre and I had been living in France, so I had no one to really talk to, to speak English with. No one to share the grief with, and when Hari was born, no one to share the joy. I was angry at Andre for dying. I was angry at God. I wrote in my journal, "Why couldn't he wait? Why couldn't he wait to see our beautiful boy?"

I just wanted to share it all with Andre. No Andre. There was nothing in the world I could do about that. It's a futile feeling. There's nothing anyone can do about death. I would be holding Hari in my arms and crying at the same time.

So happy. So sad. Bonding was incredible. I could not believe the immediate bond between Hari and me, and there's been nothing else like it in my whole life.

I really wanted my mom to come; she couldn't make the trip. My mother- and father-in-law stayed with me for a month. They cooked, cleaned, baby-sat. Thank goodness they were there. They didn't know me, the American daughter-in-law, and I'm not sure if they really liked me, but they were nice to me, they helped me. They were glad to have a grandson.

Two wonderful women, the nurse and the doctor who were part of Andre's cancer support group, were with me so much. They were with me at Andre's death and Hari's birth.

Physically I was fine. I always knew I'd have children, so birthing felt like the most natural thing in the world. I lived up three flights of stairs. When I went into labor, I walked down, to the midwife's house. I wanted to do most of it at home, so I went back. When she came over, three hours later, I was ready to go to the clinic. I made a great deal of noise when I was laboring at home. I'm sure if I had gone to the clinic right away, I would have been "constipated" vocally. I did a lot of walking, standing…but it was the noise, the groaning and grunting I was doing, that helped me the most.

I pushed for one and a half hours and my contractions were not powerful enough in the end. The hospital staff wanted to use some sort of suction method. The doctor was called. I was so intent on not letting Hari be vacuumed out of me that I jumped off the table and squatted. It still didn't work so the midwife gave me a small episiotomy. Then Hari came out right away. He had to be cleaned up, but he was fine. I was so excited he was a boy.

Afterward I had stitches; it was hard to walk and I was constipated. My nipples were sore and cracked. Fortunately in France all my medical expense was covered, so I stayed in the clinic for a week. France has socialized medical care. No one goes without medical attention for lack of money. I knew I was under a great deal of stress and a long hospital stay seemed like the best way to rest and recuperate. What was there at home for me? In the clinic, I was treated royally. It was better than being in a nice hotel. All my little immediate postpartum needs were met.

Hari was so awake that people would say, *"très éveillé,"* very awake.

Postpartum was a time when I had to make all the decisions in my life, myself. When I left the clinic with Hari, either my in-laws or friends stayed with me at my house at night. The daytime was fine, but I didn't want to be alone at night.

I cried a lot after I had my baby. I'm not sure how much of it was postpartum blues and how much of it was just what was going on at the time. It was both. Andre and I had a mutual magic. It was so strong. We used to give each other baths. Even when he was in the hospital, he would massage me! In my diary, I wrote, "I miss Andre a lot. Sometimes it's very difficult. I want to cuddle. I want to hug him. I want to snuggle. It's not very good when I think like this, but it's necessary."

People ask me how I cope, how I go on. You just do, the daily goings-on, the reality. I didn't break down. When Andre and I were in Bali, a man told us why Balinese funerals were not so sad, but more like festivals. He said, "When you hold on to a dead loved one, you hold them back so they can't go, they can't fly away." You have to let go.

But, you know, as low as I got, I've been that high. I knew at the time, when it was really hard, that farther down the road I'd arrive at a place that I'd never have gotten if I hadn't gone through the rough spots. Love, pregnancy, death, birthing, life—I've had my fill in the last two years. Now I acknowledge my power. I'm a stronger, richer person. I had an idealized image; I wanted my little family. I didn't get it just so. When I was able to accept our family, Hari and I, our situation, I was much happier. No more fighting life, fighting reality.

Tina...After the Ninth Baby

Postpartum the ninth time was facilitated—thanks to friends and a supportive mate. They helped me most by having a baby shower and housecleaning party before the baby came. This gave me the emotional boost I needed to tackle the demands of such a large household.

I got a massage the day before I gave birth, which allowed me to assist Alana with her birth. [Tina is a primary care midwife.] I also received a massage twelve hours after birthing, which helped me reclaim my body.

I went to see Alana for her first-day postpartum check. As I stood over the exact spot where she had given birth the day before, I had my first big contraction. I knew this was it. I made it home. One hour and eight minutes later, I had my ninth baby.

It was interesting to me to see which of the children were present at the birth of this baby. The two oldest were home, but they went to bed. My two middle girls sat together in a chair and watched. The younger children woke up with the baby's first cry and witnessed the placenta being delivered.

I had anticipated postpartum cramping, but I had none. I lost about two teaspoons of blood while giving birth this time. Though there is some concern that women who have had lots of babies tend to hemorrhage, I didn't at all. I drank postpartum brew for four days. (See Maui Midwives' Postpartum Brew, page 158.) I did almost nothing for four full days, and my bleeding stopped in four days.

I cooked my placenta. Everyone in the family had a taste. I felt restored by it.

It took Chico, my partner, and me a while to bond after the birth of this baby. On my second day postpartum, a friend brought a beautiful salad from her garden. Chico and I were upstairs, alone with our baby. Carrie brought up the food and served both of us. That was the first time anyone acknowledged Chico for being the father, and it felt good.

My emotions were mostly high. Oh yes, and once the baby was born there was a feeling, instantly, of finality. No more babies. Because both Chico and I are committed to this child being our last, there was an impressive switch in our sexuality. Fear of pregnancy has affected my sexual drive. It's very sporadic, which may be due in part to the fact that I have a very demanding baby. She plugs in [breastfeeds] so often. If I didn't have a mate around, I don't think I'd think of lovemaking much.

Before I knew it, I was doing my own laundry again. My standards of cleanliness have relaxed considerably. The children's rooms are their domains. The older children, age ten and up, do their own laundry. I usually have a room full of clean laundry waiting to be folded.

My baby is twenty months old now, and I still feel the effects of being postpartum. She's still nursing, so my psyche is in my breasts. I still feel my milk let down when she needs me. This is the longest I've had to wait to lose the excess weight. I'm usually ten pounds lighter. Each of my children has his or her own personality, and it's an emotional load dealing with all of it. My extra weight serves as a buffer. If I were chewed to the bone, I'd probably be in the loony bin!

Rebecca...Lotus Birth

After seeing Inti enter the world all bruised, blue, and misshapen from squeezing through a passage so tight, my heart had no question about letting him keep his placenta until he was ready to part from it. It felt right deep-down that there should not be any unnecessary procedures performed on his little body. Indeed, his cord and placenta were then still a part of his body. He had enough work to do, getting used to his body. Scott and I felt that if there was even a chance that his attached cord and placenta could make him feel whole, then so be it.

My only preparation, for the ritual of leaving our newborn son's cord intact, was to read a few essays written by Jeannine Parvati Baker about lotus birth.

Jeannine wrote from a spiritual perspective. Her words conveyed a connectedness with and a peacefulness in her own babies, who were left intact. But I was not really prepared for the practical side of it. How do you dress your "connected" baby? How do we nurse and swaddle our boy, while he's still connected to his pla-centa?

We started out by washing the blood from the placenta. We then generously applied ground rosemary, even putting the fragrant herb in all the folds. We wrapped the placenta in a disposable diaper and placed it in a basket, just beside us. We were always aware, careful not to move too quickly or pull the cord, which was still a part of our baby.

The next day Scott came up with lovingly wrapping the placenta in a cloth diaper and pinning it securely closed. Each day we would unwrap it and change the diaper; doing this we experienced a silent awe—the miracle of life. We *felt* the importance of the placenta to his health and well-being, the feeling was…"Oh, he's still being protected and taken care of by his soul brother."

Surreal, our six-year-old daughter, would gather close to us, to watch the dia-pering of her little brother's placenta. She loved to help, and we gave her the important task of lifting the placenta when we were moving Inti from one place to another. She felt so important and so connected. She seemed to understand deeply the reason for leaving her brother's placenta attached. She asked questions about her own placenta. She dreamed of visiting "her" at the tree "she" was plant-ed under. She slipped into the greater mythology of where babies come from. She told me the story of how she chose me to be her mother and of how she was once an angel with beautiful wings. She understood where Inti was before he entered this world. So, I would say for Sister Surreal, it gave her a connection, through her vast subconscious placenta memories, to her brother…a connection that would last forever. Also, Surreal would not leave the house while Inti's placenta was still attached. Not even for a tempting play with her friend next door. She didn't want to miss anything and was happy to play quietly while Inti and I slept and recovered from our tumultuous birth. Perhaps, in these quiet play times with her dolls, she was rebirthing herself. Maybe she was weaving magical spells to pro-tect her brother. Maybe she was dreaming of her own soul's placenta. Who knows?

We found that swaddling was the best way to care for the connected cord, so Inti didn't wear clothes for the three days and nights he was still connected. While the placenta wore a diaper, Inti did not, as we did not want anything to rub against the site where his cord was attached. It had dried out within the first twelve hours. It began to curl and shape itself into a dance frozen in time. The brittleness of the cord worried me, rubbing up against the baby's fresh skin. So we found ways to swaddle him so that the cord was directed away from his belly. Our only criticism of the lotus birth was that we couldn't easily swoop him up and cuddle him against our naked skin, without worrying about the cord being pulled. It was three days of total mindfulness.

What did Inti think of being connected? Or how did he feel? Only he knows, but I could say that he was calm and peaceful in the transition into his earthly body. As his cord dried up and the placenta slept in the land "between," Inti slept, he dreamt, he grew.

Alesia...Postpartum and Ayurveda

The birth of my daughter, Shanti, was an incredible experience. I was swept away into a one-hour-and-six-minute labor. Upon waking at 4:15 in the morning with labor pains, I instinctually headed for my bathtub. I had planned all along to have my baby at home and I was grateful for the immediate relief the warm water and aromatherapy candle brought me.

Sardined inside my tiny bathroom was my husband, my midwife, her assistant, and a close friend who was holding my angel-eyed son, Charan. It was cozy and homey just as I had hoped. The labor went so fast, I don't think anyone could even believe it, least of all me who had had a good ten-hour labor with my son at home just four years ago.

I was left in awe as my midwife and my husband delivered my new baby into my arms. The hour I labored seemed like only minutes and I swear I didn't even push my daughter out, instead it seemed as though she literally floated out on her own. After the birth, my midwife looked at me, and holding back tears, told me that my baby was born completely inside her water bag, and that in many countries where she had previously delivered babies, this was considered very auspicious. I am so glad that she did not break the bag as is done too often in hospitals, but rather she let nature take its course. Looking back I can't remember any pain, only bliss, the sheer ecstatic bliss of giving birth.

My postpartum days were equally full of bliss. Since the birth of my first son, I had discovered the enormous health benefits of Ayurveda, an ancient Indian tradition of health care that emphasizes the wholeness of mind, body and spirit. As a part of my Ayurvedic lifestyle, I also learned transcendental meditation and found that it offered me what I was always looking for—a deeper contact with the infinite reservoir of energy that connects all of us. During pregnancy, my meditations helped me remain calm and focused on the idea of having the best birth possible. My meditations were also a time when I felt even more connected with the growing life inside of me; it was a special and peaceful bond we both shared inside my body. During postpartum, meditating gave me a chance to spend some quiet time with myself, so that the rest of the time I spent with my new baby was calm and nourishing; this was critical especially in a time when getting enough rest at night wasn't always guaranteed.

Armed with a fair amount of knowledge of Ayurveda, and the desire to practice it, I maneuvered through my pregnancy and postpartum health with more comfort and ease than I had known the first time. I know that I was able to appease the harsh empty feelings, both physical and emotional, that can often accompany the postpartum experience with a few pearls of Ayurvedic knowledge: what to eat, when to eat, the best time to rest, the best time to be active, a few herbal recommendations and daily abyhangas (oil massage). It seems like these little things wouldn't make that big a difference in the face of modern Western science and its infinite discoveries, but it is amazing what a little "back to nature" can do. Ayurveda acknowledges that birth and postpartum is a very special time for a woman, the ideal time for the new mother to realign her physiology with nature.

During labor, the digestion shuts down so that the body can use all its energy to birth. After birth, it is critical for the woman to nourish her fragile and often weak digestion. She does this both for the good of herself and for the good of her new baby who is to take in her milk—just as the mother's digestion is fragile, so too is the new baby's. Simply eating the right foods at the right time can make the biggest difference in the world. For instance, paying attention to what you eat and how you eat it can significantly reduce the amount of painful gas that babies often experience. If you eat a meal that is easy to digest in a calm and peaceful environment, then the milk you produce will be calming and nourishing as well.

Also, one of the perks of an Ayurvedic routine is a daily abyhanga—both for the mother and the baby. It is an ideal way to dissolve away the stresses of pregnancy and postpartum, and it is also an excellent way to encourage skin-to-skin contact, which so nourishes us all. If you are lucky enough, as I was, to have a trained Ayurvedic technician give you a postpartum massage a few days after birth, I guarantee you will experience a level of bliss that you never knew possible in your postpartum days. Your baby too will thank you with her coos and stretches as you massage her tiny body that had been held snugly so long in your body.

I know my most recent experience of birth and postpartum isn't the norm. For weeks after my birth, I literally had tingling sensations of bliss throughout my whole body. When I relived the labor in my mind, these sensations would become even more pronounced and my then-empty womb still seem comfortably full. I was happy and knew that my only responsibility at this time was to rest and to take care of my new baby. For the first time in my life, I left errands up to my husband and allowed myself to rely on friends for favors and meals. I remember thinking that I wished that all women everywhere could experience birth and the postpartum transition as I did. To me it felt natural and easy—the way it probably is meant to.

For this I am grateful to Mother Nature, Ayurveda, and to Maharishi Mahesh Yogi who brought out its precious knowledge.

Nyoman Masni...Postpartum in Bali

My baby's birth was not as difficult as I had thought it would be. It was *Purnana* (full moon) and my husband went to get Ibu Robin and Ibu June. Once I saw that my midwives, my *mertua* (mother-in-love) and my *adik* (younger sister) had all gathered beside me, I felt, "Yes, I can do this. I am strong."

Immediately after my daughter was born, my midwives put her right up on my belly. I held her and looked into her eyes, and looked at my husband, who was also so happy. Right away I breastfed my child, and she was a very strong eater. About an hour later, my husband cut the cord. Along with his father and his brothers, he washed the *ari-ari* (placenta), put it in a coconut shell, with offerings of flowers, prayers, a pinch of rice. Then they buried it here by our house-door.

Next the grandmothers of our family came and washed the baby. They bundled her up and threw some offering flowers and ancient coins under the bed. Then they put the baby three times under the bed, saying, *"Mati, mati jani. Hidup, hidup jani."* (If you must die, die now, if you live, live long.) This is our tradition.

My mother is a priestess, and traditionally, as it is the season of holy rituals called *Galungan,* she was supposed to wait until the holy days had passed before coming to see me. She could not wait, so here she came by my side, the other priests and priestesses had to do her jobs. She took me to the *mandi* to bathe. My midwives advised me not to go alone for at least two days, so I would not fall down. I was lucky as I did not lose much blood, but they wanted to be certain I would be safe.

In our culture, we do not wash our hair after childbirth until the baby's cord has fallen away. During this time, we also do not go into our kitchen. In fact, the entire extended family does not attend Temple, nor do they go to parties or wedding celebrations, until the cord is released. The women in my family cooked for me and served me in every way. I was expected to just rest and breastfeed my baby, for at least forty-two days. Even after that time, for the first 105 days of the baby's life, until her *Nyabutan*—the ritual in which she touches the *Ibu Pertiwi* (Mother Earth) for the first time—new mothers mostly rest.

My first postpartum meal was *bur-bur biam,* which is a thin rice gruel made with leafy green vegetables and a little bit of chicken. I was so hungry, I ate two bowls, which made the grandmothers here very happy.

After my baby's birth, the women of our family did everything for me—washed my clothing, even cared for the baby, except, of course, for breastfeeding. The baby's daily bath and massage is a time when the big family gathers, as everyone wants to help. My mother came and slept in my bed with the baby and me, on the other side of us my *mertua* slept. My poor husband had to be content to sleep on the floor of our room. This is how his father slept when he was new in the world. After our baby's birth, my husband got a haircut, because for the entire time one's wife is pregnant in Bali, he must not cut his hair.

Joy Alcos...After My Birth in the Philippines
Each time I had a baby, my mother, who is a *hilot* (healer, midwife), came to live with me and helped in all ways with my family. My younger sister came too. We usually have a few members of our big family staying here. However, after the birth of a baby, special caring help is all around me.

My mother was very close to this last baby, a daughter born breech. It is said that a breech baby or one who is born in the sack will be a healer. Naturally my mother knew that our little Natzuki would follow after her and become a healer.

We are mountain people who grow our own red rice without chemical sprays. We also eat a lot of *kamote* (sweet potatoes) while pregnant and breastfeeding. *Kamote* is medicine for the uterus.

Every day my mother would massage and bathe the baby. She was always telling me not to do too much work; even simple things around the house, she did for me. My sister did all of our washing and cared for the other three children.

After forty days, many family members from all around the mountains came to make a big *fiesta* for Natzuki's baptism.

It is modern times, and so I will sometime go back to work teaching. This means that my younger sisters will stay with the children. They will bring the baby to me at the school several times a day, so she may breastfeed. My mother feels it is better if I can just stay home all the time and be a mother. Perhaps she is right, as I am happiest when I am a mother at home.

Lonica Halley...My Baby Did Breastfeed!
When I was a baby, my mother had me wear a button that said, "I'm a breastfed baby." I grew up thinking that everyone breastfed their babies. Naturally I planned on nursing my own children until at least two years of age as I had been.

When I was six months pregnant with my first child, I attended my very first La Leche League meeting. I was amazed to find that when I returned home, my breasts were dripping milk (colostrum). The bonding experience of breastfeeding was something I was very much looking forward to.

My husband, Michael, and I carefully planned to have a water-birth at home with my midwife, Robin. I could see that Michael was a budding superinvolved father. He was planning on catching the baby, and more than once he said to me, "I want to do half of everything for our baby." I joked, "That's fine with me, except for the breastfeeding, of course."

My due date was May 7th, and I had hoped that I would have our baby before Mother's Day, which was Sunday, May 14th. Sure enough, on Mother's Day in the evening, I began having contractions. Four days later, on Thursday morning, Lily was finally born. It had been a long and somewhat difficult labor. It had taken "everyone's bag of tricks," as my midwife said later. This included Robin, another great midwife named Kathy, Marie (a wise woman—see chapter 18), my mother, Leslie, and, of course, Michael. I was proud of myself for going through seventy-two hours of contractions and still delivering naturally at home in the water-birthing tank in our bedroom. It had been hard, but it was all worth it. We had a beautiful seven-pound girl! Our precious baby was in our arms!

Lily came to my breast immediately after birth. To my surprise, after she briefly attempted to latch on, she gave up and continued crying. I tried again and again, and each time it was the same; she would put her lips onto my nipple, then pull away and cry loudly, her mouth opening very wide. I remember I kept saying how her mouth looked so big to me on the inside—it just seemed overly big. (Later I would realize this was an early warning sign of things to come.) Eventually Lily fell asleep, exhausted from crying, but not having nursed at all. Everyone assured me to just keep trying, and that she would get it next time.

I tried again when she woke up. In fact, my mother and I spent all day trying. We tried every possible breastfeeding position; the cradle hold, football hold, clutch hold, and it was always the same. Lily would try to latch on unsuccessfully, then cry and scream loudly. I vividly remember that the only position that seemed to work at all involved Lily lying on her back on the bed and me crouching over her on all fours, with my mother kneeling beside us, holding my breast firmly into Lily's mouth. It was acrobatic to say the least, and even in this ridiculous position, she would only nurse for a few seconds at best. I just kept thinking, "This can't be right; it is so unnatural that breastfeeding should be so hard." I intuitively felt that there had to be something wrong.

Over the next few days, we had visits from every La Leche League leader and lactation consultant in town, which we were fortunate to have a lot of. They all assured me that I was doing everything right, and just to keep trying. I genuinely appreciated all of the time and advice everyone gave. However, I felt that no one seemed to be concerned that Lily hadn't nursed at all. [In actuality, the La Leche League Leaders and the midwives were so concerned that they were unable to sleep. They felt awful because they could not figure out what the problem was. They were concerned that Lily was becoming dehydrated, while they could see Lonica was doing everything she could.]

I knew and agreed with the fact that La Leche League recommended never giving a breastfed baby a bottle, because then the baby would prefer the bottle's nipple and not latch on properly, or refuse to nurse. The second day after the birth, my milk came in fully and I was painfully engorged. If I had known better at the time, I would have pumped some milk. However, I was running around with two little glass jars, catching a few drops of milk every time I felt a letdown of milk. It seemed ridiculous and it felt desperate, but every little bit made a difference in those first few days. We fed Lily the small amount of milk I collected with a tiny one-inch eyedropper. She ate hungrily, and I felt even sadder knowing that she wanted more.

Then the worst part came. Because Lily wasn't really nursing, my milk supply diminished. And instead of the first few days with my new baby being filled with joy and wonder, it was mostly frustration and worrying. I felt rejected by Lily, and yet I knew she was trying hard to nurse, but it wasn't working.

On the fifth day, Monday, we called our pediatrician, and he made a special house call. After examining Lily thoroughly, and watching me attempt to nurse her, he shook his head and said, "Well, there is nothing wrong with her, and you are doing everything right. Just keep trying."

My heart sunk as he turned to leave, as I felt that this could not be the way people learn to nurse their babies, with so much crying and suffering. Intuitively I knew there was something wrong. "Could you please just look at her mouth again?"

He turned and said, "Let me see if she will suck on my finger. Yes, she has her tongue in the right position, but the suction keeps breaking at the back. Why is it breaking?" By this time, Lily had started to cry loudly, as she always did after my attempts to nurse her. He peered into her mouth with a light, and in order to keep her mouth open, I had to let Lily keep screaming. Then he said excitedly, "Oh I've got it! Do you see that hole? That is not supposed to be there!"

He showed me the inside of her throat, which I had already seen so many times and had described to people as "so big, why is it so big?" It looked like an open archway instead of an archway with a long dangly thing (which I now know is called an uvula) hanging down the middle.

I comforted Lily, and he began to explain. Confused by his excitement, I listened with a sinking feeling as he said, "She has a birth defect called soft cleft palate. I have heard of it before, but I've never seen one. It means that she cannot hold suction to keep the breast in her mouth. It takes a minor surgical procedure to sew it up, but it's no big deal."

The words "minor surgical procedure" were still echoing in my head as he called the hospital sixty miles away to make arrangements. Then he assured Michael and me that we would be in and out of there in a flash, not to worry.

We waited a couple of hours for the hospital to call us back, using the time to explain the situation to family and to cuddle with our precious little one, who as my husband said was "still perfect." We hated to think of taking our delicate baby all the way to the hospital and going through surgery. Every parent instinctively wants to protect their baby from any unpleasant experiences, and we felt sad that Lily would have to start off her young life with this one. But we knew that it was necessary, and tried to console ourselves with the thought that soon we would all be home again, and Lily would be happily nursing, getting that most important first nourishment right from my breast.

When the phone call came, I sat on the edge of my seat (literally) while I listened to everything the nurse said. She carefully explained again that cleft palate was a birth defect occurring in about one in one thousand babies and has no known cause. Essentially the baby has an opening in the roof of the mouth, and in these cases, they recommend a specially shaped nipple and bottle for feeding. She offered to send one in the mail to me, and then told me that the soonest they could see Lily would be in two weeks.

So I quickly told the nurse that our pediatrician had assured us that this was a quick, simple procedure that we could have done right away. The nurse tentatively responded by saying that this appointment in two weeks was only to see Lily, and that the surgery could not take place until she was eleven months old. This was, she explained, because any earlier and the growth of the facial bones and muscles could be stunted.

The nurse could not have known what Lily and I had been through the last week, or how the impact of what she had just said affected me. It was all I could do to listen to the rest of what she was saying: Cleft Palate Support Foundations, special feeding instruction booklets, amounts of ounces of milk or formula to be consumed per pound of body weight per day, number of minutes to consume a certain amount of ounces, timing the feedings so that the baby didn't get exhausted trying to drink, the likelihood of frequent ear infections, nasal regurgitation, and so much more. I scribbled notes, using every ounce of control I had left. All I could think about was that I could not breastfeed my daughter. We could not enjoy the bonding experience I had looked forward to so much. Of course I still had to give her my breast milk—I felt it was essential for her health.

When I hung up the phone, I tried to relate all of this to my family, but burst into tears after a few words. In my mind, the next eleven months stretched out in front of me like a terrible eternity.

Fortunately for me, my family members sprung into action. They all left to gather the needed items. A breast hand-pump was brought over, and I began struggling with it. By then I had regained my composure, but a couple of attempts with the hand-pump, and I lost it again. Hand-pumping took as much muscle as doing pushups, and after fifty or so, I had only a few drops of milk. I sat in the kitchen sobbing, trying to get the strength to pump more, knowing my baby was hungry. Michael came in and helped by milking my breasts like a dairy cow, but still the output was very little.

My father's wife arranged to pick up the special feeding nipples and bottles at the hospital, and an electric breast pump she was able to rent just before the place closed. But it would take a few hours before she returned with the pump. I was very grateful for my family's efforts. But I knew that Lily was hungry now, and I wanted to do something.

My sister's friend Stacey had an eight-month-old boy. Stacey had just been telling my sister how she was painfully engorged because her son was eating more and nursing less. She had had to pump some milk out just to be comfortable, and was storing it in her fridge, but she didn't know what to do with it. In our tiny town, this was our saving grace.

I will never forget the look on Lily's face when I put that bottle to her lips. She drank hungrily, then stopped intermittently to smile, then drank more. She must have smiled twenty times while drinking that bottle. She just kept looking at me as if saying, "Finally, you got it! You understand what I wanted!" Her happiness relieved and touched me deeply. I was and still am so grateful to Stacey for her milk. It was the first time my baby had really had a meal and been satisfied. For the very first time, Lily drank until she fell blissfully asleep. Then the breast pump arrived.

And so began my relationship with the breast pump, a double electric Medela model. The instruction booklet had drawings of a woman pumping milk who looked like she was in ecstasy. (Maybe if she had just tried hand-pumping, by comparison it would seem like that.) It was far from ecstasy. The six-ounce plastic bottles looked huge, and I was disappointed how long it took to get any significant milk. It turned out that since Lily had not been able to suck, my milk had almost completely gone away. My mother assured me that it might take a while, but that using the pump would make my milk come back. In the meantime, I would need something to feed my baby.

I was so thankful to have my mother's help so I could focus my attention on trying to pump milk. She wholeheartedly took on the difficult job of rounding up as much donor breast milk as she could find. It was amazing that in our tiny town, she actually found a total of four women who were willing to help. Still I was always anxious that we wouldn't have enough. Each time a new bottle of donor milk arrived, it looked smaller to me because of Lily's increasing appetite.

All the while I continued pumping for about forty-five minutes every two hours, around the clock. It was absolutely exhausting, especially because of everything I had been through with the long labor and the previous week of frustration. But it worked. My milk supply finally returned! After five days of giving my baby mostly other women's breast milk, I was able to feed her with all of my own. I finally felt a moment of pride. It was a huge relief to know that it would be possible for Lily to get all the benefits of my breast milk, but it was an amazing effort.

I was inundated with bottles. As an ecologically conscious person who heretofore had almost no plastic in her house, I was suddenly swimming in it. Three kinds of bottles, four kinds of nipples, lids, caps, pump attachments, sterilizing equipment, cleaning brushes, drying racks, milk storage bags, and more cluttered the kitchen. When I finally got the courage to try glass bottles, months later, I was so relieved. It was more natural, safer, and actually easier! Still nothing could change the fact that I had to wash about forty bottles every day by hand. I was really looking forward to Lily eating food.

We rescheduled Lily's initial doctor's appointment in the hopes that if she was a little older, maybe she could learn to nurse. I had gotten the idea from an article in an old La Leche League publication written by a lady named Edith Grady. She gave birth to twins, one of which was born with cleft palate. Somehow she had not only nursed one baby full time, but her baby with cleft palate would also nurse each time during the letdown. Then she would pump the rest of her milk and give it to her baby in a bottle. At three months of age, her baby had the operation to correct cleft palate, and she was then able to teach her baby to nurse. I was empowered and inspired to teach Lily to nurse. However, the key point was that this took place after the corrective surgery. Because cleft palate surgery was now only performed once a baby was eleven months old, it changed the situation dramatically, and this meant that I would need to pump every drop of milk that Lily would drink for almost a year, and very likely longer.

As my mother had said, "That pump is going to be your new best friend." For months, I pumped every four hours around the clock, even in the night. Each time I pumped it took between thirty and forty-five minutes. This left me no free time, of course, but far worse, it came out of my sleep. After rising to care for my new baby at 2:00 A.M., waiting five minutes for the bottle to heat up, all the while with Lily crying, I would spend a half an hour feeding and burping her, then soothing her back to sleep. Then instead of going back to bed myself, I would pump milk for forty-five minutes. By the time I washed out the pump, safely stored the milk, and got back to sleep, it would only be another hour before Lily would be awake again.

This intense cycle made my milk supply go down, and so I would struggle to pump more, which meant less sleep again, making it worse. Looking back on those first few months, I am so thankful that I made it through them with out having a nervous breakdown.

One day during that particularly difficult time, I was actually sitting eating breakfast at the table instead of hooked up to the pump as I had been having all of my other meals. I could see it was warm summer weather outside, though I hadn't been out in days. Crossing the street was a parade of three little boys (all under the age of five) trailing one by one, like baby ducklings, with their lovely mother right behind them. Her flowing dress moved in the breeze, and her long hair hung loose down her back. She seemed to have it all under control. How?

I almost started to cry, feeling that I would spend the rest of my life trying to get sleep, and spending all of my waking hours tied with a thirty-two-inch tube to the breast pump. All I could hear was the annoying, rhythmic wheezing sound that the pump made, which oddly enough always sounded like a human voice repeating a phrase over and over. (The most common one it seemed to be chanting was "It's fun for me, it's fun for me, it's fun for me," which was obviously ironic.)

My mother assured me that this whole experience I was having would give me the ability to help others. I wasn't sure how, but through the next few months I would be called upon for help by several nursing mothers. One woman was going to have dental surgery, and wanted to pump some milk ahead of time, so that her baby wouldn't have to have any milk that might have anesthetics in it. She needed advice on what kind of bottles and nipples, how much milk her baby would consume during a given time frame, how to store and heat up milk, and finally, to use my electric breast pump. I was only too happy to help her.

A few months later another friend called who was very sick. Her milk supply was severely affected, and so her baby was not getting enough milk. I was able to help her as well.

I reminded myself that Lily would soon be eating solid foods, and when she reached six months, Michael and I let her try them. But it was of little use. She seemed to like several things—broccoli, yams, squash—but after a couple of bites, she would usually choke a little because some was stuck in her cleft, then she would sneeze, and it would come out her nose. This experience was obviously unpleasant for her, and so she was not inclined to eat anything. (The one fortunate thing was that I was now able to go some nights without pumping. I was still waking to feed Lily, but I had enough milk so that I could go back to bed after she fell asleep.)

When we finally had the appointment with the surgeon at the hospital, we were able to get more information about Lily's situation. Michael and I were able to put our concerns to rest about the cause of Lily's birth defect. They impressed upon us that it was no one's fault, and that it was thought to be caused by a mixture of genetic and environmental factors.

We also realized how fortunate she was, as cleft palate is usually much more severe, involving a split across the entire roof of the mouth and frequently the lips as well. This is much more difficult to correct and leaves scars. Lily's cleft was only a few millimeters in the back of the roof of her mouth, and because it was the soft palate, easier to repair. But no operation is simple, or inexpensive. We were to expect a two-day hospital stay and a three-week recovery period in which she could only have food in a liquid form in a cup, and there was no alternative. The surgeon told us that if she did not have the corrective surgery, her speech could be adversely affected, and that she would continue to have food occasionally come out of her nose. So we resolved that it was something that would be difficult, but that it would be much better after.

The difficult challenges of bottle-feeding with breast milk were something I had to become accustomed to. I could not enjoy the bonding of nursing. I was not even able to soothe Lily by having her close to my breast. She would cry and push me away if I tried to comfort her by placing her near my breast. And of course, I did not have the convenience of being able to nurse her to sleep. In fact, she had to be very calm before she would even accept the bottle each time, and I would have to estimate how much milk she would drink. If it was not enough, she would run out and start crying again, wide awake while I struggled to hold her as I heated up more milk. Then I would have to calm her down again before she would continue feeding. On the other hand, sometimes she would barely drink anything from the bottle and it would all have to be thrown out.

I felt that no one understood. In an American culture where (sadly) breastfeeding is rare, the town I lived in is the opposite. Everywhere I went, people stared at us for having bottles—especially when someone would hear me say "Michael, I need the milk," because he had pockets and I didn't. Sometimes we were asked rude questions, and always the person assumed we were feeding formula, and was disgusted. Our reply became a quick, but civil "It's breast milk, because she cannot nurse." This was enough for most people, but still we didn't feel very comfortable going out to restaurants and such. It was those people who never asked anything, but just stared holes through us so it was hard to eat our meal, who really made us feel uncomfortable.

I was so sensitive to other people's attitudes that I didn't feel like going to my La Leche League meetings anymore. I was breastfeeding after all, but I was bottle-feeding too, and I felt no one understood or appreciated what I was going through. I was wrong.

On a scorching summer Sunday, we were invited to a La Leche League family potluck lunch. I saw when I arrived what I had been avoiding by not attending the meetings. Lots of happy mothers cuddling their babies close to them while they nursed. They were more relaxed than I was. It only made me sad and envious. I was running around between the fridge, my baby, and the stove, trying not to heat up too much milk so it would go to waste, and trying to meet my baby's unpredictable feeding needs that changed from minute to minute. Lily was always fed on demand like any breastfeeding baby (rather than on a rigid schedule like most bottle-feeding babies), which was difficult.

It turned out that I was honored at this meeting for "coping with the challenges of both breastfeeding and bottle-feeding every day." The women who helped me out by supplying breast milk during those critical five days were also honored. Our midwife placed flowered crowns on our heads, woven with love, from her garden outside. It really meant a lot to me to feel acknowledged.

I have now begun to feel like Lily will never eat solid foods, now that she is almost nine months old, yet I know that it is illogical. I just have to keep on with this labor of love, knowing that it will help give her a healthy immune system. I am anxious about her upcoming operation (at age eleven months), but I am hopeful that she might be able to learn to nurse after the three-week healing time. I love Lily very much and I am proud that she has been so healthy, which I feel is due to the fact that I persevered in giving her my breast milk, when it would have been so much easier to use a substitute like formula. I am thankful to my family, my midwife, Robin, and my wonderful, supportive community for under-standing the many benefits and importance of breast milk. I want to serve as an inspiring example to other women with cleft palate babies that they can do it too. I hope that someday Lily will give her baby the gift of mama's milk, just as I have given her.

I learned recently that it wasn't until last year that breastfeeding in public became legal here in the state of Iowa. So maybe my mother was a revolutionary after all, taking her baby with her on this difficult but rewarding and important journey of advocating breastfeeding. I am proud to have worn that "I'm a breast-fed baby" button when I was a baby, and even more proud that my baby can wear it now.

After a Birth in Bali

The following story comes in letter form. Mary Kroeger, CNM came to visit me in Bali. I was working as a home-birth midwife in the villages. She had been working as a World Bank consultant/midwife in a Safe Motherhood project in Java. She arrived at my house as I was leaving to receive a baby; Mary came along to help. The birth was magical. What followed is detailed in this letter from me to Mary, written in 1997, Nyuh Kuning Village, Bali, Indonesia.

Dear Mary,

Our little baby boy in Singakerta village is growing like a weed! I have been keeping a close eye on him and have said many prayers of thanks for his life and that you were there to help me receive him. I feel you were called, and the story following will convince you.

Wayan Sekarini and Budiartha [the new mom and dad] have asked me to share their story with you. It gives our work a perspective, which too often is ignored or invisible in the West.

On the twelfth day of life, Balinese families go to a *dukun* (seer/healer/priest or priestess). The dukun receives simple offerings and prays for the child. Often he or she "receives" spiritual/psychic information that the family is happy to receive so they can nurture the baby according to his soul's needs in this life. If the dukun has *Lontars* (ancient holy books written on palm leaf, bound between bamboo), the *Lontar* page for the baby's day of birth will also be read.

This was what happened when the family of the baby we received went to the dukun:

Right away the dukun said, "He had a very hard time taking his first breath." The parents of the baby were surprised and said that it was so. [This was a baby with Apgars of two at one minute, two at five minutes, and finally eight when he reached ten minutes of life.] The dukun then told them why: "There were three other souls trying to get into this boy's body at the moment of birth. It was a war. Two of the souls are past and future members of your family, but do not have *ijin* (permission) to take birth yet. They are coming later but must first learn patience.

"Only this child you have has God's permission to be born to you at this time. There was one soul who is *jahat* (fierce) who was the most dangerous one. He very much wanted this birth, this body. His intentions were not good. You see, this boy will be a shadow puppet master. His father is very gifted and must pass the knowledge on to his son. The place of a *Dalang* (puppet master) is powerful, he lives between shadow and light and commits to memory the stories of *Adat* (culture). In this way, he helps the people learn and keep the morals and ethics of Bali Hindu Dharma. It must be kept by a pure heart. The fierce one craves the power of knowledge but is not meant to have it. In the wrong hands, the knowledge could be twisted and passed along to the people in ways that would undermine the culture of Bali.

"So the baby you have was watching the war, doing what he could to get in, and needing the help that he had from the midwives. It was very fortunate that he survived and that it is truly him who occupies this body.

"His name in this incarnation should be I. Wayan Windu Phalouna. In his previous birth, his name was I. Wayan Tampil. He was also a puppet master from your family (later confirmed by the family). He died in 1939 and was seventy-nine years old. He could have lived longer, as he was healthy. However, black magic was done on him, as this war that ended with his successful rebirth had begun long ago."

In Bali everyone believes in past and future lives. They have many experiences like this one, which confirm their belief in reincarnation. Pregnancy, birth, and postpartum are acknowledged as times when the veil between the physical and spirit worlds is very thin. For this reason, the new mother and baby are nurtured and protected by the entire extended family.

Priya K Chhalliyil...Home Birth and a Blissful Postpartum, with the Help of My Parents

My pregnancy and delivery of Pranav Chhalliyil was a spiritual experience. Conception, according to me, should not be an accident during sex. Instead it should be understood as God's gift. My husband and myself chose an auspicious day in end of April 2000. We spent the whole day in meditation and prayers. I could really feel the conception event taking place in my body the next day.

Throughout my pregnancy, I had morning sickness but took it to be a positive sign that my body was balancing the new change. I took only healthy and natural diets (mostly organic). I did not take any medications, not even vitamins and supplements. All my nutrition was derived from natural foods. I did take organic milk and very rarely eggs. For proteins and other nutrients, I included lot of pulses [mung beans, lentils, chickpeas, dahl, etc.] in my diet. I took fruits abundantly. I did not use any processed food. I used no leftover foods and no foods prepared in a microwave oven. I did not use any cosmetics either.

We did meditation and prayers regularly, and only read spiritual books and watched spiritual videos. I and my husband talked to the baby, sang songs, and maintained a peaceful atmosphere. I also talked to and read books aloud to my baby. After the conception, we maintained celibacy because we felt that would be supportive to his growing life.

I worked till the end of seventh month as a computer programmer, and during work I tried to avoid too much stress. In the seventh month, my husband and a few friends gathered in Chicago Aurora Temple and performed the traditional Hindu rituals for a pregnant woman. I was given sweets and dresses in the temple and glass bangles. It is considered that the mind of the developing child (psyche) develops in the seventh month and so the pregnant women should always be cheerful and optimistic and enjoy nice and pleasant moments. The pleasant glass bangles gives the baby the sense of sound. In India, the pregnant mom would be invited by neighbors and relatives and friends who would cook food of her choice. My friends here in Fairfield were very kind to provide lunches and dinner for me.

In India, usually in the seventh month, the girl goes to her parents' home and returns only after the third or fourth month postpartum. Since I had visa problems to go back to India, my parents came to take care of me at the beginning of the ninth month.

After my parents arrived in the United States, the atmosphere was more relaxing and fun. We were going to regular hospital checkups. We wanted a home delivery with help of a midwife. We dropped the idea because our parents would be worried, and they would think that we are crazy and taking a big risk.

By the third of January 2001, our hospital visits were unpleasant and it so happened that we thought of having home delivery with a midwife. After I started getting contractions, my husband called Robin Lim. She immediately came and did a wonderful job as a midwife. She was well equipped and did everything like a mom. She helped me to deliver Pranav and made the whole delivery a spiritual event. She joined us in chanting prayers throughout the process. She followed the Hindu tradition in doing the rituals too. It was amazing that she was also, like us, a devotee of Mata Amritanandamayi Devi, the holy saint from India. Robin made a water bath, which eased the pain. In every step, she prayed for help from the Holy Mother and used her holy ash and holy water. Robin asked my dad to let Ammachi [the holy saint mother] know that I was in labor. Ammachi was in India and my dad talked over phone with her disciple and passed on the message.

Pranav was born after midnight of 22 January 2001. He came out and cried just once and started looking at us. We did not believe in the statistics of weight and let nature decide the weight of our child. We were happy that Pranav weighed 5.8 lbs. and was 21 inches long. He had an Apgar score of 10. The most wonderful thing Robin suggested was not to cut the umbilical cord or separate our baby from his placenta. First I felt it was strange and unheard of. Robin said some traditional cultures never cut the cord and let it drop naturally. Our child was not separated from me after birth. He was just wrapped in a warm cloth (warm by keeping it inside the shirt of my dad) and laid on my breast.

We called our brothers and in-laws and let everyone know the good news. We all then slept and to our amazement he did not cry at all. He slept peacefully through the night. Next day morning Robin with her friend Marie came and cleaned the placenta and wrapped it in a diaper with herbal powder. Pranav was given a bath and was made to suck my breast. On the second day, colostrum appeared and till then he was not given anything. He did not become dehydrated and was very peaceful. My parents and husband were amazed to see the peaceful boy. It's usual that babies cry and make a big mess. I feel that did not happen because of Robin's suggestion of not cutting the cord and not separating our baby from me. Therefore this home delivery did not give stress to the mom or the baby.

It was initially inconvenient to have the placenta with him. But later we did not find it as a problem at all. Since he lived with the placenta for ten moons, butchering after birth would be violence and a great loss for our baby. All these violent practices started with modern medicine. There was no pus or pain in the placenta. The cord started to dry like a strong cable wire. On the sixth day, my mom was holding the placenta bag in her palm while Pranav was nursing. She felt pulse inside the placenta when he suckled. When he stopped, the pulse also stopped. This was incredible for my husband (he has a Ph.D. in biochemistry) to feel. He said it's so true that the placenta is still alive and was supporting the baby's mind and body. On the eighth day, the placenta dropped and did not cause any pain to Pranav. There was no infection and the whole event was very pleasant. Robin suggested we bury the placenta in the traditional way, back in India. My husband and myself were both born at home and both our placentas were buried with due homage according to the Hindu tradition. We wanted Pranav to have his roots in India and so took the dried placenta to India to be in its roots.

Robin with Marie also helped me to breastfeed my child. I did not give Pranav any formula food. My parents coming to help me was the best thing in the post-partum period. Without them, it would have been very stressful for us. My mom took care of the baby always and allowed me to take lot of rest. I was just feeding him and eating and sleeping. My dad and husband took care of home and of me. This was the most wonderful thing. I felt I was in India and had a very peaceful postpartum period. I feel every pregnant woman should have physical help from her parents instead of getting just gifts and monetary help.

Baby Pranav is very calm and does not cry unnecessarily. He cries only when he wets the cloth diapers and for hunger. He continues to be very peaceful with lots of love and affection from everyone and blessings from God.

Sophia…Postpartum in Holland

When I had my first child seven years ago, we were living in Indonesia. We had a beautiful home and my husband provided us with two helpers to take care of us and all the mundane stuff like dirty nappies and cooking meals. It was warm and beautiful like a dream. But my husband died, and things changed.

This time I was pregnant in Holland—a single mom with a seven-year-old daughter. My boyfriend had left us, and I was nervous about the birth and the sleepless nights to follow. It was ten days before Christmas when my waters broke as I was standing in line at the cash register in the supermarket.

I guess the C-section was as beautiful a birth as one can ever hope a C-section to be, but I had hoped for things to go normally.

The first four days after the operation I was in hospital, but a shortage of beds and capacity forced the hospitals to check their patients out in the least possible time. I could barely walk and looked bloated like a balloon, but the baby was fine and I had to go.

My sister picked us up. It was freezing cold outside and we had packed the baby in a little basket. We drove to the center of the old town where we live in a house with a narrow steep staircase to enter. To this day, I don't know how I got up those stairs—backwards I think—but I remember the welcoming scent of the Christmas tree and the hyacinths that I had bought the Saturday before, and which were now blooming abundantly. I remember registering the mess as we worked our way to the bedroom. Clothes were spread all over the floor, dishes all over the apartment, and my plants had dried out. My neighbors had taken care of my daughter, but she had hopped in every now and then for a change of clothes or toys, leaving the kind of mess any seven-year-old would when home alone for five days.

At this point, any single mom's postpartum story would turn into a total disaster, but I happened to be in Holland. It is regulation in Holland for insurance companies to provide a trained nurse for one week to women who have just given birth. It is up to the parents to decide how they will take advantage of this service and can take anything from two hours a day to eight hours a day to have the nurse come around. She can show a new mother how to take care of her baby and she will watch the mother's health closely.

The nurse that came to help me was a very gentle young woman who had just finished her education. She was an angel directly sent from the heavens. She cleaned and washed, did the shopping, and received the visitors whom she offered coffee. She was gentle, kind and full of valuable practical suggestions that she never imposed on me. She was the very reason I recovered at all.

Rather than the Netherlands being an incredible, humane society, I guess part of this practice is a simple math calculation: it is no doubt more economical to provide simple postpartum care than it is to treat the kind of complications that can arise from exhaustion or maltreatment out of neglect.

In my case, the simple reality was that this nurse made it possible for me to actually look at my baby, getting to know him and getting to love him. I am so grateful!

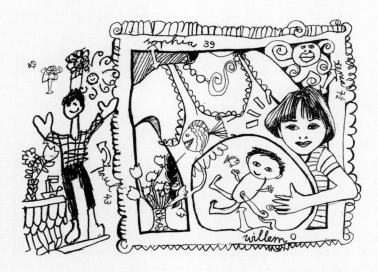

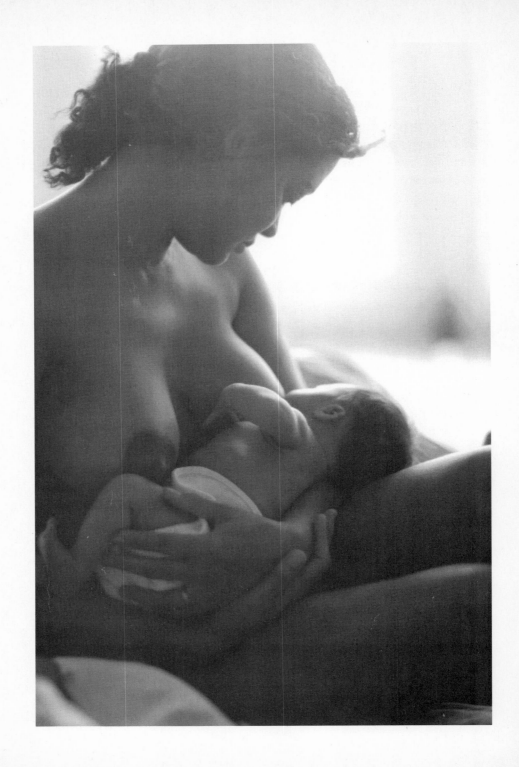

CHAPTER 18

Family Planning...An Overview

Having a baby has reinvented your family, all aspects of your life have been renewed. This is a good time to take a fresh look at family planning.

The *Merriam-Webster Dictionary* says, **Con.tra.cep.tion** n: *intentional prevention of conception.*

Such a short definition for such a huge issue. Now that you have a new baby, it is natural for you to want to avoid pregnancy. Perhaps you just wish to wait so you can breastfeed this baby in your arms for a good long time. Realistically your body needs time to reinvent herself. Perhaps your family feels complete—for now anyway. All of your reasons—personal, spiritual, political, even financial—for carefully planning your family are valid.

Some of the most commonly asked postpartum questions I hear are these: What about family planning? What can we do that is safe for my body and will not hurt my breastfeeding baby? Is there a natural form of birth control that is also dependable?

I have discovered that *birth control* and *family planning* are two very different things. Birth control (emphasis on control) is an aggressive approach, employing artificial devices or pharmaceuticals, which alters or blocks the natural state of fertility. All artificial birth control comes with side effects. A woman needs a great deal of information in order to make a wise choice for herself. A breastfeeding mother needs to make a wise choice for herself *and* her baby. *Informed choice* is the foundation of true family planning. Later in this chapter, I will share the knowledge I have gathered about Natural Family Planning (NFP). To be fair, I must tell you that what I'm about to write is my bias, based on my personal struggle with birth control and on the challenges that I have seen many women face in my years as a midwife.

> Natural Family Planning (NFP) is a cooperative, nonviolent approach to avoiding, postponing, or achieving pregnancy. Inherently NFP allows for choice within the natural boundaries of healthy living.

Let's first explore *birth control*…what is it? The political downside of *birth control* is something I refer to as *contraceptive terrorism.* In the so-called "developing world," wealthier countries, like ours, have implemented population control programs that, in my opinion, deny individual women their reproductive rights.

There is a valid argument that our Mother Earth is simply overpopulated, that she can no longer bear the strain of so many people on her natural resources. However, regarding the world's annual resource consumption, 6 percent of the world's population (people living in the United States) uses 40 percent of the resources. The wealthiest 20 percent of the world's population accounts for 80 percent of the resource use.[1] (That means a few folks at the top are using up the grain, the oil, the gas, the paper and wood products, the water, and even the food; the list goes on.) Since all living things need air, water, and food, someone thought it best to control the number of living things we create on Earth. Good thinking. I wonder why the poorer 80 percent of our world's population, who use only about 20 percent of the available resources, are being forced to bear the burden of population control?

When I say burden, I speak of concentrated population control efforts, funded by the developed countries and implemented in countries where the United States has special strategic interests: Bangladesh, Brazil, Colombia, Egypt, Ethiopia, Guatemala, India, Indonesia, Mexico, Nigeria, Pakistan, the Philippines, Thailand, and Turkey, to name a few. In 1974, a human rights issue of historic proportion was born. That was the year when the U.S. Secretary of State and National Security Council head, Henry Kissinger, drafted National Security Study Memorandum 200. It outlined "Implications of Population Growth for U.S. Security and Overseas Interests." It argued that rapid population growth could lead to unrest, which would pose a threat to the United States' access to poor countries' mineral resources. Furthermore, increased population in these countries could subtract from the success of U.S.-owned business interests and investments.[2] Translation: From one of the highest offices of our nation comes the decree to aggressively impose state control over the number of children people are permitted to have.

Having lived and served as a mother, a midwife, and teacher of Natural Family Planning in Indonesia and the Philippines, I can testify to the damage done to individual lives by this policy. The facts are not pretty. Nevertheless, I do not believe that new mothers are "too fragile" to want the facts. Forgive me if my observations concerning contraception are not pleasant.

In Indonesia and the Philippines, I have met women who cannot bear children because they were injected as girls with tetanus toxiod vaccine laced with human chorionic gonadotrophin (HCG).[3] The result is that each pregnancy they achieve ends in miscarriage as their bodies reject the developing embryo once the HCG level rises. The developed countries of the world have successfully developed a vaccine to prevent the poor from having children. This has been used on girls and women without their knowledge or consent. Many lives have been shattered as a result.[4] Clearly, in my eyes, this looks like a form of economic racial imperialism.

In 1989, Norplant 2 (which has two rods instead of six tubes) was withdrawn from the world market because there was concern about the "teratogenicity and carcinogenicity" of the Norplant rods. Prior to that date Norplant 2 was implanted in about 3,500 women. Women in India have stated that they were unaware that they were participating in an experiment.[5] I personally know a young African American woman in Chicago who was offered four hundred dollars cash by a government-subsidized clinic, if she would agree to have Norplant surgically inserted in her forearm. Friends of hers had experienced menstrual irregularities, hair loss, loss of vision, bulging painful eyes, and difficulty getting the rods removed. Fortunately for her, she decided against Norplant.

In Indonesia, I found women fitted with IUDs that had no string. One woman, who was hemorrhaging because of her IUD, went to five doctors (paying each one along the way) before one was successful in taking the device out. The doctor ridiculed her for wanting to be rid of the IUD, calling her "a stupid woman, who did not know anything." In protest, this brave woman became a teacher of Natural Family Planning.

Also, in Indonesia it is illegal for veterinarians to inject dogs with the same Depo-Provera routinely administered to women. This harmful contraceptive is injected into women who are not medically screened to determine if their health can tolerate the many potential side effects. No informed consent is sought from these women, who clearly have limited, if any, access to quality health care, should the contraception harm them and cause them to need medical assistance.

Family planning, unlike birth control or population control, is a cooperative lifestyle. I acknowledge that there are women in this world, indeed women I have known and cared about, who are not in cooperative marriages. There are women who cannot embrace natural methods of family planning because their husband and/or their culture will not allow it. For these women, it is a blessing to sneak off to the clinic and obtain a Depo-Provera injection to prevent pregnancies that could be life threatening. Every minute on Earth at least one woman dies from complications of pregnancy and childbirth. Many women make necessary compromises regarding their health to protect their well-being.

Couples employing natural methods of family planning are fortunate to be able to choose their own path rather than having that choice dictated by health officials of the state or by pharmaceutical corporations. They are free from the threat of physical side effects. The methods they use are completely reversible; Natural Family Planning methods can be employed to avoid or achieve pregnancy.

In a perfect world, no one would need to compromise. Methods of avoiding pregnancy would all be healthy; free of side effects, risk, and reactions; and affordable by all. In the cafeteria of birth-control options, Natural Family Planning has been underserved. In fact, it isn't even a side dish. It's represented

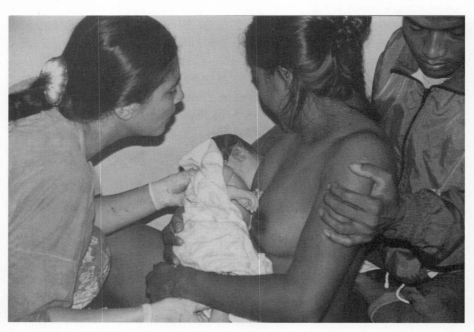

more like a sprig of parsley. For most of my reproductive life, I did not consider it a real option. This, I feel, was due to the sad fact that I did not trust my body. I became convinced that my fertility was out to kidnap me away from my "real" life. This mistrust is not something a girl is born with; I learned it in school and from my friends. Advertising paid for by pharmaceutical companies helped drill it into my belief structure. As I grew older and wiser, I began to understand that my fertility was a magnificent gift. I pray today that my daughters perceive their fertility as just that—a gift.

The intention of this chapter is to share with you knowledge gathered from many years of teaching NFP to couples in many countries. This method involves observing and charting your fertile signs and abstaining during those times of possible fertility. Like any method used to avoid pregnancy, the dependability and effectiveness of NFP will have a lot to do with you. If you depend on the "Pill" as your birth-control method and you forget to take it, you know you risk unintended pregnancy. If you choose NFP but do not observe, chart, and follow the simple rules, pregnancy will likely result. Because you must abstain during times of fertility, *this method demands cooperation, commitment, and discipline. Abstention means no genital contact. None.*

Both in Asia and in the United States, I have been told by couples that the cooperation necessary to make NFP work improves their communication with each other. This enhancement in communication naturally benefits their relationship. It has been my observation that better relationships are a positive side effect of using a cooperative method of natural family planning. On the other hand, using a method about which you don't feel good, or in which you do not have confidence, can adversely affect your relationship. *So enter these waters with care.* NFP is not for everyone, but for those couples who do work together well and who can embrace NFP as a cooperative lifestyle, the information in this chapter will be a gift.

Ask yourselves: What if we do get pregnant? Among our hundreds of NFP students, pregnancies have occurred. Less than 1 percent have been method related. This means that the couple either did not chart regularly or simply broke/bent the rules. Some did not fully understand the rules, usually because they did not fully follow up with us, or they did not take the time (or were too shy) to ask their questions and were confused about their signs of fertility. Statistically somewhere between .5 and 3 women per 100 per year of use have pregnancies related to failure of NFP methods.[6]

Clearly women run great health risks whenever a conception has taken place. It has been argued that the risks from pregnancy terminations, pregnancy complications, and birth itself are much higher than the health risks caused by the harmful side effects of the artificial methods and devices of birth control. This is true. Again I must tell you that every minute on Earth more than one woman dies from a complication of pregnancy or childbirth.

NFP is not a quick fix. You must decide if NFP is for you. I do not offer to teach women and their partners NFP because of a certain religious agenda. I consider myself a full participant in the religion of gratitude. I look for the blessing in all circumstances, and usually I find it. Families I have taught who have had unplanned pregnancies have shared with me the feeling that this child is a special blessing. I hope that all of you who choose to take the road less traveled, by using this cooperative method of Natural Family Planning, will carefully consider any unplanned pregnancies the blessing they well may be. I like to think that there are no unwanted children. Most of us were surely unplanned. The decision to have a baby will change your life forever. Also, the decision to terminate a pregnancy will change your life forever.

You can get pregnant again very soon after childbirth. Some women return to fertility immediately, especially if they bottle-feed the baby. Others go many months before ovulating. If you're not having your moons (menstrual periods) yet, be warned: You could ovulate and get pregnant before the onset of your first postnatal menstruation. To avoid this predicament, follow the Lactation Amenorrhea criteria outlined next.

LAM…Nature's Own Child Spacing

Breastfeeding suppresses fertility. This is called the **Lactation Amenorrhea Method (LAM)**. To be a dependable method of child spacing, the following three criteria must be met:

• Your menstrual periods have *not* returned.
• Your baby is fully and ecologically (see sidebar page 341) breastfed.
• Your baby is less than six months old.

Somewhere between .5 and 3 women in 100 per year get pregnant using LAM. All three of the above criteria must be met or your chances of unintended pregnancy are much greater.

I feel it's best to learn Natural Family Planning (instructions begin on page 337) during the first few months of breastfeeding, while ovulation is naturally suppressed. This gives couples time to become confident in their ability to observe, record, and interpret their signs of possible fertility before they develop fears of unintended pregnancy. LAM is nature's way of giving us a break, so we can better learn how to dance with our fertility. If you meet the above three criteria, it is quite unlikely you will become pregnant.

I've heard many stories from women that go something like this: "I was breastfeeding my son, and my moons [menstruation] had not returned. Then when my baby was seven months old, he got his first tooth, and he began to eat a little food. I was so busy I didn't even think about my fertility. The next thing you know, I was pregnant again!" This mother's menstruation had not yet returned. *However,* her baby was no longer *fully* breastfeeding and the baby was no longer *less than six months old.* She must have become pregnant as soon as her fertility returned, the first time she ovulated after childbirth.

You may wish to space your children farther apart than the mother in the story. Enjoy your time of Lactation Amenorrhea, but be on the lookout for signs that your fertility is returning. Believe me, it *is* going to come back. The only sure way to do this is to observe and chart your fertile signs and follow the rules for naturally avoiding pregnancy (see pages 337 to 349). Plan ahead to avoid unintended pregnancy. Study, learn the signs and the rules, start keeping a chart while you still meet all the LAM criteria. This will greatly reduce your anxiety. A beautiful book on this subject is *Breastfeeding and Natural Child Spacing: The Ecology of Natural Mothering* by Sheila Kippley (see Reading and Resources).

Other Natural Methods of Spacing Out...

WITHDRAWAL

Don't laugh, you've probably tried this. Among typical couples using withdrawal, about 19 percent will experience an accidental pregnancy in the first year.[7] That does not sound like very good statistics, but it's better than nothing. It's always an option and it's free. Nearly everyone I have asked has admitted that they have used withdrawal at some time in their lives.

Depending on withdrawal as a form of contraception may greatly add to a couple's stress level, causing gray hairs. The man may worry, Will I get out in time? The woman will worry, Is he really going to withdraw in time? The man must withdraw before he ejaculates, or there is no contraceptive benefit. This concern may decrease enjoyment of sex. There are also other disadvantages:

Sperm may be present in the arousal fluid that comes out of the penis before ejaculation. Withdrawal provides no protection against sexually transmitted infections, including HIV (the AIDS virus). Unless both the man and the woman are HIV-free and both monogamous (not participating in sex with other people), it is recommended that you use condoms for your protection. Withdrawal is better than nothing at all.

CHANCE
Of one hundred women who leave conception up to chance, 85 percent of them will experience pregnancy within one year.[8]

OUTERCOURSE
Sexual intimacy that does not involve the penis entering the vagina. This includes holding hands, hugging, snuggling, kissing, mutual masturbation, oral-genital contact, lots of touching. It takes discipline as the contraceptive and infection prevention benefits are lost if the couple engages in genital-to-genital contact. It's always an option and it's free.

ABSTINENCE
Not having sexual intercourse. For some people, it feels really okay to abstain from sexual relations for some times in their lives. If you are in a partnership (are a couple), it is important that both of you are honest and open with one another about abstinence. If one member of a couple is dissatisfied, communication must take place or the partnership may be at risk. This is particularly important if you are parents; children do benefit from clear communication between their parents. Abstinence has advantages: It's free, and it's effective in preventing pregnancy and infection. It can help some couples develop a deep connection aside from sex.

Caution! In the heat of arousal, which can happen at any time, a couple may change their mind about abstinence. If they don't want to get pregnant, they should have another method of contraception on hand. If abstinence is frustrating, it may not be for you.

The Lens-Fertility Magnifier *written by Jeannine Parvati Baker*
After *Conscious Conception* (1986) (see Reading and Resources) became the pioneer work in the field of integrative fertility awareness, I was sent one of the first field microscopes promoted as an ovulation indicator. The importer had arranged for the PG-53 model from Spain to come to the United States and I was designated as a potential endorser of the new product. Like a few other times in my

life, I was initially repulsed by what was to eventually become one of my best allies—the round plastic microscope with the words on it: Posibilidad de Embarazada Hoy? Si `o No? [Possibility of pregnancy today? Yes or no?]

Indeed, the Lens does demonstrate where in the cycle of fertility I am at any given moment. Like the cervical mucus changes, saliva indicates approaching and waning fertility. This information had lain buried in the gynecological literature for at least a half century when in the 1950s a Spanish researcher demonstrated how predictable ovulation is through saliva sampling. Among the many advantages I soon discovered with the saliva tester was that I always had saliva, whereas, sometimes in my various seasons of fertility, I didn't have cervical mucus (literally) handy to sample. And with the Lens, I could even take samples in public!

Since that time, I have sampled at least a half dozen other models and found some variance in the visual acuity based on design, stain to the lens, and power of magnification. From the round, "birth control device" look of the first model I used, to the lipstick-shaped model I presently use, they have all served the same goal: to highlight hormonal changes and to augment a thorough fertility awareness program. In postpartum in particular, as well as in menarche and menopause, this device is a real boon as "regularity" may not be a given. Any way to foretell ovulation is important when there are many long days of shifting fertility.

Author's note: To order a Lens, see Reading and Resources (page 366). I have found that to use the Lens effectively, charting one's findings daily, along with external mucus signs and/or along with the signs of the cervix (as taught in this chapter), is essential.

My youngest daughter has grown up with her mother licking her Lens each day and viewing the microscopic mysteries therein. When she first tried one herself, at the age of nine years or so, she exclaimed in prophetic tones, "I will have four children." She then proceeded to count out loud and when I looked in the Lens to see her first sample, there were four distinct cells she was counting, like ripening egg follicles in her mind's eye. I loved this image: my youngest of four daughters looking into the scrying device to see her future family and knowing that she needn't be a victim of her fertility. With the Lens, we have a potent tool to free ourselves from ignorance and help to make every baby conceived a welcomed baby from the beginning!

For All the Babies, *Jeannine Parvati Baker*

Using the Lens does have some, though few, disadvantages. Like all methods of natural child spacing, it requires a daily devotion to observing and recording (charting). This takes time, not a lot, but one must really do it. The viewing of one's possible signs of fertility in the Lens takes focus. It's a little device, with a tiny viewing lens. It takes patience, time, and practice to interpret what you see in the Lens. I enjoy observing my external mucus and cervical signs (NFP), doing the Lens, and charting *all* my signs on the same page. The personal charts provided at the end of this chapter have enough space to record all these possible signs of fertility.

The Artificial Methods

CONDOMS

Apart from abstention, condoms are the best method of preventing sexually transmitted infections, including HIV and AIDS. If you are in a relationship in which there is any risk at all of contacting the HIV/AIDS virus, use condoms, please.

Condoms have a relatively high effectiveness rate, 14 pregnancies per 100 women per year of typical use.[9]

Couples using condoms (prophylactics) should use them in combination with contraceptive foam containing spermicide. The incidence of pregnancy when the two are used together is considerably lower. But don't use spermicide with this (or any other) method of birth control until your cervix is closed (minimum of six weeks postpartum, and all postpartum bleeding must have stopped) as you may be especially sensitive and have a negative reaction to it.

Any genital-to-genital contact can result in pregnancy. This means that you must be very careful to ensure that no arousal fluid or semen comes into contact with your vagina. In other words, put the condom on before you begin lovemaking or as part of foreplay.

Couples must be careful not to puncture the condom or allow semen to leak into or around the vagina. It must be removed very soon after intercourse because it slips off easily as the erection diminishes. Hold onto it as you pull away. Do not use oil-based lubricants like Vaseline, whipped cream, or massage oil: These products will put holes in a latex condom within seconds. If you are allergic to latex, natural membrane (skin) condoms are available. They are more expensive than the latex condoms, less effective in preventing pregnancy, and sexually transmitted diseases *can* be transmitted through the skin condoms.

Condoms are easy to use, but they aren't foolproof. Even if you are very careful, condoms can break during intercourse—1 breakage per 161 acts of intercourse.[10] Condoms and foam have been considered unsatisfactory by some couples because they reduce the sensation for the man and for some women. Friction from insufficiently lubricated condoms can cause irritation of the lining of the vagina. Foam can be messy and inconvenient, and some couples develop rashes due to the foam or the lubricant on the condom. The synthetic material of the condoms may also be irritating or offensive to some individuals. Bottom line: Condoms are easy to find and a much wiser choice than unprotected sex.

"I give my patients condoms at their six-week postpartum check. I know how fertility can sneak up on you. I myself got pregnant again on my first fertile cycle. I didn't even suspect I was ovulating."

Joanne, a midwife

Condoms, along with vasectomy and withdrawal, are methods of birth control that place some of the responsibility of contraception on the man.

Female Condoms: They are lubricated plastic (polyurethane, not latex) sheaths with rings at each end, designed to be worn inside the woman's vagina during intercourse. The condom can be inserted up to eight hours before intercourse. With typical use, 21 percent of women experience an unintended pregnancy within the first year of use.[11] The good news is that they give women more control: You don't need to see a health practitioner or have a prescription to get it. It does guard against sexually transmitted infections.

On the downside, they are big and funny looking. If the man's penis becomes inserted between the female condom and the vaginal wall, all potential benefits are lost. They are harder to find and about three times more expensive than male condoms. Some women say the female condom squeaks during intercourse.

VAGINAL CONTRACEPTIVE FILM (VCF)

A 2 by 2-inch paper-thin sheet that contains a chemical called nonoxynol-9 that kills sperm. It is inserted in the vagina, placed on or near the cervix, where it dissolves. Among typical couples who use VCF, about 25 percent will experience an unintended or accidental pregnancy in the first year.

Advantages: VCF is easy to use, easy to find at drugstores, and you need no prescription to obtain it.

Disadvantages: You need a new VCF for each act of intercourse. Some people find they are sensitive to the VCF and for them it causes irritation. It is not effective in preventing HIV/AIDS. Remember: If you try it, wash and dry your hands well before inserting it, or the film will stick.

DIAPHRAGM

If you choose the diaphragm as your method of contraception, remember that using a diaphragm means *using* a diaphragm; it will do you no good tucked in its case. (My first daughter was the happy result of not unpacking the diaphragm when we got to France!) The diaphragm is a rubber disk that the woman places into her vagina so that it covers her cervix, blocking the man's semen. Spermicide must be placed inside the diaphragm for it to be effective in preventing conception.

If you used a diaphragm previously, your old size may not be the size you need now after having had a baby. A new fitting may be necessary after having a miscarriage, or an abortion, or a baby, or if one gains or loses fifteen pounds or more. Some women find the spermicidal gel, which must be used for the diaphragm to be effective, is irritating. If you are using a diaphragm and suffer from recurrent vaginal infections, make sure you wash and dry your diaphragm thoroughly between uses. If the vaginal infections persist, you will need to choose another method of birth control. Use of the diaphragm increases one's risk of urinary tract infections. If left in too long, the diaphragm increases the risk for toxic shock syndrome.

Women who are not good candidates for the diaphragm are those who have chronic bladder infections, cystoceles (bladder hernias), and postpartum women who have a prolapsed or displaced uterus. (Over time, by doing kegel exercises—see pages 132–33—a woman can restore the proper position of her uterus and cervix making it possible to use a diaphragm.) Your health-care provider can help you determine if the diaphragm is a good choice for you now.

Among typical couples who initiate use of the diaphragm, about 20 percent will experience an accidental or unintended pregnancy in the first year. If the diaphragm is consistently and correctly used, about 6 percent will become pregnant.[12]

Of the couples using the diaphragm, only 35 percent continue to use it after the first six months. To be an effective contraceptive device, the diaphragm must be *correctly* inserted before there is any genital contact. Many people feel this disrupts the spontaneity of lovemaking; others are fine with it. To be effective as a contraceptive, the diaphragm must be left in place for six hours after the last act of intercourse. Spermicide must be reapplied with each act of intercourse.

CERVICAL CAP

The cervical cap, a barrier method, similar to the diaphragm (but smaller with a tall dome), has been approved by the FDA for use in the United States and has become increasingly more available. As with the diaphragm, to be effective it must be used with spermicidal gel. Women who have given birth recently (six to twelve weeks) should not use the cap as it will not be effective for them. Other women who should stay away from this form of birth control are those who have chronic urinary tract infections, are allergic to latex, have cervical erosion, malformation or infection of the cervix, and those with a history of toxic shock syndrome. The cervical cap may predispose some women to cervical and uterine infections. Studies report 8 to 27 pregnancies per 100 users per year.[13]

BIRTH CONTROL PILLS

Also called "combination oral contraceptives," these pills are man-made versions of estrogen and progestin; taken daily, they block one's normal hormone messages. No ovum are permitted to mature and conception is prevented. Breastfeeding mothers who wish to take oral contraceptives, or "the Pill," should give this issue careful thought. The *Physicians' Desk Reference* (55th edition) says: "Small amounts of oral-contraceptive steroids have been identified in the milk of nursing mothers, and a few adverse effects have been reported, including jaundice and breast enlargement. In addition, oral contraceptives given in the postpartum period may interfere with lactation by decreasing the quantity and quality of breast milk. If possible, the nursing mother should be advised not to use oral contraceptives but to use other forms of contraception until she has completely weaned her child."[14]

If taken exactly as directed, the Pill is highly effective: less than 1 in 100 women become pregnant per year. In actuality, the statistic is 6 to 8 pregnancies per 100 women a year.[15] Another source states: "Among typical couples who initiate use of combined pills about 5% will experience an accidental pregnancy in the first year."[16]

"Mini Pills," also called "progestin only pills" (POP), which contain no estrogen and have a lower dose of progestin than the combined birth control pills, are also available. They are not as potent and therefore are less effective; the user must be very careful not to forget to take her pill *at the same time every day.* Keep in mind that use of the Mini Pill has been significantly linked to an increased risk of ectopic pregnancy (an extremely dangerous pregnancy in which the egg implants inside a fallopian tube rather than the uterine cavity and can be fatal). [17]

If you feel you must take oral contraceptives and you are breastfeeding, the "Mini Pill" may be recommended by your doctor.

The fourth edition of *Drugs in Pregnancy and Lactation* rates the risk factor of oral contraceptives as X. This means that "[s]tudies in animal or human beings have demonstrated fetal abnormalities, or there is evidence of fetal risk based on human experience, or both, and the risk of the use of the drug in pregnant women clearly outweighs any possible benefit. The drug is contraindicated in women who are or may become pregnant." About oral contraceptives, the book goes on to say that "[b]oth estrogens and progestins cross into milk.... If breastfeeding is desired, the lowest effective dose of oral contraceptives should be chosen."[18]

> "Hormones contained in the pill have been shown to enter breast milk, and thus they may be absorbed by the breastfed baby. Synthetic progesterone is known to act on the hypothalamus-an important brain center. What effect this has on the developing infant is not yet established."
>
> -Dr. Evelyn Billings & Ann Westmore[19]

A Short List of Potential Side Effects of the Oral Contraceptive Pill[20]

- Increased risk of cancer of the reproductive organs
- Possible link with breast cancer
- Menstrual irregularities, in some women periods stop altogether
- Infertility after the Pill is discontinued
- Failure to menstruate within six months of coming off the Pill
- Adverse effects on bone growth of adolescent girls taking the Pill
- Reduced blood levels of several essential vitamins and minerals
- Aggravation of genital herpes and thrush infections
- Weight gain due to altered carbohydrate metabolism
- Migraine headaches (Discontinue use immediately if this happens!)
- Nausea
- Changes in blood insulin levels, risk for diabetes
- Depression—the longer you use it, the more "down" you may feel
- Loss of libido and irritability

Use of oral contraceptives does not offer any protection from sexually transmitted diseases including HIV/AIDS.

> Cigarette smoking increases the risk of serious adverse effects on the heart and blood vessels from oral-contraceptive use. This risk increases with age and with heavy smoking (15 or more cigarettes per day) and is quite marked in women over 35 years of age. Women who use oral contraceptives should not smoke.
> *-The Physicians' Desk Reference* (55th edition)

IUD (INTRAUTERINE DEVICE)

A small device that is placed into the uterine cavity for the purpose of contraception. The IUD irritates the uterine wall preventing fertilized eggs from implanting. Some IUDs contain copper, which stops sperm from making their way up through the uterus into the fallopian tubes, thus preventing fertilization. Other IUDs contain hormones to thicken the cervical mucus to prevent fertilization. Discuss the benefits, precautions, potential adverse reactions, and risks with your doctor, midwife, or nurse practitioner well ahead of time.

The advantage of an IUD is that the spontaneity of intercourse is not interrupted because you do not have to think about birth control—it is always in place. The rate of effectiveness is 1 to 6 pregnancies per 100 users per year of use.[21] If you do become pregnant while an IUD is in place, medical problems can arise and you should see your doctor right away.

Warnings for the IUD listed in the 2001 *Physicians' Desk Reference* (55th edition) include:

- Septic abortion, reports indicate an increased incidence of septic abortion with septicemia, septic shock, and death in patients becoming pregnant with an IUD in place.
- Increased risk of spontaneous abortion and sepsis should patient elect to continue pregnancy with IUD in place.
- Increased risk of ectopic pregnancy for patients who have a history of ectopic pregnancy.
- Pelvic inflammatory disease, IUDs have been associated with an increased risk of PID. PID can necessitate hysterectomy and can also lead to tubo-ovarian abscesses, tubal occlusion and infertility, and tubal damage that can predispose to ectopic pregnancy. PID can result in peritonitis and, infrequently, in death.
- Embedment of the IUD in the endometrium or myometrium, resulting in difficult removal. In some cases this can result in breakage of the IUD, necessitating surgical removal.
- Partial or total perforation of the uterine wall, particularly during lactation, is a risk, as is the possibility of migration of the device after insertion.
- IUDs do not offer any protection from sexually transmitted diseases, including HIV/AIDS.

DEPO-PROVERA (MEDROXY-PROGESTERONE)

An injectable form of contraception used widely in both developed and developing countries. The advantages are that nothing needs to be taken daily or used at the time of intercourse. It is very effective as contraception, about 3 in 1,000 users will experience an unintended pregnancy in the first year. Women may use it in privacy; no one need know, except the health-care provider who administers it. Depo-Provera does not offer any protection from sexually transmitted diseases including HIV/AIDS. Normally a Depo-Provera injection is administered once every three months.

NORPLANT IMPLANTS

Six matchstick-size contraceptive rods containing long-acting progesterone. The rods are inserted by a doctor or a health-care provider under the skin of the woman's upper arm. Only about 1 in 1,000 women using Norplant implants will experience an accidental pregnancy in the first year.[22] Norplant inhibits ovulation and thickens the cervical mucus, preventing penetration by sperm.

Advantages: There is nothing you must do on a daily basis or at the time of intercourse to prevent pregnancy once the Norplant System is in place. Only one regular check up per year with a health-care provider is required.

The Norplant System does not offer any protection from sexually transmitted diseases, including HIV/AIDS.

A surgical incision is required to insert Norplant System. Complications related to insertion include pain, edema, bruising (sometimes rash), infections, blistering, ulcerations, sloughing, excessive scarring, phlebitis, and hyperpigmentation at the insertion site. Removal is also a surgical procedure and may take longer, be more difficult, and/or cause more pain than insertion, and may be associated with difficulty locating capsules.[23]

TUBAL STERILIZATION

An operation that blocks the fallopian tubes, which normally carry a woman's ovum (egg) to her uterus. After the operation, sperm cannot reach the ovum nor can the ovum reach the uterus. Tubal sterilization should be considered permanent. Please be absolutely certain you do not wish to deliver more children before taking this step. It is very expensive to attempt to reverse a tubal sterilization, and less than 50 percent of reversals are successful. It's a good idea when considering this option to speak with other women who have done it. Ask them if they have regrets and why. Be aware that sterilization does not offer any protection from sexually transmitted diseases, including HIV/AIDS.

Health risks and adverse reactions associated with Depo-Provera, listed in the 2001 *Physicians' Desk Reference* (55th edition) include:

- Menstrual irregularities
- Weight changes
- Headaches
- Nervousness
- Abdominal pain or discomfort
- Dizziness
- Asthenia (weakness or fatigue)
- Decreased libido or anorgasmia
- Backache
- Leg cramps
- Depression
- Nausea
- Insomnia
- Leukorrhea (whitish discharge fr. vagina)
- Acne
- Vaginitis
- Pelvic pain
- Breast pain
- No hair growth or alopecia
- Bloating
- Rash
- Edema
- Hot flashes
- Arthralgia (joint pain)

Fewer than 1% of the women experienced:

- Galactorrhea (excessive secretion of the mammary glands)
- Melasma (dark pigmentation of the skin)
- Chloasma (hyperpigmentation of the skin)
- Convulsions
- Changes in appetite
- Gastrointestinal disturbances
- Jaundice
- Genitourinary infections
- Vaginal cysts
- Dyspareunia (painful coitus)
- Paresthesia (abnormal sensation due to disorder of the sensory nervous system)
- Chest pain
- Pulmonary embolus (lung obstruction)
- Allergic reactions
- Anemia
- Drowsiness
- Syncope (sudden loss of strength or suspension of consciousness due to cerebral anemia)
- Dyspnea (labored difficult breathing) and asthma

- Tachycardia (abnormally rapid heart rate)
- Fever
- Excessive sweating and body odor
- Dry skin
- Chills
- Increased libido
- Excessive thirst
- Hoarseness
- Pain at injection site
- Blood dyscrasia (abnormal or pathologic condition of the blood)
- Rectal bleeding
- Changes in breast size
- Breast lumps or nipple bleeding
- Axillary (armpit) swelling
- Breast cancer
- Prevention of lactation
- Sensation of pregnancy
- Lack of return to fertility
- Paralysis
- Facial palsy
- Scleroderma (a chronic disorder of progressive collagenous fibrosis)
- Osteoporosis (abnormal rarefaction of the bone)
- Uterine hyperplasia (increase in volume of the organ)
- Cervical cancer
- Varicose veins
- Dysmenorrhea (painful menstruation)
- Hirsutism (abnormal growth of hair)
- Thrombophlebitis (development of venous thrombi in the presence of inflammatory changes)
- Unexpected pregnancy—An increased risk of low birth weight, significant increase in incidence of polysyndactyly (webbing between adjacent digits of hands or feet) and chromosomal anomalies was observed among infants of users of Depo-Provera contraceptive injection.
- Deep vein thrombosis (clots)
- Reports of anaphylaxis (exaggerated reaction of an organism to a foreign protein) and anaphylactoid reaction to Depo-Provera injection

---

The *Physicians' Desk Reference* (55th edition) reports the following warnings and precautions for Norplant Implants:

- Headache
- Nervousness/Anxiety
- Nausea/Vomiting
- Dizziness
- Adnexal (appendages; accessory organs) enlargement
- Dermatitis/Rash
- Acne
- Change of appetite
- Mastalgia (pain in the breasts)
- Weight gain
- Hirsutism (abnormal hair growth), hypertrichosis, and scalp hair loss
- Breast discharge
- Cervicitis (inflammation of the cervix)
- Musculoskeletal pain
- Abdominal discomfort
- Leukorrhea (whitish discharge from the vagina)
- Vaginitis (inflammation of the vagina)
- Emotional lability
- Idiopatic (occurring without known cause) intracranial (within the cranium) hypertension (abnormally increased blood pressure)
- Induration (hardening)
- Bruising
- Dysmenorrhea (painful menstruation)
- Abscess (inflammation with pus), cellulitis (spreading between layers of involved tissue)
- Migraine
- Arm pain
- Numbness
- Tingling
- Depression
- Excessive scarring
- Hyperpigmentation
- Nerve injury
- Congenital anomalies
- Pulmonary (pertaining to the lungs) embolism (impaction in a blood vessel of any undissolved material)
- Superficial venous thrombosis (clotting)
- Deep-vein thrombosis (clotting)
- Myocardial infarction (heart stoppage)
- Blistering, ulcerations, and sloughing
- Thrombotic thrombocytopenic purpura (associated with a decrease in the number of platelets in the blood)
- Stroke
- Pruritus (itching)
- Urticaria (raised itchy patches)
- Asthenia (fatigue/weakness)
- Phlebitis (inflammation of a vein)

Regret after sterilization is greater if the woman divorces, remarries, is under twenty-five, or if her child dies. It is *not* a good idea to seek tubal sterilization if you have just had a baby or an abortion. You can expect to mourn the babies you will never have if you choose this option.

Advantages: It is effective. After tubal sterilization, one need not worry about taking a contraceptive precaution and sexual intercourse is not interrupted.

The operation is fairly simple; however, complications arising from the anesthesia necessary to perform the surgery can be serious.

Possible complications of tubal sterilization include pelvic infection, vaginal dryness during lovemaking, ectopic pregnancies (up to twenty times the normal risk rate), and excessive bleeding. Psychological stress disorders may become a problem if the woman suffers from regret. [24]

VASECTOMY

An operation that blocks the vas deferens, the tubes that normally carry a man's sperm to his penis.

Advantages: It is a permanent and effective form of contraception. It is less expensive and involves fewer complications than tubal ligation (female sterilization). It should be noted that vasectomy offers no protection against sexually transmitted diseases, including HIV/AIDS.

Possible complications of vasectomy include infection and hemorrhage. Suspected consequences of the body making antibodies to retained sperm include diabetes, circulatory disorders, heart disease, thyroid and joint problems. [25]

If you are absolutely certain that you won't want to have more children, no matter what, think again. Feel with your heart, not just your mind. There are other choices that are not so irreversible.

This has been a lengthy discussion about contraception, birth control, family planning, and the highly charged issues linked to sexuality. Sex is the doorway by which we all find our way to planet Earth. Through the miracle of sexual reproduction, you had your beautiful baby. With thoughtful consideration, armed with knowledge, men and women can dance gracefully with their fertility. While seeking to avoid pregnancy, please don't make an enemy of your sexuality. Study, think, feel, choose. Here I have attempted to give you, the reader, both a personal view and a global vision of the multifaceted issue of contraception. Now, with the help of Marie Zenack (who was my own Natural Family Planning teacher), I will try to shine a brighter, more positive, and very practical light on fertility.

The Signs of Fertility With Marie Zenack*

NATURAL FAMILY PLANNING—LET'S BEGIN

Mother Earth is a perfect example of the cycle of fertility alive within women in their childbearing years.

When there is no rain and the earth is dry, you may plant seeds, but they will not grow. However, when moisture is present, any seed, whether carefully planted

---

*Marie Zenack is a devoted grandmother living in the heartland of America in a small town called Fairfield, Iowa. She is a master organic gardener, an excellent whole-foods cook, and a fantastic wife to Nathan (who, by the way, is a supportive husband). Marie has taught Natural Family Planning in the United States, China, the Caribbean, Mexico, India, Indonesia, and Ottumwa, Iowa. She is a good witch in the art of healing rituals, helping us to reinvent our culture in the new millennium. She is certified as a teacher, and is an active pioneer in the home-school movement. Currently Marie is working with Robin on four books: *Celebrating the Cycle: A Guidebook for Maidens; Celebrating the Mother; Celebrating the Crone;* and *The Natural Family Planning and Sexuality Handbook: A Lifestyle of Nonviolence.*

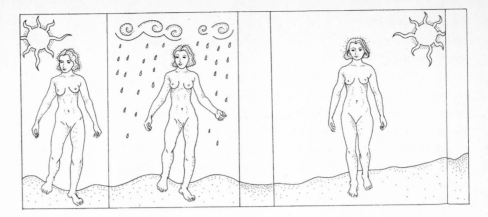

or carelessly sprinkled on the surface, may sprout. This is also true of women. Dryness indicates infertility. Wetness indicates fertility. Just as the earth's moisture may be seen on the surface or felt just below it, the moisture indicating a woman's fertility may been seen at the outlet of her yoni or felt just inside the yoni (vagina).

In this chapter, we'll suggest proven procedures for observing and accurately charting this phenomenon. We'll also discuss using cervical changes as a cross check to these observations. Taken together, external mucus observations and the cervical check can provide a proven, nonviolent method of family planning.

MOTHER EARTH—MOTHER WOMAN CONCEPT
from the book Teaching the Ovulation Method Step by Step Cycle by Cycle
by Dr. Francesca Kearns and Denis L. St. Marie
During ovarian activity (possible fertility) the cervix produces fertile-type mucus, which can be observed outside the vagina in an external exam. However, for many months after the birth of your baby, you may see and feel nothing outside the vagina. This is because your baby's suckling stimulates pro-lactin, a hormone

Natural Family Planning Side Effects
· Unintended pregnancies
· No increased risk of birth defects for the baby
· Increased body awareness
· Couple communication
· A lifestyle of nonviolence

that suppresses follicle stimulating hormone, preventing the beginning of your fertile cycle. As long as this situation continues, your ovaries are at rest, and your family planning is easy.

You can never know, however, when your fertility will return. Changes in your baby's suckling pattern, such as illness or the introduction of food or water to your baby's diet, can decrease the level of prolactin and allow the production of follicle-stimulating hormone, leading to possible fertility. Even with complete breastfeeding, many women will return to fertility while they are still hard at work caring for and breastfeeding the baby they already have.

NFP—Natural Family Planning

NFP means learning to recognize your body's signs of fertility and infertility. To avoid pregnancy, a couple abstains from all genital contact during times of possible fertility. To achieve pregnancy, they make love during the times in the woman's cycle that are possibly fertile. Teachers of NFP know that NFP cannot be taught. They can only offer orientation, information, and guidance. It is the woman herself who, through careful observing and charting of her body's unique fertile signs, discovers how to dance with her own fertility.

THE NUTS AND BOLTS OF NFP

NOTE: Abstinence is necessary for the first two to three weeks of charting, while you are learning to observe, interpret, and chart your fertile signs.

Observing and Charting the External Mucus

Pay attention to the sensations at the vulva as you go about your daily activities. Just as you are able to notice the beginning of menstrual bleeding, you will be able to notice the sensation of fertile mucus in and outside the vagina.

- Using white, unscented, and unbleached toilet paper, wipe from front to back before and after each urination or bowel movement. Notice the feeling as you wipe: Is it slippery? Is it sticky? Check the tissue for mucus—amount, appearance, and feeling of wetness or dryness.
- Chart what you feel and what you see every evening after observing all during the day. If you are dry in the morning and a little wet in the afternoon, chart wet for that day. *Always chart your most fertile sign for any given day.*

KEY: Using these international symbols chart one of the following:

ззз Bleeding or spotting—possibly **fertile**. Be careful.

ζ Spotting—possibly **fertile**. Be careful.

☰ Dry—You felt nothing and you saw nothing (looks like cracks in the dry earth).

◊ Wet—You felt something or you saw something, even slight, either externally at your vulva or internally at your cervix. **Fertile.**

◖ Slippery mucus and or really wet—You saw clear mucus or felt a slippery feeling. Feels like raw egg white or a live fish. **Fertile.**

☺ Dry but *still fertile*—Like dry soil a day or two after rain, if you dig down one
☰ inch, you find moisture. Still **fertile.**

☼ *Continuous infertile discharge*—You have a pasty or sticky, dry or wet or creamy-type mucus that is the same every day (called basic infertile pattern of mucus or infertile continuous discharge—see page 345 to establish if this is you).

☽ Sexual relations in the evening.

☀ Sexual relations in the morning or day.

☺ Baby face—Chart her along with any fertile signs.

CERVICAL CHANGES DURING ECOLOGICAL BREASTFEEDING

External mucus observations are the key to monitoring your fertility. However, cervical changes can help confirm your state of fertility or infertility. By using both these indicators you can greatly increase your success at NFP.

As long as infertility continues during breastfeeding, your cervix remains *low*, and *easy to reach within the vagina*. It is firm, like the tip of your nose, closed, and dry. (If mucus is always present, see page 345, on continuous discharge.)

As possible fertility approaches, the cervical os (opening of the cervix) *opens* slightly and the cervix becomes *softer*, more like the lips of the mouth, and *rises inside the vagina,* making it difficult to reach. It also becomes slippery from the presence of cervical mucus.

Useful Vocabulary...

Corpus Luteum The empty egg sack. After the release of an ovum, this is the yellow structure formed and left behind on the ovary. If the egg is fertilized, the corpus luteum produces hormones (progesterone) that support the pregnancy. If fertilization does not take place, it degenerates and is reabsorbed.

Estrogen A hormone, chiefly produced by the ovaries, that is responsible for our female characteristics and is essential for ovulation.

Fertility The ability to reproduce.

Follicle Stimulating Hormone (FSH) Produced by the pituitary gland, this hormone stimulates the ovaries to ripen and mature an ovum. It also inspires the production of estrogen hormone.

Luteinising Hormone (LH) This hormone from the pituitary gland (in your brain) stimulates ovulation and the formation of the corpus luteum.

Mucus, Cervical The secretion from the lining cells of the cervix.

Ovary The female sex organ, which contains our egg cells, and where hormones that influence fertility are produced.

Ovulation The release of an egg from the ovary.

Oxytocin Known as the hormone of love. Oxytocin is present when people share a meal or a lively conversation. When a couple makes love, oxytocin is there. It causes the uterus to expel the baby during childbirth and is responsible for the letdown of breast milk during lactation.

Preovulatory Phase The time in a woman's cycle between the first day of menstruation and ovulation.

Progesterone A female hormone produced by the corpus luteum when ovulation has taken place. It is necessary to support pregnancy.

Prolactin A hormone, manufactured by the pituitary gland, that stimulates breast milk production.

Ecological breastfeeding means...

- Your baby is fed only at your breast.
- No supplemental bottles of milk or infant formula are given.
- Baby is not yet eating solid foods.
- Baby is not being given a pacifier.
- Baby is not being breastfed by another woman.

THE CERVIX

As the possible fertile time passes, the cervix quickly changes back to its infertile state. The os closes, and the cervix becomes firm, moves lower, and is easier to reach. The absence of mucus makes the cervix feel less slippery compared to the fertile cervix. To make the observations of the cervix, stand on the floor and raise one foot up onto the toilet or chair. (Make sure your hands and nails are clean.) Insert two fingers into the vagina and feel for the cervix, which will be at the top of the vagina, toward the front. (See illustration.) Open the two fingers around the cervix and gently draw them together again, rubbing slightly over the surface of the cervix. If any cervical mucus is present, it will gather between the fingers. Keep the two fingers together as you remove them from the vagina. Check the mucus, if there is any, for amount, elasticity, sensation, appearance.

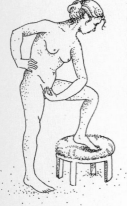

Cervix check

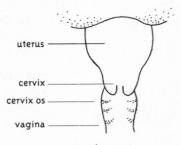

uterus

cervix

cervix os

vagina

Fertile cervix:
high, open, soft like lips

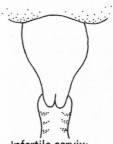

Infertile cervix:
low, closed, firmer like a nose.

CHARTING THE SIGNS OF THE CERVIX

The presence or absence of cervical mucus at the cervix can be charted using the international symbols. (See page 340.) The size and position of the cervix can be charted by a simple drawing/diagram. Like this:

o = open soft cervix   • = closed firm cervix

In addition, you can also use letters to indicate firm (F) or soft (S).

You may very well notice changes in the cervix before your mucus discharge begins, partly because your mucus is slightly less obvious during breastfeeding, but especially because you are pretty busy during breastfeeding!

Charting your cervical changes is a good cross-check to your mucus observations, giving you more confidence in your observations. Abstain at any sign of fertility. Don't average your observation or discount one sign of fertility because other observations didn't confirm it.

WHY THE CERVICAL CHECK?

Many schools of Natural Family Planning teach only the external mucus observation and charting. However, during breastfeeding the external mucus is less obvious. As a breastfeeding mother, you feel highly motivated to space your children, so the baby you now have in your arms may derive the maximum benefit from extended breastfeeding. By observing and charting *both* the external mucus and the cervical signs, you will feel more confident of your observations.

The reason couples get confused and end up with unplanned pregnancies is this: External signs of fertility can be subtle. Particularly when a woman is breastfeeding or premenopausal, she needs more information to determine the status of her fertility at any given time. We know that it is harder to get confused when you have this intimate and ever present relationship with your fertile signs. This is the beauty of adding the signs of the cervix to your personal observations.

Occasionally a woman feels uncomfortable checking her cervix. We encourage you to keep trying. It is in there.[26] Usually within a short time, the cervical check becomes easy and comfortable.

WHEN TO START YOUR MUCUS AND CERVIX CHARTING

If you are motivated to avoid pregnancy, start your external mucus observations after your postpartum discharge (lochia) has stopped. Start the observations of the cervix, once a day in the evening, when your baby is two and a half months old.

Many women enjoy a long period of uninterrupted infertility for about the first six months after their baby's birth. Eventually, however, fertility returns. Often the return is gradual, and proceeds with many stops and starts before settling into a regular pattern. This is never an easy time. Patches of mucus and periods of cervical change seem to come again and again with little, if any, clearly infertile time in between. This is a time to be grateful for the previous months of infertility. It is also a time to be extremely careful and to maintain your sense of humor. This difficult time sometimes lasts about three months. But it does not last forever. When mucus patches are frequent or cervical changes erratic, or you have a bleed, abstain until you feel secure about your signs of fertility.

A Few Words to the Wise

A word about that first ovulation: We have seen several couples observe and chart and follow rules devotedly for up to two years of breastfeeding and weaning only to decide to have relations at the time of the first ovulation! That urge to have relations at the time of the first real fertility can be irresistible. If you have been faithfully charting through weeks/months of infertility and begin to find yourself trying to rationalize away signs of fertility or starting to play one observation off against another, this suggests increased desire on the woman's part, a sure sign of the return of fertility.

THE RULES FOR AVOIDING PREGNANCY DURING BREASTFEEDING

1. Chart your mucus and your cervical signs every night. Observation alone is not an effective way to plan your family. If you don't chart, you should prepare for the possibility of an unplanned pregnancy.

2. During dry days with a low, firm, dry, closed cervix, consider the evenings only, but not consecutive evenings, *open for relations* (lovemaking).

3. If you see or feel a change in sensation (wetness, mucus, or bleeding) or the cervix changes (rises, opens, or softens), *abstain during all of these changes plus four full days*. That means abstain from all genital contact until the evening of the fourth dry day of low, firm, closed, and dry cervix. At that time you may consider evenings only, but not consecutive evenings, available for relations. Don't play one sign against the other. *Even one fertile sign means possible fertility.* This method depends upon accurate observation and charting of your most fertile sign.

Continue these simple rules until you have weaned your baby and have had *three consecutive normal cycles.** If you have bleeding, don't be fooled into thinking you have menstruated. *Bleeding during breastfeeding, especially your first bleed, is very likely to be hiding fertility.* Observe carefully. Follow the rules carefully. Abstain during all bleeding, as well as all mucus patches or cervical changes, plus four dry days with a low, closed, firm, dry cervix.

IF YOU EXPERIENCE MUCUS PATCHES DURING BREASTFEEDING

While you are fully breastfeeding, the frequent suckling of your little one keeps your level of oxytocin and prolactin high, which in turn puts the brake on your follicle stimulating hormone (FSH). If you begin to observe frequent wetness or mucus patches, and/or changes in the cervix, it means that more FSH is being produced, causing some follicles to begin the ripening process and produce estrogen. *Practically speaking, it means that your fertility may return at any moment.*

If you want to extend your natural infertility during breastfeeding, try taking a little extra rest and nursing a little more frequently. This doesn't mean breast-feeding your child more, just more often. These more frequent feedings will repress the FSH. With luck, your dry days of low, firm, closed, dry cervix will return. Remember, no pacifiers! Whenever your baby sucks anything other than your breasts, your hormones begin to allow your fertility to return.

If your child is growing up and interested in food, you may be ready to allow your fertility to return. Let her join in the family's healthy table food, and decrease the number of breastfeedings. Observe and chart carefully. Follow the rules. If the wet patches increase, you are in a very unpredictably fertile time. Resign yourselves to abstinence until you again feel confident of your fertile and infertile times.

Even when your cycles return, remain on the breastfeeding rules until your child is completely weaned. The rules are:

- Consider as available for lovemaking, evenings only, and not consecutive evenings, of dry days with low, closed, firm, dry cervix.
- Abstain during all bleeding, spotting, wetness, mucus patches, or cervical changes, plus four more days.

Beginning the evening of the fourth dry day with a low, closed, firm, dry cervix, consider alternate evenings again open for lovemaking.

If your child is completely weaned, and you have had three consecutive normal cycles, you may consider your cycles back to normal.*

IF YOU HAVE CONTINUOUS DISCHARGE...

If you observe wetness or mucus all the time, first ask yourself if the discharge is accompanied by irritation or pain in the vaginal area. Also observe if the odor is different from your normal body odor, or if there is a green or gray coloring. Any of these things indicates an infection that needs attention. Please see your health-care provider if you suspect you have an infection.

If you do not have an infection, observe the mucus/wetness carefully for at least two weeks. Note the amount, what it looks like, and what it feels like. Two weeks (minimum) of wetness that is the same in amount, appearance, and sensation suggests an infertile pattern of wetness. Be sure to confirm the infertile mucus pattern by checking for a low, closed, firm cervix.

---

*Definition of "normal cycle": A cycle with an obvious mucus pattern with cervical changes followed by a bleed, eleven to sixteen days later.

Once you are confident of your infertile pattern of wetness, begin treating these days of infertile wetness as "dry" days. That means, consider days of the infertile pattern of wetness to be open to relations in the evening, but not on consecutive evenings. If there is *any* change in the amount, appearance (color, clarity, elasticity), or sensation, or if there is any change in the position or firmness or opening of the cervix, abstain during the change plus four days of infertile pattern

---

The Rules for Normal Cycles

Follow these rules only if your baby is weaned and you have had three consecutive normal cycles.

A normal cycle is defined as an obvious mucus pattern with cervical changes followed by bleeding eleven to sixteen days later. If you are new to Natural Family Planning and do not want to conceive, plan to abstain until after ovulation (see sample charts page 350) for two or three cycles, until you have learned to recognize your fertile signs with confidence.

REMEMBER TO...

- **Observe** your wet, dry, or bleeding signs of fertility at the vulva (what you see and what you feel), all day, every day, even during your moon time (menstruation).
- **Check cervical changes** as soon as the menstrual flow has stopped, or has been reduced to only a little spotting that does not interfere with observations. Do this once a day, before going to bed or before making love.
- **Chart**—if you don't keep a chart you are not employing any family planning. Nothing makes one as forgetful or as "ditzy" as being fertile. If you don't have a chart, in plain sight, that is a constant reminder of your fertile status, you will mess up. Chart mucus and cervix every evening. Begin a new line of charting with the onset of your menstrual flow.

1–2–3... THE EARLY DAYS RULES

1. **Abstain during menstruation.** Fertile mucus can begin at any time. There is no way to observe the fertile signs during your moon time

with closed, firm, low cervix. Beginning the evening of the fourth dry day with low, firm, closed, cervix, again consider alternate evenings open for lovemaking.

WHEN YOU HAVE YOUR FIRST BLEED AFTER HAVING A BABY

You can no longer trust that your continual wetness means infertility. Abstain again for two weeks or longer—until you are again certain of your infertile pat-

---

because the mucus is masked by the menstrual flow and the cervix is open and soft to allow for menstruation.

2. **On dry days** with a low, closed, firm, dry cervix, have relations in the evening only, and not on consecutive evenings. (Evenings only gives you all day to observe the mucus signs. Alternate evenings guards against confusing fertile mucus with seminal and arousal fluid.)

3. **Abstain during all times of possible fertility** until the evening of the fourth day of dryness with a low, closed, firm, dry cervix. Possible fertility means that you see or feel something other than dryness, or your cervix raises, opens, or softens.

4. **Postovulatory bonus:** After you do observe your normal ovulatory pattern, you may consider yourself infertile, morning or evening, beginning on the evening of the fourth dry day with a low, closed, firm, dry cervix until the start of the next menstruation (usually about eight to twelve days).

This means that from the evening of the fourth dry day until the onset of your next moon you may fool around morning, noon, and night. Have fun. But don't throw caution to the wind. If slippery mucus or cervical changes return, go back to 1–2–3...THE EARLY DAYS RULES.

Adhere to observing all day and charting every night, regardless of where you are in your cycle.

PLEASE: Do not take the postovulatory bonus unless you have weaned your child and have had three consecutive normal cycles. A normal cycle has an obvious mucus pattern with cervical changes followed by menstruation eleven to sixteen days later.

tern. Be very careful. If you are returning to cycling, two weeks may take you right up to ovulation! Be patient. *By observing* (what you see and what you feel) *carefully every day, all day, and charting every evening,* you will again become certain of your fertile and infertile times.

IS NATURAL FAMILY PLANNING CULTURALLY APPROPRIATE?

Between the two of us, we have taught couples and made teachers of NFP in the United States, China, Central and South America, Indonesia, and the Philippines. Christian, Catholic, Hindu, Muslim, and Animist people, of all social and economic circumstances, have embraced this method and felt it dovetailed with the teachings of their faiths.

...Oops

A wise midwife[27] who helped many Amish women who were not permitted by their religion to chart their fertile signs to avoid pregnancy (not all Amish people have this conflict, only some of the sects forbid all forms of contraception, even natural) has fantastic advice for women. She taught the women to pay attention to their subtle feelings of arousal. For example, you are a busy mother, you have just put up forty quarts of tomato sauce today. While you are still cleaning the kitchen and preparing the evening meal, your husband comes home. *If* he looks exceptionally fine to you, *if* making love is suddenly your idea, you are fertile. Be careful!

DETAILS OF THE "EARLY DAYS" OR PREOVULATORY RULES

Fall back on the "early days" rules when you're just not feeling certain that you have had a true ovulation. If you're not sure how to interpret your fertile signs, abstain and continue to observe and chart. Ask yourself if you are observing your normal pattern of mucus and your normal ovulatory changes in the cervix.

If you have had a few days of fertile signs, then a return to dryness, then again observe mucus or cervical changes, abstain during those changes until the fourth day of dryness with low, closed, dry, firm cervix.

In any given cycle, if you are not sure that you have observed your normal pattern of ovulation, abstain during all bleeding and spotting, plus four days of dryness. *Do this even if the bleeding seems in every way like a true menstruation.* If the mucus/cervical pattern before the bleed was not normal, the bleed could actually be associated with ovulation. Stay on these "early days" rules until you are sure you have observed your normal ovulatory pattern of mucus and cervical changes.

DON'T GET DISCOURAGED

This is a time in your life that is child-led. It is always wise to take "baby steps" when learning something new. Step by step you'll catch on. Be patient with one another, a lifestyle of nonviolence is well worth striving for.

We also felt confused when we were learning how to dance with our fertility. We felt insecure and afraid. Read and reread these pages. Make your observations and keep your chart, even when you are unsure. Abstain if you are in doubt. It is worth the time and the diligence you must invest as a couple to practice family planning without doing any violence to your bodies or our planet.

Good Advice

Douching confuses the mucus signs of fertility. It also disrupts the friendly flora of your yoni, causing vaginal infections. Please do not douche.

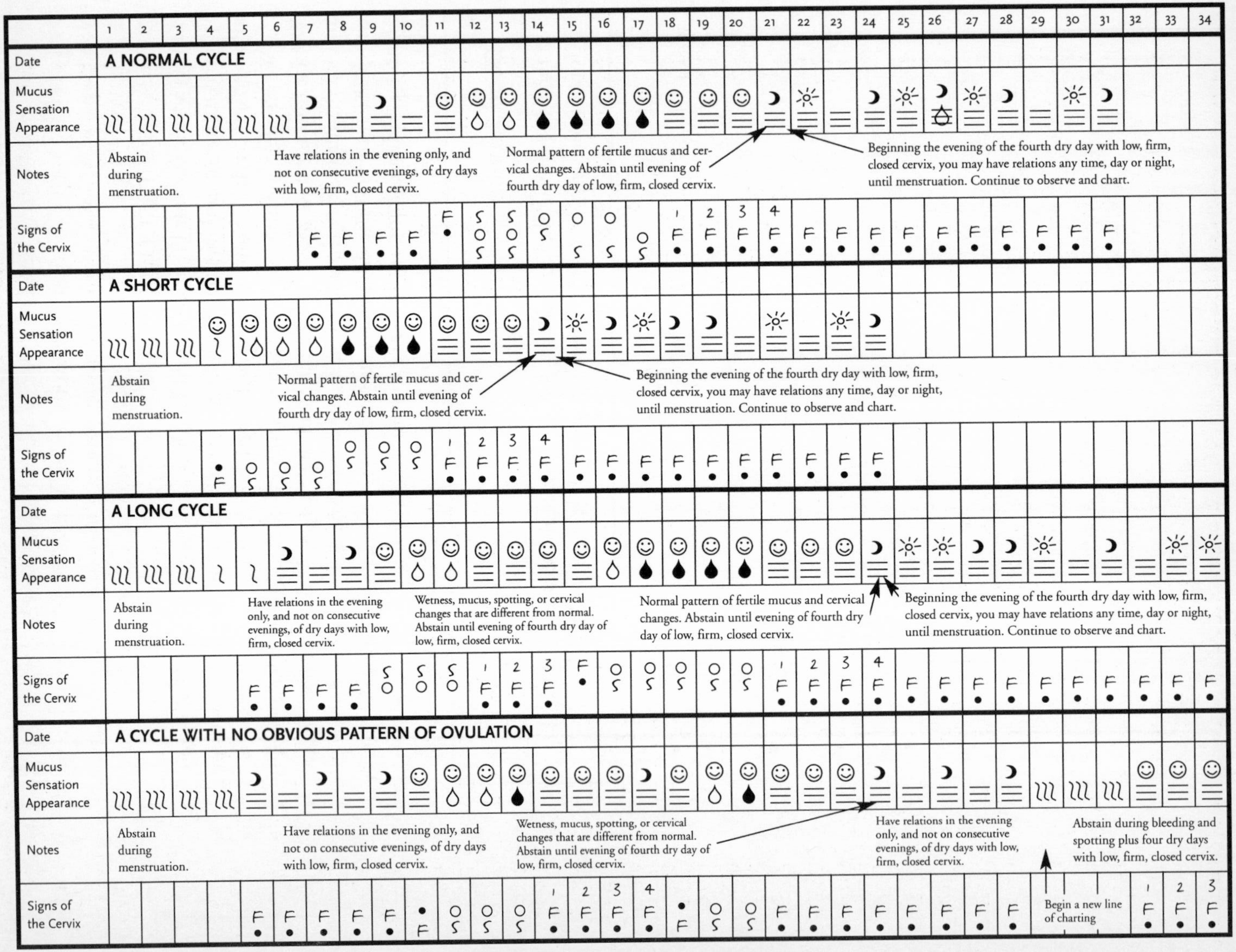

Avoiding Pregnancy in Normal Circumstances

350

Columns numbered 1–34.

A NORMAL CYCLE

Row labels: Date | Mucus (Sensation / Appearance) | Notes | Signs of the Cervix

Notes:
- Abstain during menstruation.
- Have relations in the evening only, and not on consecutive evenings, of dry days with low, firm, closed cervix.
- Normal pattern of fertile mucus and cervical changes. Abstain until evening of fourth dry day of low, firm, closed cervix.
- Beginning the evening of the fourth dry day with low, firm, closed cervix, you may have relations any time, day or night, until menstruation. Continue to observe and chart.

A SHORT CYCLE

Row labels: Date | Mucus (Sensation / Appearance) | Notes | Signs of the Cervix

Notes:
- Abstain during menstruation.
- Normal pattern of fertile mucus and cervical changes. Abstain until evening of fourth dry day of low, firm, closed cervix.
- Beginning the evening of the fourth dry day with low, firm, closed cervix, you may have relations any time, day or night, until menstruation. Continue to observe and chart.

A LONG CYCLE

Row labels: Date | Mucus (Sensation / Appearance) | Notes | Signs of the Cervix

Notes:
- Abstain during menstruation.
- Have relations in the evening only, and not on consecutive evenings, of dry days with low, firm, closed cervix.
- Wetness, mucus, spotting, or cervical changes that are different from normal. Abstain until evening of fourth dry day of low, firm, closed cervix.
- Normal pattern of fertile mucus and cervical changes. Abstain until evening of fourth dry day of low, firm, closed cervix.
- Beginning the evening of fourth dry day with low, firm, closed cervix, you may have relations any time, day or night, until menstruation. Continue to observe and chart.

A CYCLE WITH NO OBVIOUS PATTERN OF OVULATION

Row labels: Date | Mucus (Sensation / Appearance) | Notes | Signs of the Cervix

Notes:
- Abstain during menstruation.
- Have relations in the evening only, and not on consecutive evenings, of dry days with low, firm, closed cervix.
- Wetness, mucus, spotting, or cervical changes that are different from normal. Abstain until evening of fourth dry day of low, firm, closed cervix.
- Have relations in the evening only, and not on consecutive evenings, of dry days with low, firm, closed cervix.
- Abstain during bleeding and spotting plus four dry days with low, firm, closed cervix.
- Begin a new line of charting

Date | 1 2 3 ... 34

Row group 1

Mucus — Sensation / Appearance

Signs of the Cervix

Notes: The previous cycle not normal. Abstain during bleeding and spotting plus four dry days with low, firm, closed cervix.

Sticky

Normal pattern of fertile mucus and cervical changes. Abstain until evening of fourth dry day of low, firm, closed cervix.

Beginning the evening of the fourth dry day with low, firm, closed cervix, you may have relations any time, day or night, until menstruation. Continue to observe and chart.

Row group 2

Date

Mucus — Sensation / Appearance

Signs of the Cervix

Notes: Abstain during menstruation.

Sticky

Normal pattern of fertile mucus and cervical changes. Abstain until evening of fourth dry day of low, firm, closed cervix.

Beginning the evening of the fourth dry day with low, firm, closed cervix, you may have relations any time, day or night, until menstruation. Continue to observe and chart.

Row group 3

Date

Mucus — Sensation / Appearance

Signs of the Cervix

Notes: Have relations in the evening only, and not on consecutive evenings, of dry days with low, firm, closed cervix.

Sticky

Normal pattern of fertile mucus and cervical changes. Abstain until evening of fourth dry day of low, firm, closed cervix.

Beginning the evening of the fourth dry day with low, firm, closed cervix, you may have relations any time, day or night, until menstruation. Continue to observe and chart.

Luteal phase (Time between last wet day and menstruation, is less than 11 days. Cycle not normal.

Row group 4

Date

Mucus — Sensation / Appearance

Signs of the Cervix

Notes: The previous cycle not normal. Abstain during bleeding and spotting plus four dry days with low, firm, closed cervix.

Sticky

Normal pattern of fertile mucus and cervical changes. Abstain until evening of fourth dry day of low, firm, closed cervix.

Beginning the evening of the fourth dry day with low, firm, closed cervix, you may have relations any time, day or night, until menstruation. Continue to observe and chart.

Avoiding Pregnancy in Normal Circumstances (cont.)

Avoiding Pregnancy for Women Who Are Breast Feeding

Date | 1 | 2 | 3 | 4 | 5 | 6 | 7 | 8 | 9 | 10 | 11 | 12 | 13 | 14 | 15 | 16 | 17 | 18 | 19 | 20 | 21 | 22 | 23 | 24 | 25 | 26 | 27 | 28 | 29 | 30 | 31 | 32 | 33 | 34

Mucus — Sensation, Appearance

Notes: This basic infertile pattern may go on for weeks or months if you are ecologically breast feeding. Have relations only in the evening, and not on consecutive evenings, of dry days with a low, firm, closed cervix. Abstain during wetness, mucus, bleeding, or spotting, (whether external or at the cervix) and during any rising, softening or opening of the cervix, plus four dry days with a low, closed, firm cervix.

Signs of the Cervix

Notes: Patch of wetness and cervical changes. Abstain until evening of fourth dry day of low, firm, closed cervix.

Beginning the evening of the fourth dry day with low, firm, closed cervix, you may have relations only on alternate evenings with low, firm, closed cervix.

Beginning the evening of the fourth dry day with low, firm, closed cervix, you may have relations only on alternate evenings with low, firm, closed cervix.

Sporting. Abstain until evening of fourth dry day of low, firm, closed cervix.

Notes: Long pattern of fertile type mucus and cervical changes. Abstain until evening of fourth dry day of low, firm, closed cervix.

Beginning the evening of the fourth dry day with low, firm, closed cervix, you may have relations only on alternate evenings with low, firm, closed cervix.

Notes: Abstain during bleeding and spotting plus four dry days with low, firm, closed cervix.

Uncertain time. Abstain.

Normal pattern of fertile mucus and cervical changes. Abstain until evening of fourth dry day of low, firm, closed cervix.

cervix rising

	1	2	3	4	5	6	7	8	9	10	11	12	13	14	15	16	17	18	19	20	21	22	23	24	25	26	27	28	29	30	31	32	33	34

Date

Mucus — Sensation / Appearance

Signs of the Cervix

Notes

- Bleeding may mask fertility. Abstain plus four dry days with low, firm, closed cervix.
- Uncertain time. Abstain.
- Normal pattern of fertile mucus and cervical changes. Abstain until evening of fourth dry day of low, firm, closed cervix.
- Beginning the evening of the fourth dry day with low, firm, closed cervix, you may have relations only on alternate evenings with low, firm, closed cervix.

Date

Mucus — Sensation / Appearance

Signs of the Cervix

Notes

- Bleeding may mask fertility. Abstain plus four dry days with low, firm, closed cervix.
- Uncertain time. Abstain.
- Normal pattern of fertile mucus and cervical changes. Abstain until evening of fourth dry day of low, firm, closed cervix.
- Beginning the evening of the fourth dry day with low, firm, closed cervix, you may have relations only on alternate evenings with low, firm, closed cervix.

Date

Mucus — Sensation / Appearance

Signs of the Cervix

Notes

- Bleeding may mask fertility. Abstain plus four dry days with low, firm, closed cervix.
- Beginning the evening of the fourth dry day with low, firm, closed cervix, you may have relations any time, day or night, until menstruation. Continue to observe and chart.
- Normal pattern of fertile mucus and cervical changes. Abstain until evening of fourth dry day of low, firm, closed cervix.

Date

Mucus — Sensation / Appearance

Signs of the Cervix

Notes

- Bleeding may mask fertility. Abstain plus four dry days with low, firm, closed cervix.
- Beginning the evening of the fourth dry day with low, firm, closed cervix, you may have relations any time, day or night, until menstruation. Continue to observe and chart.
- Normal pattern of fertile mucus and cervical changes. Abstain until evening of fourth dry.

Date

Mucus — Sensation / Appearance

Signs of the Cervix

Notes

cervix rising

Avoiding Pregnancy for Women Who Are Breast Feeding or Weaning

	1	2	3	4	5	6	7	8	9	10	11	12	13	14	15	16	17	18	19	20	21	22	23	24	25	26	27	28	29	30	31	32	33	34
Date																																		
Mucus Sensation Appearance																																		
Notes																																		
Signs of the Cervix																																		
Date																																		
Mucus Sensation Appearance																																		
Notes																																		
Signs of the Cervix																																		

KEY: Using these international symbols chart one of the following:

≋ Bleeding or spotting—possibly **fertile**. Be careful.

~ Spotting—possibly **fertile**. Be careful.

≡ Dry—You felt nothing and you saw nothing (looks like cracks in the dry earth).

◊ Wet—You felt something or you saw nothing, even slight, either externally at your vulva or internally at your cervix. **Fertile.**

● Slippery mucus and or really wet—You saw clear mucus or felt a slippery feeling. Feels like raw egg white or a live fish. **Fertile.**

☺ Dry but *still fertile*—Like dry soil a day or two after rain, if you dig down one inch, you find moisture. Still **fertile.**

≣ *Continuous infertile discharge*—You have a pasty or sticky, dry or wet or creamy-type mucus that is the same every day (called basic infertile pattern of mucus or infertile continuous discharge—see page 345 to establish if this is you).

☽ Sexual relations in the evening.

☼ Sexual relations in the morning or day.

☺ Baby face-Chart her along with any fertile signs.

• Observe mucus signs all day
• Check cervix in evening or before making love
• Chart every evening
• Communicate

The size and position of the cervix can be charted by a simple drawing/diagram. Like this:

O = open soft cervix   • = closed firm cervix

In addition, you can also use letters to indicate firm (F) or soft (S).

Personal Fertility Chart (photocopy as needed)

	1	2	3	4	5	6	7	8	9	10	11	12	13	14	15	16	17	18	19	20	21	22	23	24	25	26	27	28	29	30	31	32	33	34
Date																																		
Mucus Appearance																																		
Mucus Sensation																																		
Signs of the Cervix																																		
Notes																																		
Date																																		
Mucus Appearance																																		
Mucus Sensation																																		
Signs of the Cervix																																		
Notes																																		
Date																																		
Mucus Appearance																																		
Mucus Sensation																																		
Signs of the Cervix																																		
Notes																																		
Date																																		
Mucus Appearance																																		
Mucus Sensation																																		
Signs of the Cervix																																		

Endnotes

ACKNOWLEDGMENTS

1. World Health Organization/UNICEF /World Bank, "Reduction of Maternal Mortality: A Joint WHO/UNICEF/ World Bank Statement," World Health Organization, Geneva. Report 10 of the Council on Scientific Affairs, (1999): 1–99.

CHAPTER 3—THE FIRST DAYS POSTPARTUM

1. American Medical Association, "Neonatal Circumcision" (an AMA policy statement). *American Medical Association Resources,* http://www.ama-assn.org/ama/pub/article/2036-2511.html (17 May, 2001). The American Medical Association calls neonatal circumcision a "non-therapeutic" procedure, which is performed for social reasons. Risks and adverse effects "mitigate" any possible medical benefit.

CHAPTER 4—POSTPARTUM PRIMER

1. Ellen, Kleiner. "The Disposable Diaper: A Misnomer," *Mothering* 51 (Spring 1989): 83.

CHAPTER 5—BREASTFEEDING, BOTTLE-BEEDING, AND BREAST CARE

1. "Breastfeeding and the Use of Human Milk," American Academy of Pediatrics Policy Statement (RE9729), vol. 100, no. 6, (Dec. 1997): 1–7.
2. Ibid.
3. S. Chua, S. Arulkumaran, I. Lim, et al., "Influence of Breastfeeding and Nipple Stimulation on Postpartum Uterine Activity," *British Journal of Obstetrics and Gynaecology* 101 (1994): 804–805
4. K. I. Kennedy and C. M. Visness, "Contraceptive Efficacy of Lactational Amenorrhoea," *Lancet* 339 (1992): 227–30. See also R. H. Gray, O. M. Campbell, R. Apelo, et al., "Risk of Ovulation during Lactation," *Lancet* 335 (1990) 25–29, and M. H. Labbock and C. Colie, "Puerperium and Breastfeeding," *Current Opinions in Obstetrics and Gynecology* 4 (1992): 818–25.
5. K. G. Dewey, M. J. Heinig, and L. A. Nommsen, "Maternal Weight-Loss Patterns during Prolonged Lactation," *American Journal of Clinical Nutrition* 58 (1993): 162–66.
6. L. J. Melton, S. C. Bryant, H. W. Wahner, et al., "Influence of Breastfeeding and Other Reproductive Factors on Bone Mass Later in Life," *Osteoporosis International* 3 (1993): 76–83.
7. R. G. Cumming and R. J. Klineberg, "Breastfeeding and Other Reproductive Factors and the Risk of Hip Fractures in Elderly Women," *International Journal of Epidemiology* 22 (1993): 684–91.
8. K. A. Rosenblatt and D. B. Thomas, "WHO Collaborative Study of Neoplasia and Steroid Contraceptives," *International Journal of Epidemiology* 22 (1993): 192–97.
9. P. A. Newcomb, B. E. Storer, M. P. Longnecker, et al., "Lactation and a Reduced Risk of Premenopausal Breast Cancer," *New England Journal of Medicine* 330 (1994): 81–87.
10. D. Montgomery and P. Splett, "Economic Benefit of Breast-Feeding Infants Enrolled in WIC," *Journal of the American Dietary Association* 97 (1997): 379–85. See also C. R. Tuttle and K. G. Dewey, "Potential Cost Savings for Medi-Cal, AFDC, Food Stamps, and WIC Programs Associated with Increasing Breast-Feeding among Low-Income Hmong Women in California," *Journal of the American Dietary Association* 96 (1996): 885–90.
11. L. Righar and Mo Alade, "Effect of Delivery Room Routines on Success of Breastfeeding," *Lancet* 336 (1990): 1105–1107.

12. Mary Kroeger, C.N.M., M.P.H., "Labor and Delivery Practices: The Eleventh Step to Successful Breastfeeding?" (paper presented at the 23rd Congress of Midwives, Vancouver, British Columbia, Canada, May 1993): 1–11.
13. American Academy of Pediatrics, "Pacifiers Linked to a Decrease in Breastfeeding." *American Academy of Pediatrics,* (1 March 1999) http://www.pediatrics.org.
14. Mary Renfrew, Chloe Fisher, and Suzanne Arms, *Bestfeeding: Getting Breastfeeding Right for You* (Berkeley, CA: Celestial Arts, 2000).
15. K. Dewey et al., "Growth Patterns of Breastfed Infants during the First Year of Life: The Darling Study," *American Journal of Clinical Nutrition* 57 (1993): 140–145.
16. Elizabeth Hormann, "Breastfeeding in a Polluted World," *Mothering,* May/June 2000. See also Jack Newman, "Mother's Milk Maligned but Breast Is Best," *Mothering,* May/June 2000, 62–70.
17. J. M. Alexander, A. M. Grant, et al., "Randomized Control Trial of Breast Shells and Hoffman's Exercises for Inverted or Non-Projectile Nipples," *British Medical Journal* 304 (1990): 1030.
18. Newcomb, Storer, Longnecker, et al., "Lactation and a Reduced Risk," 81–87.
19. Dewey et al., "Growth Patterns of Breastfed Infants," American Journal of Clinical Nutrition 57 (1993): 140–145.
20. Nancy Mohrbacher, IBCLC, and Julie Stock, B.A., IBCLC, *The Breastfeeding Answer Book* (Schaumburg, IL: La Leche League International, 1997) 113–114.
21. Ibid., 188.
22. Michal Ann Young, M.D., FAAP, "Press Statement on Breastfeeding on Federal Property," *American Academy of Pediatrics,* 25 September 1998, http://www.aap.org/advocacy/washing/92598pre.html.
23. "Breastfeeding and the Use of Human Milk," American Academy of Pediatrics Policy Statement (RE9729), vol. 100, no. 6, (Dec. 1997): 3.
24. Press Statement: Breastfeeding Improves Cognitive and Academic Outcomes into Adolescence. *Pediatrics Electronic Pages* (5 Jan. 1998) http://www.pediatrics.org.

CHAPTER 6—POSTPARTUM PELVIC HEALTH

1. Elizabeth Bruce, "Saying No to Episiotomy . . . Getting through Labor and Delivery in One Piece," *Mothering,* January/February 2001, 55.
2. Sheila Kitzinger, *Episiotomy and the Second Stage of Labor* (Seattle: Pennypress, 1990).

CHAPTER 16—ISSUES OF THE HEART

1. Lawrence Krukman and Susan Smith, "An Introduction to Postpartum Illness," *Postpartum Support International* (1998): http://www.postpartum.net.
2. Ibid.
3. Ibid.
4. Hendrick, L. L. Altshuler, and R. Suri, "Hormonal Changes in the Postpartum and Implications for Postpartum Depression." *Psychosomatics* 39 (1998): 93–101.
5. B. Harris, L. Lovett, J. Smith, G. Read, R. Walker, and R. Newcombe, "Postnatal Depression at 5 to 6 Weeks Postpartum, and Its Hormonal Correlates across the Peripartum Period" (Cardiff puerperal mood and hormone study III), *British Journal of Psychiatry* 168 (1996): 739–744.
6. J. Fisher, J. Astbury and A. Smith, "Adverse Psychological Impact of Operative Obstetric Interventions: A Prospective Longitudinal Study," *Australian and New Zealand Journal of Psychiatry* 31 (1997): 728–738.
7. M. Righetti-Veltema, E. Conne-Perreard, A. Bousquet., and J. Manzano, "Risk Factors and Predictive Signs of Postpartum Depression," *Journal of Affective Disorders* 49: 167–180.
8. L. Krukman, "Ritual as Prevention: The Case of Postpartum Depression," *Paper Presented at the 14th International Congress for Anthropological and Ethnological Sciences,* College of William and Mary (1998).
9. Ibid.
10. R. Lim, "Childbirth in Bali," *Field Research for Earthwatch Foundation* (1996).
11. Krukman and Smith, "An Introduction to Postpartum Illness," http://www.postpartum.net: (1998).
12. Ibid.

13. Ibid.
14. Ibid.

CHAPTER 18—FAMILY PLANNING...AN OVERVIEW

1. Danielle Knight, "Seeing beyond the Numbers: The Human Costs of Population Control in Brazil." *The Parecon Site,* Sept. 1996. http://www.zmag.org/zmag/articles/sept96knight.htm (31 Jan. 2001).
2. Carole J. L. Collins, "Women as Hidden Casualties of War," *Ms.,* November/December 1992, 14–15.
3. *The Witness Series,* "The Human Laboratory," produced by the British Broadcasting Corporation, 1996.
4. James A. Miller, "Baby-Killing Vaccine: Is It Being Stealth Tested?" *HLI Reports,* June/July (1995): 1.
5. Joseph, Ammu, "India's Population 'Bomb' Explodes over Women," *Ms.,* November/December 1992, 12–14.
6. Mercedes Arzu Wilson, *Love & Fertility,* (Dunkirk, MD: Family of the Americas Foundation, 1998): 71–80.
7. Emory University, R. Hatcher, M.D., M.P.H., Choosing a Contraceptive Homepage, "Withdrawal: Coitus Interruptus or 'Pulling Out,'" http://www.emory.edu/WHSC/MED/FAMPLAN/choices.html.
8. J. Trussel et al, "A Guide to Interpreting Contraceptive Efficacy," *Obstetrics and Gynecology* 76 (Sept. 1990): 565.
9. Ibid.
10. R. Hatcher, M.D., M.P.H., et al, *Contraceptive Technology,* 15th edition (New York: Irvington Publishers, 1992) 167.
11. R. Hatcher, M.D., M.P.H., Choosing a Contraceptive Homepage, "The Reality of Female Condoms," http://www.emory.edu/WHSC/MED/FAMPLAN/reality.html.
12. R. Hatcher, M.D., M.P.H., Choosing a Contraceptive Homepage, "The Diaphragm," http://www.emory.edu/WHSC/MED/FAMPLAN/diaphragm.html.
13. R. Hatcher, M.D., M.P.H., et al, *Contraceptive Technology,* 15th edition (New York: Irvington Publishers, 1992) 204.
14. *Physicians' Desk Reference,* 55th ed. (Montvale, NJ: Medical Economics Co., 2001) 3001, 3281, 3337.
15. "FAQ Sheet 3," Linkages Project, Academy for Educational Development.
16. R. Hatcher, M.D., M.P.H., Choosing a Contraceptive Homepage, "Combined Oral Contraceptives—The Pill,'" http://www.emory.edu/WHSC/MED/FAMPLAN/pills.html.
17. Dr. Evelyn Billings and Ann Westmore, *The Billings Method: Controlling Fertility without Drugs or Devices* (Melbourne, Australia: Anne O'Donovan, 1980), 173.
18. G. G. Briggs, R. K. Freeman, and R. J. Yaffe, *Drugs in Pregnancy and Lactation,* 4th ed. (Baltimore, Maryland: Williams and Wilkins, 1994), 644–645.
19. Dr. Evelyn Billings and Ann Westmore, *The Billings Method: Controlling Fertility without Drugs or Devices* (Melbourne, Australia: Anne O'Donovan, 1980), 173.
20. *Physicians' Desk Reference,* 55th ed. (Montvale, NJ: Medical Economics Co., 2001) 2361–2362. See also Billings and Westmore, *The Billings Method,* 168–177.
21. R. Hatcher, M.D., M.P.H., et al, *Contraceptive Technology,* 15th edition (New York: Irvington Publishers, 1992) 357.
22. R. Hatcher, M.D., M.P.H., Choosing a Contraceptive Homepage, "Norplant Implants." http://www.emory.edu/WHSC/MED/FAMPLAN/norplant.html.
23. Physicians' Desk Reference, 3407–3409.
24. Dr. Evelyn Billings and Ann Westmore, *The Billings Method: Controlling Fertility without Drugs or Devices* (Melbourne, Australia: Anne O'Donovan, 1980), 188.
25. Ibid., 189.
26. Margaret Nifzinger, *Signs of Fertility* (Deetsville, AL: MND Publishing Inc. 1998), 27.
27. "I'd like to thank Sandra Morningstar for giving me her wise counsel regarding women, arousal, and fertility. I'll always remember that day in November of 2000, over tea at my kitchen table."

Reading and Resources

PREGNANCY AND BIRTHING BOOKS AND VIDEOS

Active Birth: The New Approach to Giving Birth Naturally by Janet Balaskas (Boston: Harvard Common Press, 1992). Janet answers that so often asked question: What's wrong with obstetrically managed birth? The diagrams of the physiology of pregnancy and birth are excellent.

The American Way of Birth by Jessica Mitford (New York: Penguin Group, 1992).

Artemis Speaks: V.B.A.C. Stories and Natural Childbirth Information by Nan Koehler (available from the author at 13140 Frati Lane, Sebastopol, CA 95472). This book was my own favorite pregnancy guide, many times over. I really love it.

Birth, revised and updated, by Caterine Milinaire (New York: Harmony Books, 1974). This is the book that changed how we have babies.

Birth as an American Rite of Passage by Robbie Davis-Floyd (Berkeley, CA: University of California Press, 1992). Turning over stones for us, that's what Robbie is so good at.

The Birth Book by Raven Lang (CA: Genesis Press, 1972). The beautiful photos and inspiring words in this book helped me decide to become a mother.

Birthing from Within: An Extra-Ordinary Guide to Childbirth Preparation by Pam England, C.N.M., M.A. and Rob Horowitz, Ph.D. (Albuquerque, NM: Partera Press, 1998). This beautiful book gives expectant couples so much. It addresses the many issues they will be facing, shining light and offering practical solutions as well as honest answers. To order, call (800) 888-4741.

The Birth Partner: Everything You Need to Know to Help a Woman through Childbirth by Penny Simpkin, P.T. (Boston: Harvard Common Press, 1989). The role of being a birth partner (father-to-be, friend, relation, doula, whoever stays with and advocates for the laboring woman) is huge. Penny has written a manual to steer you through these waters. With her help, birth partners can help make wise, informed choices regarding hospital technology while maintaining the ever-important protective power of love and touch.

Birth Reborn by Michel Odent (New York: Pantheon Books, 1986). The miracle of antiobstetrics as practiced (or not) by Doctor Odent. See photos of the pregnant women of Prithers, France, singing as prenatal care—beautiful.

Birth without Violence by Frederick Leboyer (New York: Knopf, 1975). This classic will warm the hearts of all expectant parents.

A Book for Midwives by Susan Klein (Palo Alto, CA: Hesperian Foundation, 1995). Available through Hesperian Foundation, P.O. Box 1692, Palo Alto, CA 94302.

Complete Book of Pregnancy and Childbirth, revised and expanded edition, by Sheila Kitzinger (New York: Knopf, 1989). Excellent drawings, photos, and answers to your pregnancy questions.

Conscious Conception: Elemental Journey through the Labyrinth of Sexuality by Jeannine Parvati Baker and Frederick Baker (Berkeley, CA: North Atlantic Books and Monroe, UT: Freestone Publishing, 1986). This is one of the most important books you'll ever lay hands on. If you are interested in bringing the "possible" human Earth-side, please read and reread *Conscious Conception.*

Cosmic Cradle: Souls Waiting in the Wings for Birth by Elizabeth M. Carman and Neil J. Carman, Ph.D. (Fairfield, IA: Sunstar Publishing, 1999). Do you remember choosing your parents? Many people do. The Carmans have interviewed them and share their inspirational stories in their book. A scholarly look at where babies come from.

Encyclopedia of Childbearing by Barbara Katz Rothman (Phoenix: Oryx Press, 1993). So much knowledge at your fingertips.

Energetic Pregnancy by Elizabeth Davis (Berkeley, CA: Celestial Arts, 1988). Full of information for first-time and veteran mothers.

Essential Exercises for the Childbearing Years: A Guide Health and Comfort before and after Your Baby Is Born by Elizabeth Noble (Boston: Houghton Mifflin, 1988). One of those valuable books that every expectant woman could use. Women recovering from cesarean birth will benefit greatly from Elizabeth's words.

Experience of Childbirth, 5th ed., by Sheila Kitzinger (New York: Penguin Books, 1984). Personal accounts and childbirth facts make this book well worth reading.

The Five Standards of Safe Childbirth, fully revised, by David Stewart. Available through NAPSAC (see Organizations, this section). An excellent book.

A Guide to Effective Care in Pregnancy and Childbirth, 3rd ed., by Murray Enkin et al. (Oxford and New York: Oxford University Press, 1989).

Giving Birth: Challenges & Choices by Suzanne Arms. (Video 35 minutes, Durango, CO, Birthing the Future, www.BirthingtheFuture.com). Suzanne has long been the pioneer and champion of normal birth. This is a great way to introduce your extended family to the benefits of natural childbirth. I highly recommend it.

Having Twins: A Parent's Guide to Pregnancy, Birth and Early Childhood, 2nd ed. by Elizabeth Noble (Boston: Houghton Mifflin, 1991). Tips for having healthy full-term twins and all that follows.

Heart & Hands: A Midwife's Guide to Pregnancy and Birth, 3rd ed. by Elizabeth Davis (Berkeley, CA: Celestial Arts, 1997).

Holistic Midwifery: A Comprehensive Textbook for Midwives in Homebirth Practice, Vol. I, *Care During Pregnancy* by Anne Frye. This book is essential reading for all midwives and obstetricians. Anne dedicates her amazing book to her sister healers, witches, wise women, and midwives. Reading this and using it for reference has made me a better midwife. Also by Anne Frye: *Understanding Diagnostic Tests in the Childbearing Year; Healing Passage: A Midwife's Guide to the Care and Repair of the Tissues Involved in Birth; Suturing Techniques for Midwives,* (a two-hour video) and *Quick Reference Cards for Newborns with Problems* (set of seven laminated, color-coded cards). One may obtain Anne's excellent books by contacting: Labrys Press, 7528 NE Oregon St., Portland, OR 97213-6271, (503) 255-3378, Fax (503) 255-1474, E-mail: info@midwiferybooks.com, www.midwiferybooks.com

Hypnobirthing: The Celebration of Life by Marie Mongam (Concord, NH: Rivertree, 1992).

Immaculate Deception II: Myth, Magic & Birth by Suzanne Arms (Berkeley, CA: Celestial Arts, 1994). Suzanne made history and changed maternity care in the United States with this book.

Lotus Birth compiled by Shivam Rachana (Yarra Glen, Victoria, Australia, Greenwood Press 2000). All expectant families would be wise to read about and consider lotus birth. It will take courage to question the medical ritual of umbilical cord cutting, Shivam Rachana can help arm you with knowledge. *Lotus Birth* contains many case histories, writings by authorities on natural birth, and photographic illustrations. "This book is destined to be a classic in the conscious birth literature," says Jeannine Parvati Baker, a contributor. If you would like to purchase a copy of the book, please forward a check (specify you want the *Lotus Birth* book) for $19.95 + $5.05 postage and handling ($25) and your address to: 40 North State Street, Joseph, UT 84739.

The Miraculous World of Your Unborn Baby by Nikki Bradford (NTC, 1998) Does your baby remember being in the womb? What about those amazing pregnancy dreams you had? Does your unborn baby learn, feel, play? Stunning photos and illustrations.

Mothering the Mother: How a Doula Can Help You Have a Shorter, Easier and Healthier Birth by Klaus Marshall, M.D., Phyllis Klaus, C.S.W., and John H. Kennell, M.D. (Reading, MA: Addison-Wesley, 1993). After reading this, wise couples will have a doula with them at their hospital births. A fantastic book.

Obstetric Myths vs. Research Realities by Henci Goer (New York: Bergin and Garvey, 1994). Also by Ms. Goer is *The Sinking Woman's Guide to a Better Birth.*

Open Season: A Survival Guide for Natural Childbirth by Nancy Cohen (Westport, CT: Greenwood Publishing Co., 1991).

Pregnant Feelings: Developing Trust in Birth by Rahima Baldwin and Terra Palmarini Richardson (Berkeley, CA: Celestial Arts, 1986). A beautiful workbook for pregnant women and their partners.

Pregnancy, Childbirth and the Newborn by Penny Simpkin, Janet Whalley, and Ann Keppler (Deerhaven, MN: Meadowbrook Press, 1991).

Prenatal Yoga and Natural Birth, revised edition, by Jeannine Parvati Baker (Berkeley, CA: North Atlantic Books, 1986). A milestone book that introduced yoga for pregnant women to the West. Jeannine is a pioneer, wise woman, and blessed being.

Pursuing the Birth Machine by Marsden Wagner (Camperdown, NSW, Australia: ACE Graphics, 1994). Highly recommended, a fantastic book.

Resexualizing Childbirth by Leilah McCracken (1999, see Leilah's Web site at http://www.birthlove.com). A radically beautiful look at pregnancy and birth.

The Scientification of Love by Michel Odent, M.D. (London/NY: Free Association Books, 1999). Here at last is the book that cites the research that says what all women know, that love is important, in fact essential to human survival.

Silent Knife by Nancy Wainer Cohen and Lois Estner (New York: Bergin and Garvey Publishers, Inc., 1983). Every midwife and doula must read this book about the cesarean epidemic. All cesarean mothers will find solace here.

Special Delivery: The Complete Guide to Informed Birth by Rahima Baldwin (Berkeley, CA: Celestial Arts, 1987). A reader-interactive dream book for expectant families.

Spiritual Midwifery 3rd ed. by Ina Mae Gaskin (Summertown, TN: The Book Publishing Company, 1990). Every expectant woman would be wise to read this book. All five times I was pregnant, I read and reread it—even found it in a used bookstore in Indonesia! Each time I felt it speak to me fresh from the heart.

CHILDREARING & BREASTFEEDING

Adoption: A Handful of Hope by Suzanne Arms (Berkeley, CA: Celestial Arts, 1990). A beautiful book for adoptive families and for mothers who have relinquished babies.

Babies, Breastfeeding & Bonding by Ina Mae Gaskin (South Hadley, MA, Bergin & Garvey Publishers, Inc., 1987). From the heart of a mother and a midwife, so well done.

Bestfeeding: Getting Breastfeeding Right for You by Mary Renfrew, Chloe Fisher, and Suzanne Arms (Berkeley, CA: Celestial Arts, 2000). A clear straightforward and complete guide to the best way to feed your baby.

Breastfeeding and Natural Child Spacing: The Ecology of Natural Mothering by Sheila Kippley (New York, NY: Penguin Books, 1978). A beautiful book, one of my favorites over the years.

Car Seat Safety, Injoy Productions and Cosco Video, 1998 (15 minutes). At last, a guide for the proper safety precautions for babies and children riding in vehicles.

Circumcision: What Every Parent Should Know by Anne Briggs (Earlysville, VA: Birth & Parenting Publications, 1985). Includes the history of circumcision, description with photographs of the procedure and discussion of risks. Also how to care for your intact boy.

Continuum Concept by Jean Liedloff (Reading, MA: Addison-Wesley, 1986). Based on the well-founded belief that life outside the womb is a continuum of the intimacy of life before birth.

Everyday Pediatrics for Parents by Elmer R. Grossman, M.D. (Berkeley, CA: Celestial Arts, 1996). A thoughtful guide for today's families.

Liberated Parents, Liberated Children: Your Guide to a Happier Family by Adel Faber and Elaine Mazlish (New York: Avon Books, 1990). A practical guide to communicating with your children. Also by the same authors: *How to Talk So Kids Will Listen and Listen So Kids Will Talk.*

Loving Hands: The Traditional Art of Baby Massage by Frederick Leboyer (New York: Newmarket Press, 1977). Dr. Leboyer's beautiful photos will inspire all families to massage their babies. Inspirational.

Magical Child by Joseph Chilton Pearce (New York: Bantam Books, 1981). Insight on the importance of bonding through all the developmental stages of life.

Mothering Multiples, 2nd ed., by Karen Gromada (Franklin Park, IL: La Leche League International, 1985). Advice from a mother who had single births before the birth of her twins.

Natural Family Living: The Mothering Magazine Guide to Parenting by Peggy O'Mara with Jane McConnell (New York: Pocket Books, 2000). This is the book so many of us have been waiting for. Under one cover: All-natural approaches to pregnancy and birth; current research on eating, sleeping, circumcision, vaccinations, diapering, weaning, crying; innovative ways to handle divorce, loss, and change; tips for integrating technology, plus time-out for parents.

Natural Healing for Babies and Children by Aviva Jill Romm (Freedom, CA: The Crossing Press). Also by Aviva: *The Natural Pregnancy Book.*

Our Babies, Ourselves: How Biology and Culture Shape the Way We Parent by Meredith Small (New York: Anchor Books, 1998). Which behaviors sustain our babies and which prepare them for living in society? Anthropologist Meredith Small evaluates and enlightens us.

Questioning Circumcision: A Jewish Perspective by Ronald Goldman, Ph.D. with a foreward by Rabbi Raymond Singer, Ph.D. (Boston: Vanguard Publications, 1998). This book sheds light on the history, risks, unrecognized consequences, research, personal experiences, and the conflicts and the questions regarding circumcision that Jewish families must face today.

Say No to Circumcision! 40 Compelling Reasons by Thomas J. Ritter, M.D. and George C. Denniston, M.D. (Aptos, CA, Hourglass Book Publishing, 1996). The unvarnished medical facts about foreskin amputation.

Vaccination: The Issue of Our Times edited by Peggy O'Mara. (Santa Fe, NM: Mothering Resource Library, 1997). Parents questioning vaccination will find a wealth of information and resources in these pages. To order, write P.O. Box 1690, Santa Fe, NM 87504 or call (888) 984-8116.

The Womanly Art of Breastfeeding by Judy Torgus (Franklin Park, IL: La Leche League International 1997). This is a fantastic, dependable guide to breastfeeding. It answers all the questions you can think of, and then some. Every mother needs this one.

You Are Your Child's First Teacher by Rahima Baldwin (Berkeley, CA: Celestial Arts, 1989) Education begins at conception (or maybe sooner). Rahima brings this profound knowledge home to parents.

Your Baby and Child, rev. ed. by Penelope Leach (New York: Knopf, 1989). This is a terrific gift for new parents. Very helpful.

WOMEN'S PHYSICAL AND EMOTIONAL HEALTH

Ayurveda, The Science of Self-Healing: A Practical Guide by Vasant Lad (Wilmont, WI: Lotus Light Publications, 1984). Helps the reader gain a basic working knowledge of the Ayurvedic system of health.

Cooking for Life: Ayurvedic Recipes for Good Food and Good Health by Linda Banchek (New York: Harmony Books, 1989). This cookbook features and entire section on cooking for Vata, perfect for postpartum women. Gourmet section, wonderful. Try the egg-free oatmeal cookies!

Courage to Heal: A Guide for Woman Survivors of Child Sexual Abuse by Ellen Bass and Laura Davis (New York: Harper Trade Books, 1988). An important book for women in the healing process.

Herbal Healing for Women: Simple Home Remedies for Women of All Ages by Rosemary Gladstar (New York: Fireside Book/Simon & Schuster, 1993). A how-to book for women interested in building a home apothecary—all natural and from the heart. Rosemary is so deeply good for sharing her wisdom with us in a way we can use it.

The Menopause Self-Help Book, 4th rev. ed. by Susan M. Lark, M.D. (Berkeley, CA: Celestial Arts, 1998). A guide to feeling wonderful for the second half of life. A practical, all-natural plan for relieving and preventing every symptom of menopause. Also by Susan M. Lark: *PMS Self-Help Book: Heavy Menstrual Flow* and *Anemia Self-Help Book; Women's Health Companion; Menstrual Cramps Self-Help Book; The Estrogen Decision Self-Help Book; Anxiety & Stress Self-Help Book.* All are very reader-friendly and helpful.

Natural Alternatives to Hormone Replacement Therapy Cookbook by Marilyn Glenville (Berkeley, CA: Celestial Arts, 2000). Eat your way through menopause. The photos are as delicious as the recipes.

New Laurel's Kitchen, 2nd ed., by Laurel Robertson, Carol Flinders, and Brian Ruppenthal (Berkeley, CA: Ten Speed Press, 1986). Vegetarian cooking and nutritional knowledge. Excellent.

Our Bodies, Ourselves, rev. 2nd ed., by the Boston Women's Health Book Collective (New York: Simon & Schuster, 1976). An honest look at the multifaceted issue of women's health. Self-help suggestions. A classic guide.

Step by Step: A Guide to Organizing a Postpartum Parent Support Network in Your Community by Jane Honikman, M.S. (Santa Barbara, CA: Postpartum Support International, 2000). To order, send $20.00 to Jane at Postpartum Support International (see address under Organizations).

Tao of Balanced Diet: Secrets of a Thin and Healthy Body by Stephen T. Chang (San Francisco, CA: Tao Publishing, 1987). Eating healthy is the secret to a thin body, not dieting. Also by Dr. Chang: *The Tao of Sexology: The Book of Infinite Wisdom* and *The Complete System of Self-Healing: Internal Exercises.* All of Dr. Chang's work is excellent.

Where Women Have No Doctor by Burns, Lovich, Maxwell, and Shapiro (Palo Alto, CA: Hesperian Foundation, 1997). Available through Hesperian Foundation, P.O. Box 1692, Palo Alto, CA 94302.

Wise Woman Herbal for the Childbearing Year by Susun S. Weed (Woodstock, NY: Ash Tree Publishing, 1986). Susun offers women a wealth of useful information concerning our friends in the plant queendom.

The Yoga of Herbs: An Ayurvedic Guide to Herbal Medicine by Vasant Lad and David Frawley (Wilmot, WI: Lotus Light Publications, 1986). An easy-to-use herbal listing the plants by their western, Chinese and Sanskrit names. Traditional uses are given.

MAGAZINES

Hip Mama
> PO Box 12525
> Portland, OR 97212
> Irreverent, up to date, serious fun.
> www.hipmama.com

Midwifery Today and *Having a Baby Today*
> P.O. Box 2672
> Eugene, OR 97402
> (541) 344-7438, Fax (541) 344-1422
> Inquiries E-mail: inquiries@midwiferytoday.com
> http://www.midwiferytoday.com
> These publications will amuse you, enlighten you, and restore your faith in pregnancy, birth, and postpartum. Enjoy!

Mothering
P.O. Box 1690
> Santa Fe, NM 87504
> 800) 827-1061
> *Mothering* fiercely advocates for children and their families. This quarterly magazine is characterized by the courage to tackle the tough issues such as choosing home birth, saying "no" to circumcision, sharing the family bed, breastfeeding toddlers, and dealing with blended families, VBAC, vaccination, home schooling. Parent, child, and planet friendly.

SPECIAL CHILDREN, MISCARRIAGE, AND CHILDREN WHO HAVE DIED

About Handicaps by Sara Stein (New York: Walker & Co., 1984). Designed to help parents and children cope with handicaps together.

Bereaved Parent by Harriet S. Schiff (New York: Crown Books, 1987). Time opens bereaved parents to their healing process. This book can also help.

Differences in the Family: Living with a Disabled Child by Heather Featherstone (New York: Penguin Books, 1981).

Footprints on Our Hearts by Paraclete Video Productions (60 mins.) Mothers and fathers openly express their loss and share what most helped them.

Miscarriage: A Shattered Dream by Sherokee Ilse and Linda Hammer Burns (Maple Plain, MN: Wintergreen Press, 1985). Also by Sherokee Ilse: *Empty Arms: Coping with Miscarriage, Stillbirth, and Infant Loss.* The pain of miscarriage has been ignored in our society, leaving the grieving parents in isolation. These books offer much needed help. Web site: www.wintergreenpress.com. To order, write Wintergreen Press, 3630 Eileen St., Maple Plain, MN 55359 or call (952) 476-1303.

Motherhood and Mourning: Perinatal Death by Larry G. Peppers and Ronald J. Knapp (New York: Praeger Publications, 1980). When pregnancy does not end in the birth of a living child, parents may use the advice in this book to help themselves heal.

The Premature Baby Book: A Parents Guide to Coping and Caring in the First Years by Helen Harrison and Ann Kositsky (New York: St. Martin's Press, 1983). This book fills a giant need for parents who have a baby in neonatal intensive care.

Remember the Secret by Elisabeth Kübler-Ross (Berkeley, CA: Celestial Arts, 1988). A story for children of all ages, lovingly and honestly told, about dying.

When Pregnancy Fails: Families Coping with Miscarriage, Stillbirth, and Infant Death by Susan Borg and Judith Lasker (New York: Bantam Books, 1989). A sourcebook for grieving families.

ORGANIZATIONS

American Academy of Husband-Coached
    Childbirth (The Bradley Method)
    P.O. Box 5224
    Sherman Oaks, CA 91413-5224
    (800) 423-2397 or (800)-4-A-birth
    (818) 788-6662
    Web site: www.bradleybirth.com
Association for Pre- and Perinatal Psychology and
    Health (APPAH)
    P.O. Box 994
    Geyserville, CA 95441
    (707) 857-4041
    E-mail: APPPAH@aol.com
    Web site: www.birthpsychology.com
Association for Retarded Citizens of the United
    States (ARC)
    1010 Wayne Ave., Suite 650
    Silver Spring, MD 20910
    (301) 565-3842, Fax (301) 565- 5342
    E-mail: Info@thearc.org
    Web site: www.thearc.org
    Web site for autism-related resources:
    www.thearcofwinn-boone.org/autism
Birthing from Within
    (505) 254-4884
    E-mail: paterna@flash.net
    Web site: www.birthpower.com
Birth Works, Inc.
    P.O. Box 2045
    Medford, NJ 08055
    (609) 953-9380 or 888-to birth (862-4784)
    Web site: www.birthworks.org
Compassionate Friends-National Office
    P.O. Box 3696
    Oak Brook, IL 60522-3696
    (877) 969-0010 or (603) 990-0010
    Fax (603) 990- 0296
    Web site: www.compassionatefriends.org
Doulas of North America (DONA)
    1100 23rd Ave. E.
    Seattle, WA 98112
    Fax (206) 325-0472
    *"Having a Doula is the only way to end up with
    a normal birth in a hospital today."*—Dr. Eden
    Gabrielle Fromberg, Clinical Assistant
    Professor of Obstetrics and Gynecology, SUNY
    Downstate Medical Center, Brooklyn, NY
The Farm
    P.O. Box 48 (clinic) or P.O. Box 42 (publica-
    tions)
    Summertown, TN 38483

If you wish to have your baby at The Farm,
write to the clinic four to six months before
you are due. Also write to obtain a copy of
Spiritual Midwifery.
Federation for Children with Special Needs
    1135 Tremont St., Suite 420
    Boston, MA 02102
    (617) 236-7210, Fax (617) 572-2094
    Web site: www.fcsn.org
Global Maternal/Child Health Association, Water-
    birth Information and Referral Center
    P.O. Box 366
    West Linn, OR 97068
    (503) 682-3600
    Web site: www.waterbirth.org
International Cesarean Awareness Network (ICAN)
    P.O. Box 276
    Clarks Summit, PA 18411
    (717) 585-4226
    Web site:
    www.childbirth.org/section/ICAN.html
International Childbirth Education Association
    (ICEA)
    P.O. Box 20048
    Minneapolis, MN 55420-0048
    (800) 624-4934 , Fax (612) 854-8772
    Web site: www.healthy.net/pan/cso/ICEA.htm
    Interdisciplinary approach to childbirth educa-
    tion.
International Lactation Consultants Association
    (ILCA)
    1500 Sunday Drive, Suite 102
    Raleigh, NC 27607
    (919)787-5181, Fax (919) 787-4916
    E-mail: ilca@erols.com
    Web site: www.ilca.org
La Leche League International
    1400 N. Meacham Road
    Schaumburg, IL 60173-4048
    (847) 519-7730, Fax (847) 519-0035
    E-mail: lllhq@llli.org
    Web site:
    http://www.lalecheleague.org/LLLIlang.html
Midwives' Alliance of North America (MANA)
    4805 Lawrenceville Highway, Suite 116-279
    Lilburn, GA 30047
    (801) 720-3026
    Toll free (888) 923-MANA (6262)
    E-mail: info@mana.org
MotherLove, Inc.
    Debra Pascali-Bonaro, B.Ed. CCE, CD
    (DONA) president MotherLove, Inc.
    (201) 358-2703, Fax (201) 664-4405
    E-mail: MotherLove@prodigy.net

National Association of Parents and Professionals
   for Safe Alternatives in Childbirth (NAPSAC)
   Route 1, Box 646
   Marble Hill, MO 63764
   (314) 238-2010
National Organization of Mothers of Twins Clubs,
   Inc.
   P.O. Box 23188
   Albuquerque, NM 87192-1188
   (505) 275-0955
   Web site: www.nomotc.org
National Organization of Circumcision
   Information Resource Centers (NOCIRC)
   P.O. Box 2512
   San Anselmo, CA 94979-2512
   (415) 488-9883, Fax (415) 488-9660
   Web site: www.nocirc.org
   Other important Web sites regarding this issue:
   www.cirp.org and www.SexuallyMutilated
   Child.org
Nursing Mothers Council
   National referral # (605) 599-3669
   Web site: www.nursingmothers.org
Parent Care, Inc.
   9041 Colgate Street
   Indianapolis, IN 46268-1210
   (317) 872-9913
PMS Access
   429 Gammon Place
   Madison, WI 53719
   (800) 222-4767 or (800) 558-7046
   Web site: www.health.gov/nhic/scripts
   For information, support groups, advice, and
   referrals.
Postpartum Support International
   Jane Honikman, founder
   927 N. Kellogg Ave.
   Santa Barbara, CA 93111
   (805) 967-7636, Fax (805) 967-0608
   E-mail: jhonikman@earthlink.net
   Or,
   Sonia Murdock, president
   109 Udall Road
   West Islip, NY 11795
   (631) 422-2255, Fax (631) 422-1643
   E-mail: postpartum@aol.com
   Web site: www.postpartum.net
Primal Health Resource Center
   Dr. Michel Odent
   59 Roderick Road
   London NW3 2NP, England
   (071) 485-00-95

c/o Birth Works
   (609) 953-9380 or 888-to birth (862-4784)
   www.birthworks.org
SIDS Alliance
   1314 Bedford Ave., Suite 210
   Baltimore, MD 21208
   (410) 653-8226, Fax: (410) 653-8709
   E-mail: sidshq@charm.net
   Web site: www.sidsalliance.org
Tiny Treasures
   c/o Sara Matzoll-Phillips
   1272 Ironwood Lane #1
   Eagan, MN 55123
   Tiny Treasures is an organization dedicated to
   providing support and information to parents
   having experienced premature or high-risk
   birth. Online premie resources:
   majordomo@vicnet.net.au

BREAST PUMPS

NOTE: Full-size automatic electric breast pumps
   are available from many hospitals and pharma-
   cies or through your local La Leche League
   leader. Contact the following companies for
   the nearest location:
Ameda/Egnell
   765 Industrial Drive
   Cary, IL 60013
   (800) 323-8750
   From Illinois, Alaska, or Hawaii, call collect:
   (708) 693-2900
Medela
   4610 Prime Parkway
   McHenry, IL 60050
   (800) 835-5968

SUPPLIES

Baby Bunz and Co.
   (800) 67NIKKY or (800) 676-4559
   Web site: www.babybunz.com
   This is the place to order my very favorite cot-
   ton and wool diaper covers, NIKKYs.
Beverly's Gardens
   25858–292 Street
   Mount Sterling, IA 52573
   Herbalist and wise woman Beverly Francis
   makes the best herbal balms in the world.
Beyond Kegels
   Phoenix Publishing
   P.O. Box 8213
   Missoula, MT 59807
   (800) 549-8371

Beyond Kegels is a guided treatment program for women who are having problems with continence and pelvic weakness.

Birth Waves—Penny Meslo
121 Main Street North
Markham, Ontario L3P1Y2
Canada
(905) 201-8570
E-mail: penny@birthwaves.ca
Midwifery and birth supplies, inspired T-shirts, and much more.

Cascade HealthCare Products, Inc.
141 Commercial Street, NE
Salem, OR 97301
Customer service: (503) 371-4445 Orders:
(800) 443-9942
Web site: www.1cascade.com
Request their catalog for midwifery and birth supplies.

Childbirth Graphics
P.O. Box 21207
Waco, TX 76702-1207
To order or request a catalog,
call (800) 299-3366 or fax (888) 977-7653.
Beautiful teaching and learning aids for pregnancy, birth, and breastfeeding.

Danish Woolen Delight
1325 VT Rte 128
Westford, VT 05494
(802) 878-6089 , Fax (802) 878-6091
E-mail: Danishwool@aol.com
To purchase the best quality wool nursing pads and other mother/baby products.

The LENS-Fertility Magnifier, available from:
Six Directions Foundation-Freestone
Publishing
40 North State Street
Joseph, UT 84739-1207
Or,
P.O. Box 398
Monroe, UT 84754
(435) 527-3738
E-mail: freestone@hubwest.com
Web site: www.freestone.org
A not-for-profit organization devoted to the Possible Family.

Medea Books
P.O. Box 128
Bristol, VT 05443
(802) 453-3332
For a wide selection of books concerning midwifery, birth, breastfeeding, and beyond.

HERBS

Herbal Healing for Women by Rosemary Gladstar (New York: Simon & Schuster, 1993).
Herbs and Things: Jeanne Rose's Herbal by Jeanne Rose (New York: Grosset & Dunlap, 1972).
Hygieia: A Woman's Herbal by Jeannine Parvati (Monroe, UT: Freestone Publishing Company, 1979).
The Way of Herbs by Michael Tierra (New York: Pocket Books, 1988).
Wise Woman Herbal for the Childbearing Year by Susun S. Weed (Woodstock, NY: Ash Tree, 1985).
The Yoga of Herbs: An Ayurvedic Guide to Herbal Medicine by Vasant Lad and David Frawley (Wilmot, WI: Lotus Light Publications, 1986).

NATURAL FAMILY PLANNING

The Art of Natural Family Planning is available from Couple to Couple League International, Inc, P.O. Box 111184, Cincinnati, OH 45211-1184.

A Cooperative Method of Natural Birth Control and *Signs of Fertility: The Personal Science of Natural Birth Control* (Second edition) by Margaret Nofzinger. Both may be ordered by writing MND Publishing, Inc., 573 Marina Rd., Deatsville, AL 36022. Ms. Nofzinger's books teach one to observe, interpret, and chart mucus, cervical signs of fertility, and basal body temperatures. She is a pioneer in what I feel is the most promising revolution in women's health, the movement toward effective natural forms of family planning.

A Couple's Guide to Fertility, by R. J. Huneger and Rose Fuller, can be ordered from Norwest Family Services, 4805 N. El Glisan, Portland, OR 97213.

Love and Fertility by Mercedes Arzú Wilson details the Ovulation Method of Natural Family Planning, also known as the Billings Method. Ovulation Method(OM) is not Rhythm Method. It is available, along with useful kits for charting your fertility, through the Family of the Americas Foundation. Call 800-443-3395.

Index